TO
STUART
MY FRIEND
AND A PROFESSIONAL
ADMINISTRATOR
Jerry
11/3/81

AMERICAN HEALTH CARE ASSOCIATION/ CBI PUBLISHING COMPANY SERIES IN HEALTH CARE MANAGEMENT

RESIDENT CARE MANAGEMENT SYSTEMS
Erwin Rausch
Maria Menna Perper

BASIC ACCOUNTING AND BUDGETING FOR LONG-TERM CARE FACILITIES
Jerry L. Rhoads

SOCIAL WORK IN THE LONG-TERM CARE FACILITY
Shirley Conger
Kay Moore

DEVELOPMENTAL DISABILITIES: A TRAINING GUIDE
Henri Deutsch
Sheldon Bustow

Basic Accounting and Budgeting for Long-Term Care Facilities

BASIC ACCOUNTING AND BUDGETING FOR LONG-TERM CARE FACILITIES

Jerry L. Rhoads, CPA

Written for The American Health Care Association

CBI Publishing Company, Inc.
51 Sleeper Street   Boston, Massachusetts 02210

Production Editor/Becky Handler
Text Designer/Roy Howard Brown
Compositor/Haddon Craftsmen
Cover Designer/Roy Howard Brown

Library of Congress Cataloging in Publication Data

Rhoads, Jerry L 1939–
    Basic accounting and budgeting for long-term care facilities.

    Includes index.
    1. Nursing homes—United States—Accounting.
I. Title.
HF5686.N9R47   657'.8322   80-27971
ISBN 0-8436-0795-5

Copyright © 1981 by CBI Publishing Company, Inc.
All rights reserved. This book may not be reproduced in any form without written permission from the publisher.
Printed in the United States of America
Printing *(last digit):* 9 8 7 6 5 4 3 2 1

Contents

Preface *vii*
   Acknowledgments *xi*

Chapter 1 Accounting Theory *1*
   Accounting *1*
   Generally Accepted Accounting Principles *2*
   Accrual Accounting *4*
   Accounting Equation and Records *5*

Chapter 2 Accounting Control *29*
   How Accounting and Reporting Safeguard the Assets of the Nursing Home Business *29*

Chapter 3 Accounting Principles for Nursing Homes *45*
   Is Cash Position Still Important? *46*
   Billings and Accounts Receivable *48*
   Contractual Discounts (Medicare and Medicaid Accounting) *50*
   Allowance for Bad Debts *51*
   Prepaid Expenses and Deferred Charges *54*
   Purchases, Accounts Payable, and Inventories *57*
   Current Assets, Liquidity, and Noncurrent Assets *57*
   Capital (Depreciable) Assets and Construction-in-Progress *58*
   Contingent Assets *62*
   Accrued Expenses *62*
   Unpaid Income Taxes *64*
   Current Liabilities, Liquidity, and Long-Term Debt *65*
   Deferred Income, Liabilities, and Credits *67*
   Capital Stock, Contributions, and Retained Earnings *69*
   Contingent Liabilities (Loss Contingency) *70*
   Revenues *71*
   Capital Costs *75*
   Depreciation *76*
   Patient Funds *77*
   Life Care Contracts: An Accounting Nightmare *78*

Chapter 4 Operating Budget *89*
   Business Failures *89*
   Budgeting *91*
   Annual Operating Budget *96*
   Nursing Services Budget *99*
   Ancillary Services Budget *100*
   Support Services Budget *101*
   Administrative Budget *102*
   Sample Annual Operating Budget *104*
   Budget Analysis *120*
   Variance Analysis *126*

Chapter 5 Capital Budgeting *131*
How Is Capital Budgeting Used? *131*
Capital Investment Options *131*
Evaluation of Capital Investment Options *132*
Choosing an Investment *138*

Chapter 6 Cash Flow Budgeting *141*

Chapter 7 Financial Reports *149*
Objectives of Management Reporting *149*
Components of Management Reporting *149*
Stage One—Daily *150*
Stage Two—Monthly *151*
Financial Ratios *152*
Financial Analysis *185*
Stage Three—Annually *205*

Chapter 8 Cost Accounting *207*
Definition of Cost Accounting *207*
Objectives of Cost Accounting *208*
Cost Accounting Data *209*
Cost Department *210*
Cost Accounting and Other Functions *210*
Cost Accounting and Government Agencies *211*
Cost and Financial Accounting *212*
Analysis of Service Costs *213*
Cost Distribution/Cost Centers/Cost Finding *216*

Chapter 9 Cost Reimbursement *221*
Medicare and Medicaid Reimbursement *221*

Appendix 1 Chart of Accounts *228*
Uniform Expense Classification Guide *228*
Expense Classification *229*
General Ledger Chart of Accounts *243*

Appendix 2 Medicare Reimbursement *249*
Optimization of Facility Bed Size for Medicare Reimbursement Purposes *249*
Medicare Reimbursement Illustration *250*
Compliance Checklist *251*

General Accounting Terms *256*
Accounting and Finance Terms for Long-Term Care Facilities *263*

Index *269*

Preface

What is Quality Care in a Nursing Home?

Is quality care happy patients? Yes!
Is quality care happy employees? Yes!
Is quality care happy management? Yes!
Is quality care happy surveyors and purveyors? Yes!
Is quality care expensive? Yes!
Is quality care attainable? Yes!

What does this have to do with accounting, costing, and budgeting? No doubt about it, quality care is the result of many interdependent factors. For quality to be at its optimum yet economical is very difficult, to say the least. The attainment of the above objectives takes a sophisticated system of management, medical procedures, personnel policies, and a definition by the purchaser of the services considered to be necessary or not necessary. The primary hangup to quality care is accountability and cost. Nearly all the facilities I have been in, which approaches 300 by now, are capable of providing quality medical services, if they can collect a reasonable price for quality and still stay within a reasonable budget for government-financed programs. Let's speculate a little bit about quality and what it costs to provide quality. First let's define in general terms the services being provided.

Each resident receives basically the same services for housekeeping, laundry, dietary, maintenance, utilities, and administration. The only difference from patient to patient is in the degree of extra services, *support services,* required if the patient is more seriously ill. The extra services are mainly due to incontinence, special diet, and housekeeping in the room. The quality in support services is physically obvious. Is the food good? Are the rooms clean? Is the facility free of odor? Is the climate adequately regulated? Is the facility well organized?

Nursing services are more difficult to gauge. Most all residents receive a certain degree of routine nursing services. The routine nursing services in nursing homes are providing the patient with help in their activities of daily living (ADLs). These services relate to such activities as bathing, dressing, transferring, and turning. These services are fairly routine in nature and are received in about the same degree by each patient. As the degree increases the likelihood of a resident requiring skilled nursing services increases. As a resident progresses towards the need for skilled nursing services, the activities of daily living become a more time consuming requirement for the nursing staff. These services can be termed skilled routine nursing services which are of a higher degree and of a more expensive cost than the basic routine nursing services. These services require more staff, more supplies, and more rehabilitation appliances, such as, wheelchairs, hospital beds, gerichairs, feeder tables, and so on. The evaluation of quality for the routine services is also physically detectable. Is the resident clean? Is the resident well groomed? Is the resident up and about? Is the resident free of bed sores and decompensation?

Beyond the routine nursing services are the services directed towards specific patients' needs. These needs can vary based on diagnosis, clinical condition and plan of care. The variables relate to eating, mobility, behavior, rehabilitation, incontinence, enemas and douches, medication, injections, suctioning, dressing and appliances, oxygen, and ancillary services for speech therapy, laboratory, and x-ray work. Evaluation of the quality of the special nursing services gets to be more intangible.

As the patients require more care they are in the stages of physical deterioration, so it is not easy to detect physical signs of quality or poor quality care. Of course questions can be asked that will enable the trained medical reviewer to determine if adequate care is being given. Is the patient making an attempt to function as independently as would be expected considering their diagnosis, condition, and plan of care? Does the patient feed himself? Does the patient get up and transfer by himself? Is the patient psychologically responding to social services? Is the patient responding to the plan of physical therapy? Is the patient responding to a bowel and bladder training program? Is the patient responding to medications, injections, and other habilitation procedures?

The difficulty of judging quality of care in the special nursing services area becomes more apparent as you try to define it. This is because the services are responding to medical needs not easily detected by sight, sound, or touch. Quality, in this area, many times involves a physician, the resident's family, and the resident's will to improve. So should we just accept that quality is indefinable, or should we make an attempt to somehow judge the quality provided by a facility in carrying out special nursing procedures? I feel we should make an attempt. Otherwise quality will always be an elusive concept which is used or misused for political and business purposes.

Logically our work in this area must include the diagnosis, the plan of care, and the medical record keeping of the medical professional. The federal minimum standards have given us assistance in this area. They require that certain trained professionals be available to supervise, assess, and observe the plan of care in response to a particular diagnosis and clinical condition. This being the case, the paperwork documenting the carrying out of the plan of care, in response to a diagnosis, must be of a high quality if we are ever to judge the quality of the services being rendered. In other words, we need something tangible to look at so we can judge the physical activities taking place to respond to a resident's needs. So documentation seems to be the most important single factor in judging the quality of special nursing services.

As I stated before I have been in very few facilities that are not able to provide quality services to its residents. All the facilities are licensed. They must meet the minimum standards and are reviewed on a regular basis for the quality of the facility and its staff. Of course, many of these surveys and reviews are cursory in nature. However, as the documentation improves, the surveys of the medical review will be more meaningful and accountability will be established. In the past, record keeping has been more academic than productive.

Now let's get very practical. Of course all nursing homes can provide quality. All it takes is money to pay the bills for providing the services and proper management of the productive process. But as we know, adequate money is not readily available to the nursing home industry. The reasons for this are not important. The important thing is to determine how much the present long-term care dollar will buy. If it is not adequate to buy quality services, then quality services will not be made available to the residents. As long as it takes cash to pay bills, the quality of the services will seek the same level as payment. An old adage is relevant here. "You may get less than what you pay for, but very seldom do you get more than what you pay for." So to be frank, the quality of services is as much dependent on reimbursement as it is on good nurses. It takes money to pay good nurses. Regardless of the varying viewpoints, political and otherwise, looking at long-term care the overall question must be, how much can be provided for the available dollar?

I think it is high time the nursing home industry realized that its responsibility is to define the services it is going to provide. This definition should be in very explicit, detailed terms. Until this is done the buyer will continue to be suspicious and very cautious in the manner in which they pay for the services. The more the buyer knows of the product and its costs, the more likely the buyer is to pay the going price. So now is the time, nursing homes, if you expect to receive adequate payment for quality care, to define your product. You must be able to cost your product, deal with the buyers on a more sophisticated basis, and be accountable. If you fail to do this, you have failed yourself, and you have failed the residents, and you have failed the Nursing Home Industry. The task is not impossible. As a matter of fact, it is imperative. As a matter of fact, it is a very reasonable request. Effectively this is what the federal programs are asking of the nursing home industry. They are saying:

> We're paying a lot of money for long-term care. We don't know exactly what we're getting and we're concerned we may be paying for more than we're getting. So tell us what we're getting so we can determine its value. Once we're able to determine value we then can conceive of ways to finance the cost of care.

The buyer very well knows a return must be paid on the investment of the entrepreneurs in the long-term care industry. However, they will not acquiesce to speculation as to the value of the services and then approve a mark-up on an indefinable promise to deliver. There enters the patrons of accountability: accounting, costing, and budgeting.

For years I have defended the nursing home industry on many fronts; in the Offices of Public Aid, Public Health, at the legislature, and to the public. I've done this many times without adequate ammunition to fend off very difficult questions. Most of the questions relate to cost and quality of care. In the future, the nursing home industry will have to become more sophisticated in its marketing, management, and promotional efforts. If it does not, it will continue to suffer and be dominated by the governmental purchasers because it is not accountable. It would be wise for the leaders of the industry to step back and look at its status. The pattern of growth and maturity of nursing homes is very similar to hospitals. Unless nursing homes learn from the mistakes made by the hospital industry, I am afraid they will be facing the same trials and tribulations. To this day, hospitals are unable to adequately define the services they are providing, and do not accept their responsibility to be accountable. They still are not able to provide the purchaser with an effective means of gauging the cost and quality of their services. As a result they are dying a slow death. I hope this is not the epitaph of the nursing home industry.

What can you do? Basic accounting and budgeting! Take some time to write down on a piece of paper the services you are providing in a manner in which the services can be evaluated. The cost of services should also be determined, documented, and marked up to a reasonable level of profit. This reasonable level should then be compared to the reimbursement level of your governmental purchasers and any deficiencies communicated to the industry leadership. Until you take time to do this, everything is an exercise in speculation. You can also start communicating to your residents and their families the services you provide and the pains you take to make sure they are of quality. Of course quality in degree must be dealt with also. This is where we get into a matter of semantics and the use of terms such as, reasonable, adequate, minimum, standards, and so on. Frankly, in the long run I think we will find the degree of quality will relate to the amount of money available to purchase a degree of quality. If a higher degree of quality is demanded by the purchaser, then the seller of the services must be ready to tell them how much it will cost and why.

What else can you do to ensure quality? You can reduce staff turnover, you can improve inservice training, you can participate in association activities, you can subject your facility to peer review, you can become more astute in doing your job. It also does not hurt to care for the resident as a human being. For as the greatest orator of all times said, "Ye shall reap in the same proportion as ye sow." Or in modern lingo, "You will get paid, only if you're accountable," and being accountable involves accounting, costing, and budgeting.

The objective of this book is to provide a framework for gathering the information it takes to determine a fair price for a fair day's service, and in the process meet the demands of the marketplace. The framework consists of:

- Basic *accounting principles and procedures* for nursing homes. Some nursing home principles and procedures are totally unique, while others conform very closely to generally accepted accounting procedures. This book will deal with both.
- Methods of *cost accounting* and the uses of the information. This segment of accounting is the most important and the least understood. This book will communicate practical techniques in understandable terms to those responsible for cost control.
- *Budgeting* and how it is used to establish prices, control costs, and manage for profit. Budgeting is the dream everyone agrees should come true but somehow never comes true. This book will simplify budgeting so the administrator can prepare an operating budget.

Acknowledgments

I would like to thank the following organizations for their financial support and/or encouragement in my educational efforts. The writings and materials used in my lectures have all contributed to this book:

Illinois Health Care Association
American Health Care Association
National Council of Health Care Services
American College of Nursing Home Administrators
Illinois CPA Society
American Institute of CPAs
Ohio Health Care Association
Hospital Financial Management Association
Maryland Health Facilities Association
Colorado Health Care Association
Kentucky Association of Health Care Facilities
Idaho Health Facilities, Inc.
Montana Nursing Home Association
New Hampshire Association of Licensed Nursing Homes and Related Facilities
Nebraska Health Care Association
Alabama Health Care Association
Georgia Health Care Association

I would also like to thank my wife Shari and my family for their patience for two and a half years of late nights and early mornings. They are truly my inspiration. Also a special thanks to my expert speller and typist Jane Jensen.

CHAPTER 1
Accounting Theory

Accounting

DEFINITION OF ACCOUNTING

The process of accumulating economic information pertaining to the conduct of a business entity consists of recording in books of record business revenues (income), capital expenditures (outgo), and business noncash expenses (depreciation, amortization, and bad debts).

The result of this process is a compilation of information which reports the financial position of a business at a certain point in time and the results of its operations during a period of time. Bookkeeping is the process of recording the financial events in accordance with an accounting system.

OBJECTIVES OF ACCOUNTING

The objective of accounting is to arrange information pertaining to the conduct of a business entity in a manner that will enable a business manager to control assets and costs and establish prices and profit margins.

COMPONENTS OF ACCOUNTING

The accounting process records the financial events of an organization by making additions to and removals from specific classifications known as accounts. There are five general types of accounts: assets, liabilities, owners' capital, revenues, and expenses. The first three of these categories are used to describe the financial position of an organization at a point in time. Periodically, these categories are shown on a statement called a *balance sheet,* which is divided into two major sections. One section lists all of the assets of the organization, and the other lists both liabilities and owners' equity. The total shown in the asset section always equals the total shown in the liabilities and owners' capital section.

Assets are financial resources over which an organization has control and ownership. Examples of these are cash, claims to receive cash, buildings, land, equipment, and unused inventories. Generally, assets are divided into current and noncurrent portions on the balance sheet. The current portion shows the assets that are equivalent to cash or are expected to be realized in the form of cash within one operating cycle. This is usually the same period as the accounting (fiscal) year. The noncurrent portion contains assets that will not be converted to cash within one operating cycle, such as, plant, property, equipment, and investments.

Liabilities are financial obligations such as unpaid taxes, bills, outstanding mortgages, and other kinds of open debt. Liabilities are also presented in current and noncurrent terms. Current liabilities consist of obligations that will require the use of current assets in their payment, while the noncurrent liabilities will require funds from more than one operating cycle.

Owners' capital represents the excess of the assets over liabilities. Owners' capital consists of the direct financial investment of the owners plus the increase or decrease in the assets of the organization which have come about through the results of the business enterprise. For nonprofit organizations, the term for owners' capital is fund balance.

The revenue and expense categories of accounts are used to record the results of operations during the operating cycle. *Revenues* are resources earned in exchange for providing goods and services to others. *Expenses* are costs incurred during the operating cycle to provide goods and services to others.

Total revenue and expense are compared during the operating cycle. The excess of revenue over expense is referred to as profit or net income. If it is not paid out in the form of dividends it becomes retained earnings which are part of owners' capital. If expenses exceed revenue, owners' capital is reduced. Revenue, expense, and profit during or at the end of the operating cycle are presented in a financial report entitled *Statement of Income, Operating Statement,* or *P/L Statement.*

Generally Accepted Accounting Principles

Underlying the financial reports are generally accepted accounting principles (GAAP) and the fundamental concepts regarding the accounting entity, the accounting period, consistency, objective evidence, accounting estimates, and historical cost.

GAAP are the accounting techniques and procedures that have acceptance in the accounting profession and financial community. They are a result of many years of accounting research and experience documented in authoritative textbooks and literature published by professional accountants.

THE ACCOUNTING ENTITY

The accounting entity must be separate from the private or personal affairs of those who own or manage it. A corporation is an entity for both accounting and legal purposes. Sole proprietorships and partnerships, although not considered legal entities, are accounted for as separate and distinct from owners and management.

THE ACCOUNTING PERIOD

The accounting period is the operating cycle, usually one year, that is used to report financial results. Any business may choose the annual period most convenient to them, since a particular period is not required of any business. The annual period selected may be twelve monthly periods, thirteen four-week periods, or any rational accounting cycle chosen by the facility. Once a particular period has been selected by a facility, the same period is normally used from year to year. A facility must notify certain regulatory bodies, such as the Internal Revenue Service (IRS), in writing whenever the facility's fiscal year is to be changed. For internal purposes the annual period should be broken down into specific periods (usually monthly) to enable the facility to close its records on a timely basis during the operating cycle, to provide management with current information on financial status.

CONSISTENCY

Consistency is the practice of recording accounting transactions in the same manner each time they arise. Methods of recording identical transactions should be the same from one period to the next. This is necessary to permit the facility to keep its records on the accrual basis and make comparisons among different operating cycles. To permit comparisons, the methods of accounting and recording the same transactions should be consistent from one year to the next. Generally accepted accounting principles specify a single required method of accounting for a large number of transaction types.

OBJECTIVE EVIDENCE

Objective evidence refers to documents that are unbiased and subject to verification. Accounting information should be based, to the degree possible, on objectively determined, documented facts. Examples of such evidence are invoices, contracts, receiving reports, and canceled checks. In some cases objective evidence is not available and estimates must be used.

ACCOUNTING ESTIMATES

Accounting estimates are frequently required in order to properly maintain financial records in accordance with generally accepted accounting principles. They are also required in anticipating the life of depreciable assets, determining the portion of accounts receivable that is uncollectible, and determining the liability for goods and services that have been used, although the specific cost is not known because a bill has not been received. Once an estimate has been made, it should be reviewed periodically to determine if it is still valid. If a new estimate is required, an adjustment to the accounting records must be made. For example:

Cost of plant	$1,000,000
Estimated depreciable life	40 years
Actual life	35 years
(Beds were considered nonconforming and the whole facility had to be replaced.)	
Annual estimated depreciation based on a 40-year life	$25,000
Number of years in use	×35
Total depreciation	$875,000
Original cost	1,000,000
Error in depreciation	$125,000 *

*An adjustment to depreciation expense must be made in the year that the beds become nonconforming. The adjustment is spread over the remaining useful life.

HISTORICAL COST

Historical cost is the most basic of generally accepted accounting principles. It is the requirement that all assets be presented in financial statements at their acquisition cost. In recent years, one of the most discussed subjects in accounting circles is the reporting of the current market value of assets as well as the actual cost of the assets. However, generally accepted accounting principles require that assets be recorded and reported at their cost (market value at the time of acquisition). For assets that are purchased, the actual cost is taken to be the best indication of market value at the date of acquisition. For assets that are donated, the estimated fair market value of the asset at the time of donation is its cost value.

Accrual Accounting

According to the dictionary, accrue means to become an enforceable right or commitment. Therefore accrual accounting is the enforceable right to revenues as earned and the enforceable commitment for expenses as incurred, regardless of when the cash is collected or disbursed.

This means that a patient's bill for services for a particular period, even though not collected until later, becomes income to the business entity when there is an enforceable right to the money. Therefore, as the patient receives services, the business entity is provided with an enforceable right to the money. This represents an account receivable and earned revenue.

It also means that nurses' salaries for a particular period, even though not paid until payday, become an expense of the business entity when there is an enforceable commitment to pay the money. Therefore, as the nurse provides the patient services, the business entity is enforceably committed to pay that employee for that service. This represents a payable or accrued liability and an incurred expense.

For providing services the long-term care facility incurs a wide variety of expenses. For the most part, these expenses are paid from revenues provided in exchange for care furnished to its patients. It is important to note that both revenues and expenses result from the provision of services by the facility, and because of this, an attempt should be made to match these revenues and expenses. This matching concept should be shown clearly in the presentation of the financial information for the period in which the service was performed.

To present financial information in such a manner, generally accepted accounting principles require that a nursing home* maintain its records on the *accrual basis.* Under the accrual basis, revenue and expense are recognized when the service to which they relate is performed; the actual time when money is received or paid out usually has nothing to do with the recognition of revenue or expense in the accounting records. A facility that records revenue and expense when money actually changes hands is using a form of what is known as the *cash basis* of accounting. The cash basis of accounting is not in accordance with generally accepted accounting principles.

What does this mean? It means that if you bill a patient $500 for this period's services, you have earned and have an enforceable right to that $500 even though the cash has not yet been collected. Likewise, if you are employing a nurse at a salary equivalent to $200 to care for the patient during this same period, you have incurred an expense of and an enforceable obligation to pay the $200 even though payday is not until the next financial period.

---

*The terms nursing home and long-term care facility should be considered interchangeable, both here and throughout the book.

Now, let us use these two transactions and assume they are the extent of the nursing home's activities for one period. This will allow us to compare the cash basis and accrual basis of accounting:

	Cash Basis	Accrual Basis
Income (patient services)	$-0-	$500
Expense (nursing salaries)	-0-	200
Net income	$-0-	$300

Since no cash changed hands there are no cash receipts or expenditures. If you were accumulating information only as cash comes in and goes out, there would be no net income until cash changed hands. On the other hand, the service has been provided and expenses incurred, so to show no income or expense does not depict the true results; a net income of $300 has been earned and an enforceable right to it has been established. The example is quite simplistic, but realistic. If you are the owner or administrator of this nursing home, the accrual information is meaningful in determining profit or loss. The cash results are meaningful only in managing finances and cash flow.

WHY IS ACCRUAL ACCOUNTING NECESSARY?

Accrual accounting is the outgrowth of the following basic accounting assumptions:

- *Periodicity*—The economic activity of a business is continuous in nature with regard to economic input and output flows through the entity, but the enterprise has a business cycle. To be able to judge the profit or loss of the enterprise, a fiscal reporting period is established (usually twelve months) and used to evaluate the results of the business cycle.
- *Revenue recognition*—Revenue is recognized in the period in which it is earned, and when an enforceable right has been established to receive the revenue.
- *Matching*—Expenses incurred during the period in which the revenue is earned must be matched with the revenues earned during the same period, if meaningful profit and loss figures are to be produced.

When the expenses incurred for the period are matched to the revenues earned during the same period, management can determine if the desired return on the investment in goods, people, and resources is being attained. If it is not, adjustments in strategy, action, and procedures must come about immediately. So as we talk about a management information system, we will be referring to a system of records and reports that match expenses incurred with revenue earned to determine the amount of profit or loss and return on investment.

Accounting Equation and Records

The following information is designed to acquaint you with the concepts and terms of basic bookkeeping and accounting.

THE DOUBLE ENTRY ACCOUNTING EQUATION

The primary equation for double entry accounting is:

ASSETS = LIABILITIES + CAPITAL (Net Worth)

where:

ASSETS	=	Cash, accounts receivable, inventory, buildings, and equipment that are owned by the business
LIABILITIES	=	Amounts owed to creditors
CAPITAL (Net Worth)	=	Equity accumulated (represents net assets that would be distributed if the business were liquidated)

RULES FOR DEBITS AND CREDITS

In every accounting entry there is always a corresponding debit or debits for every credit; and there is always a corresponding credit or credits for every debit. The debits must always be the same amount as the credits. This concept becomes the goal of double entry accounting—to have all the debits equal the credits and thereby produce balanced books.

Debits (Left Side of Accounts)	Credits (Right Side of Accounts)
Acquisition of assets or increases in asset values	Disposal of assets or decreases in asset values
Decreases in liabilities	Increases in liabilities
Decreases in capital and retained earnings	Increases in capital and retained earnings
Decreases in revenue	Increases in revenue
Increases in expenses	Decreases in expenses

(*Note:* This account structure is known as a T account because the lines resemble the letter "T.")

BILLINGS JOURNAL

The Billings Journal (Exhibit 1-1) is designed to collect in one place all the billings resulting from the sale of supplies and services to patients.

The record is a listing of the billings. The following facts are recorded:

1. Patient name
2. Patient account number (if applicable)
3. Room number or bed number
4. DEBIT Accounts Receivable
5. CREDIT (arrange credit columns according to the chart of accounts based on the type of revenue):
   a. Room and board (by level of care and payer)
   b. Supplies
   c. Ancillary services (by type)

Posting to the Billings Journal provides totals of the bills submitted to the residents for the month and the distribution of the income into useful, informative categories. The individual patient ledger cards (Exhibit 1-2) are then posted for each charge and payment, as a perpetual record of the status of each patient's account.

Charges normally should be recorded according to a single uniform schedule of charges. Uniformity of charges is a requirement of Medicare and may be useful in determining the potential revenue that is being absorbed due to cost-related reimbursement contracts.

ACCOUNTS PAYABLE JOURNAL OR PURCHASE JOURNAL

The Accounts Payable Journal (Exhibit 1-3) is designed to collect in one record, each month, all transactions that result in a debt for purchased services and commodities to be paid on a short-term basis.

This journal is a listing of the monthly purchases. The following facts are recorded:

1. A voucher number
2. Name of the vendor
3. Date of the entry
4. Date of the invoice
5. Explanation (optional)
6. Date of payment (optional)
7. Check number (optional)
8. CREDIT Accounts Payable
9. DEBIT (arrange remaining columns according to the chart of accounts based on reason for expenditure):
   a. Expense accounts
   b. Inventory
   c. Equipment
   d. Prepaid expenses

Posting to the Accounts Payable Journal provides totals of the accounts payable and the expenditures for the month, for posting to the General Ledger accounts. Each purchase is then posted to the Accounts Payable Ledger (Exhibit 1-4) which keeps track of the amount purchased, the amount paid, and the balance due each supplier.

PAYROLL JOURNAL

The Payroll Journal (Exhibit 1-5) is designed to collect in one place all payroll checks released for the month. Since the accounting in the General Ledger requires salary expense to be recorded according to a specific cost center, the Payroll Journal must group the payroll amounts by cost centers.

Where employees divide their time between two or more cost centers, the employee should be listed and paid in the principal cost center with an allocation made to transfer a portion of the payroll expense to the appropriate cost center.

Exhibit 1-1 Billings Journal

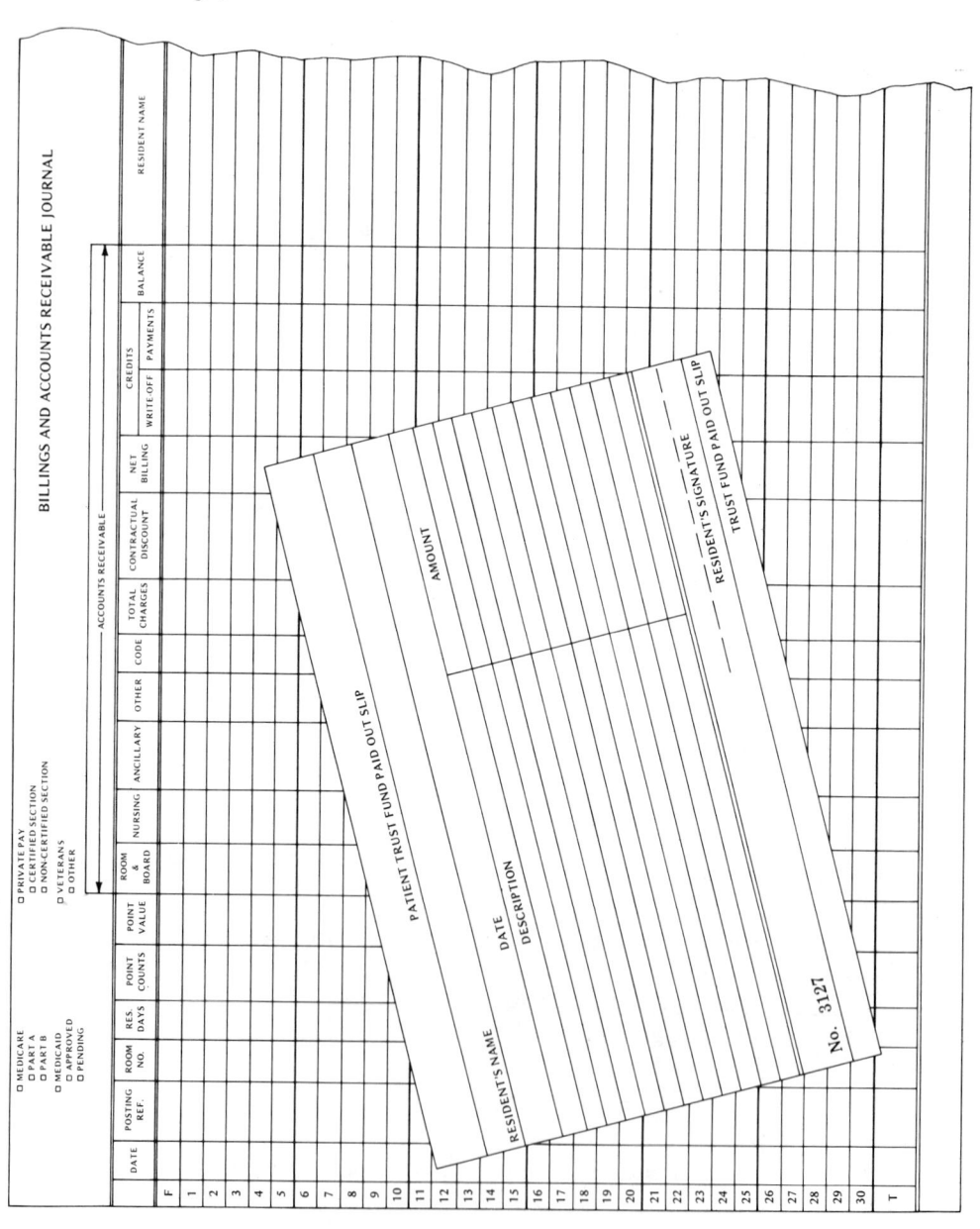

Exhibit 1-1 (cont.)

Exhibit 1-2 Patient Ledger Card

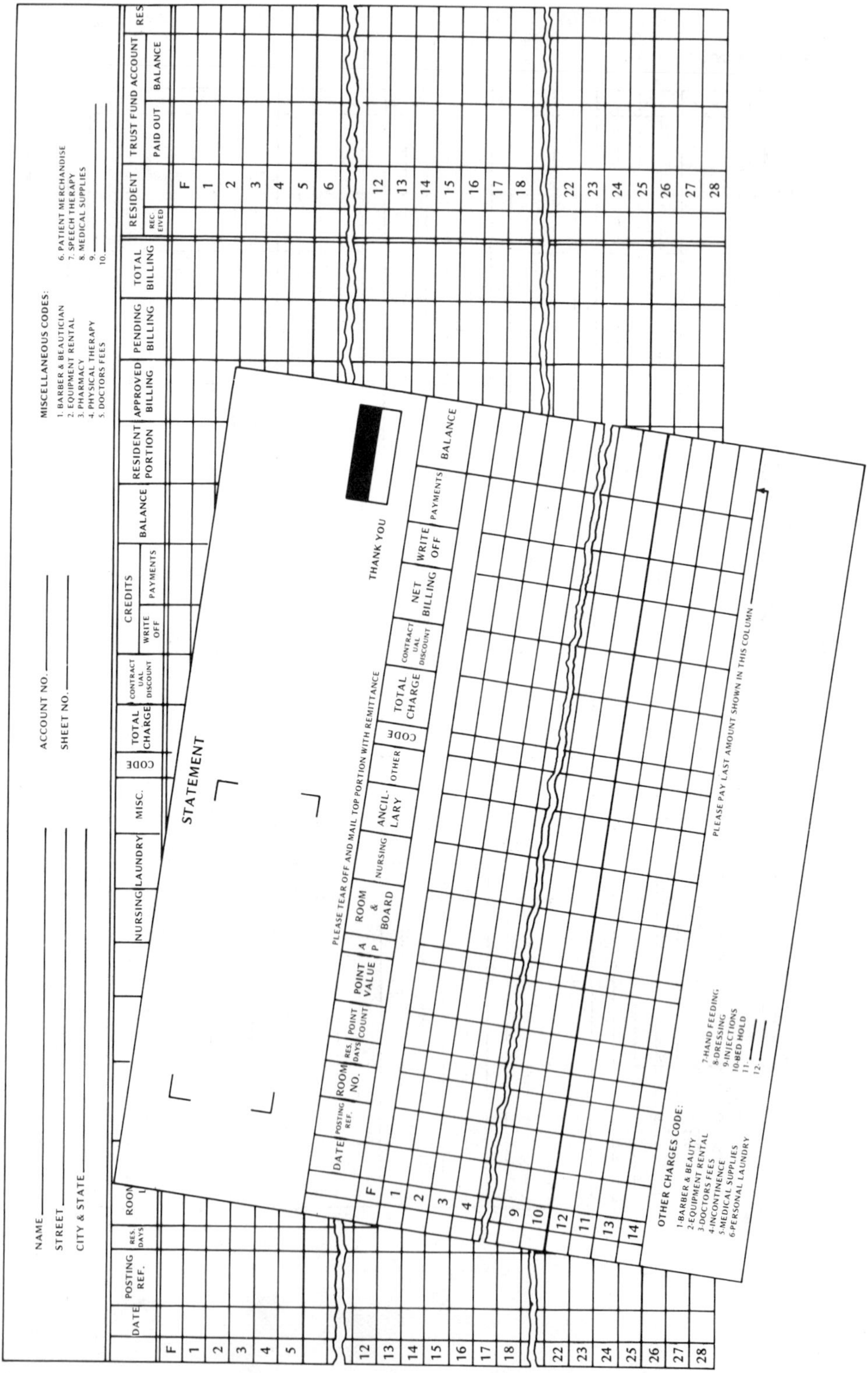

Nursing staffs that "float" between departments, for example, skilled to intermediate or certified to noncertified, should be allocated to the appropriate cost center, as the payroll is recorded, based on hours worked or according to a costed staffing plan.

In addition to obtaining the gross pay for each employee by cost center, the Social Security and unemployment compensation taxes may be gathered for each cost center. This is helpful in determining the proper distribution of the employer's cost for payroll taxes. This is the first step in cost finding.

The Payroll Journal should record information about an employee's pay by cost center. The following facts are recorded:

1. Date of the payroll
2. Name of the employee
3. Employee's record or social security number
4. Regular hours worked and pay
5. Overtime hours worked and pay
6. Sick time hours and pay
7. Vacation time hours and pay
8. Excused time hours and pay
9. GROSS PAY
10. Federal withholding tax
11. State withholding tax
12. Local withholding tax
13. Social security withholding tax
14. Other deductions (with space for a code)
15. NET PAY
16. Date of check
17. Check number

CASH RECEIPTS JOURNAL

The Cash Receipts Journal (Exhibit 1–6) is designed to collect in one place all the cash received from the sale of supplies and services to patients. It is important that all checks recorded in the Cash Receipts Journal be deposited daily intact in the bank. Checks should be endorsed "For Deposit Only" as received. The bank deposit must agree with the Cash Receipts Journal postings. (Cash payments should never be made directly from cash receipts. Disbursement should always be made by check except for those that can be made from petty cash.)

The cashier should issue a separate receipt slip for each cash item collected. Preferably, the receipt should be in triplicate—original to the payor, duplicate to the bookkeeper, and triplicate retained by the cashier. The receipt slips should be prenumbered and accounted for when making out the daily deposit slip.

When the day's receipts are deposited, have the bank teller validate two copies of the deposit slip. One copy goes to the cashier and one copy to the

Exhibit 1-3 Accounts Payable Journal (Purchase Journal)

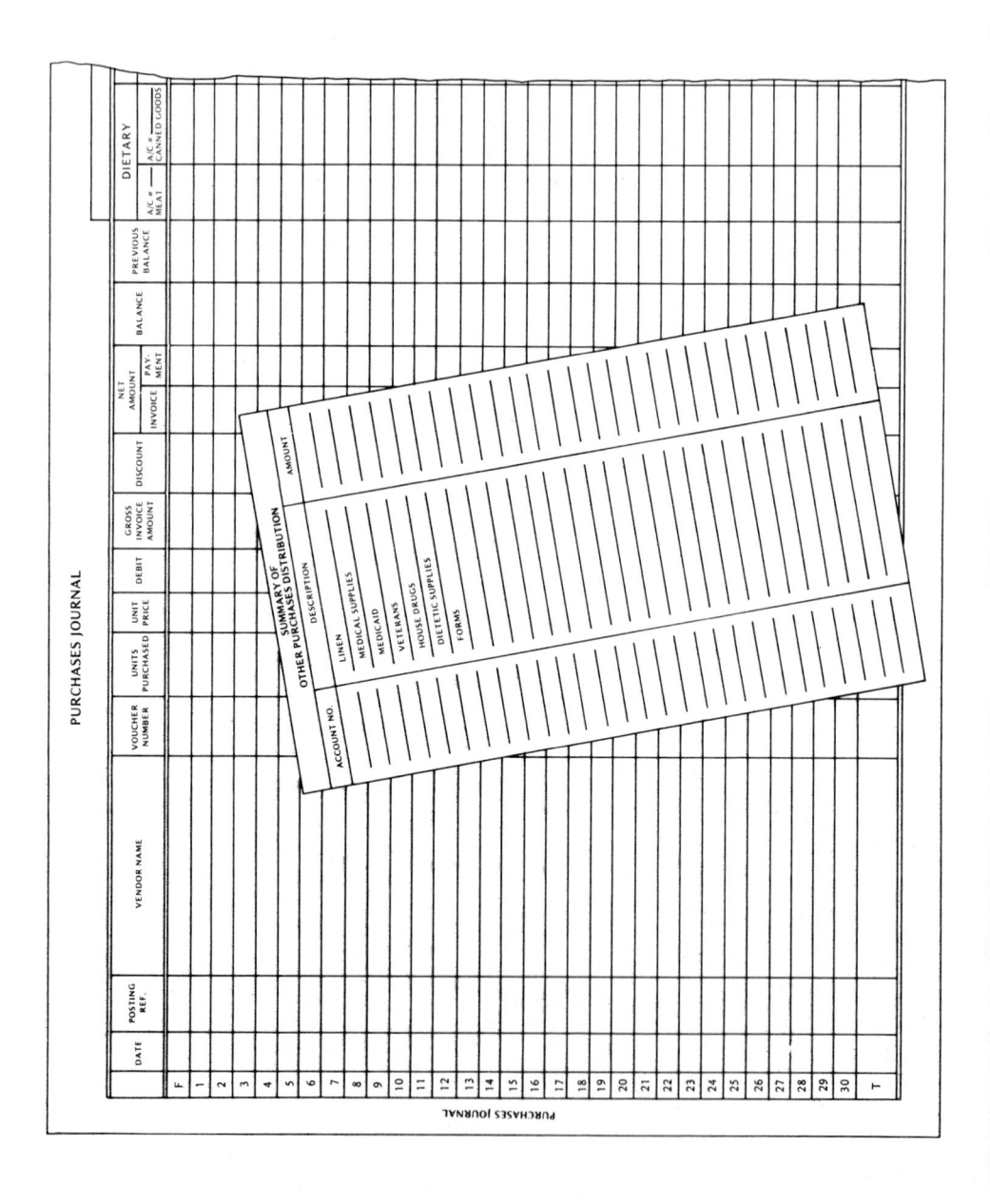

12

Exhibit 1-3 (cont.)

Exhibit 1-4 Accounts Payable Ledger

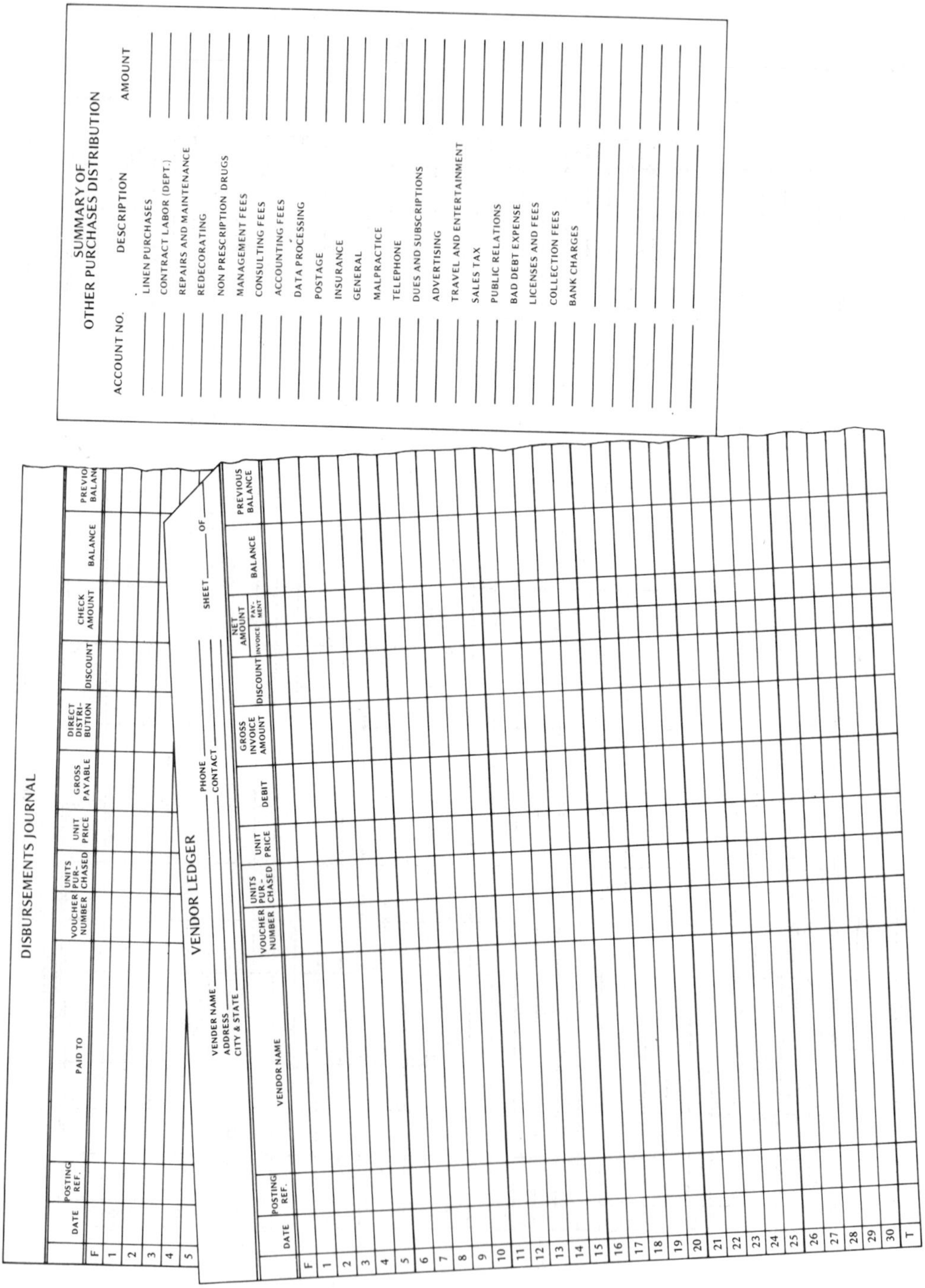

SUMMARY OF
OTHER PURCHASES DISTRIBUTION

ACCOUNT NO.	DESCRIPTION	AMOUNT
	LINEN PURCHASES	
	CONTRACT LABOR (DEPT.)	
	REPAIRS AND MAINTENANCE	
	REDECORATING	
	NON PRESCRIPTION DRUGS	
	MANAGEMENT FEES	
	CONSULTING FEES	
	ACCOUNTING FEES	
	DATA PROCESSING	
	POSTAGE	
	INSURANCE	
	GENERAL	
	MALPRACTICE	
	TELEPHONE	
	DUES AND SUBSCRIPTIONS	
	ADVERTISING	
	TRAVEL AND ENTERTAINMENT	
	SALES TAX	
	PUBLIC RELATIONS	
	BAD DEBT EXPENSE	
	LICENSES AND FEES	
	COLLECTION FEES	
	BANK CHARGES	

DISBURSEMENTS JOURNAL

	DATE	POSTING REF.	PAID TO	VOUCHER NUMBER	UNITS PUR-CHASED	UNIT PRICE	GROSS PAYABLE	DIRECT DISTRI-BUTION	DISCOUNT	CHECK AMOUNT	BALANCE	PREVIO BALAN
F												
1												
2												
3												
4												
5												

VENDOR LEDGER

VENDER NAME _____ PHONE _____ SHEET _____ OF _____
ADDRESS _____ CONTACT _____
CITY & STATE _____

	DATE	POSTING REF.	VENDOR NAME	VOUCHER NUMBER	UNITS PUR-CHASED	UNIT PRICE	DEBIT	GROSS INVOICE AMOUNT	DISCOUNT	NET AMOUNT INVOICE	NET AMOUNT PAY-MENT	BALANCE	PREVIOUS BALANCE
F													
1													
2													
3													
4													
5													
6													
7													
8													
9													
10													
11													
12													
13													
14													
15													
16													
17													
18													
19													
20													
21													
22													
23													
24													
25													
26													
27													
28													
29													
30													
T													

bookkeeper. Both should file these in date sequence. Remember to keep each day separate.

The Cash Receipts Journal should list the same information that is recorded on the cashier's receipt slip. The facts about the payment are:

1. Cashier's receipt number
2. Date of the cash collection
3. Patient's account number
4. Name of the patient
5. Name of the payor (if different from patient)
6. DEBIT Cash—Operating Account
7. CREDIT Accounts Receivable (by payor)
8. Debit contractual discount (if a third party pays a cost-related rate different than the customary charge for the noncovered portion of the billing)

Posting to the Cash Receipts Journal provides totals of the cash received and the reduction of accounts receivable for posting to the General Ledger.

CASH DISBURSEMENTS JOURNAL

The Cash Disbursements Journal or Check Register (Exhibit 1–7) is designed to collect in one place all the cash disbursed for the purchase of supplies and services to be used in rendering services to patients. The Check Register is a listing of the checks, names of the payees, and information about the payments.

It is recommended that checks be issued only on the authority of an approved invoice. The invoice must be supported by a receiving report attesting that the goods or services listed on the invoice were received satisfactorily; and, to be sure everything delivered was actually ordered, by a copy of the purchase order bearing the signatures of various responsible persons. All of this documentation is necessary to authorize the issuance of a check.

With a good purchase system, the Check Register needs very few columns. Normally there are columns for:

1. Date of check
2. Name of payee
3. Check number
4. Voucher number (accounts payable number)
5. CREDIT Cash—Operating Account
6. CREDIT Discounts Earned (if applicable)
7. DEBIT Accounts Payable—Current Month
8. DEBIT Accounts Payable—Prior Months
9. DEBIT miscellaneous accounts

Columns 6, 7, and 8 help to show how well accounts payable are being managed.

Posting to the Check Register provides totals of the cash disbursements and the reduction of accounts payable for posting to the General Ledger.

Exhibit 1-5 Payroll Journal

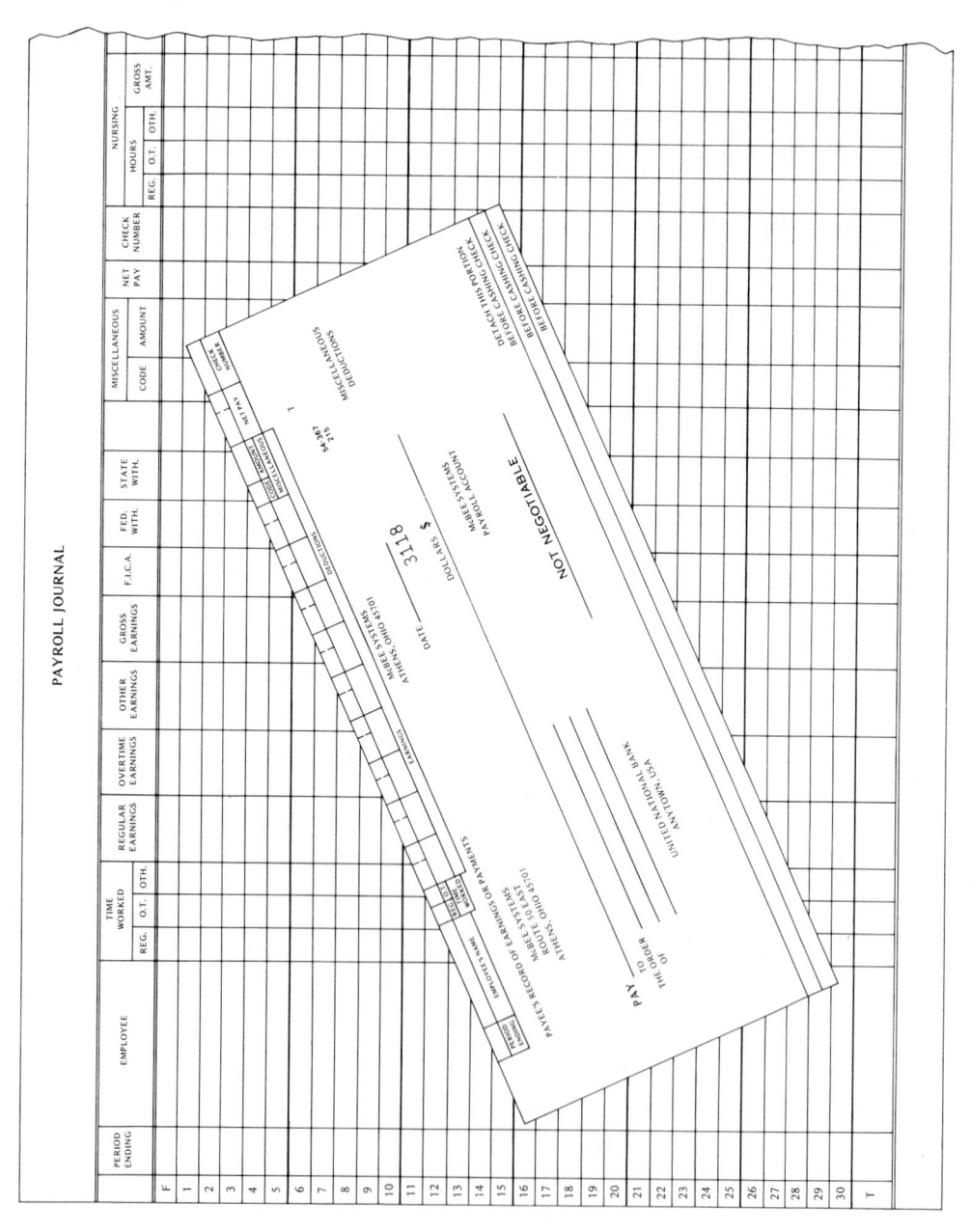

Exhibit 1-5 (cont.)

Exhibit 1-6 Cash Receipts Journal

CASH RECEIPTS JOURNAL

	DATE	POSTING REF.	ROOM NO.		WRITE OFF	PAYMENTS	BALANCE	RESIDENT TRUST FUND			ACCOUNTS RECEIVABLE (CREDIT)
								RECEIVED	PAID OUT	BALANCE	
F											
1											
2											
3											
4											
5											
6											
7											
8											
9											
10											
11											
12											
13											
14											
15											
16											
17											
18											
19											
20											
21											
22											
23											
24											
25											
26											
27											
28											
29											
30											
T											

Exhibit 1-6 (cont.)

		RESIDENT OR PAYOR NAME				OTHER CASH RECEIPTS			TOTAL DEPOSIT	RESIDENT TRUST FUND		
						DESCRIPTION	ACCT. NO.	AMOUNT		CHECK NUMBER	DEPOSIT AMOUNT	
	F											F
	1											1
	2											2
	3											3
	4											4
	5											5
	6											6
	7											7
	8											8
	9											9
	10											10
	11											11
	12											12
	13											13
	14											14
	15											15
	16											16
	17											17
	18											18
	19											19
	20											20
	21											21
	22											22
	23											23
	24											24
	25											25
	26											26
	27											27
	28											28
	29											29
	30											30
	T											T

PAGE NO.
DATE

Exhibit 1-7 Check Register

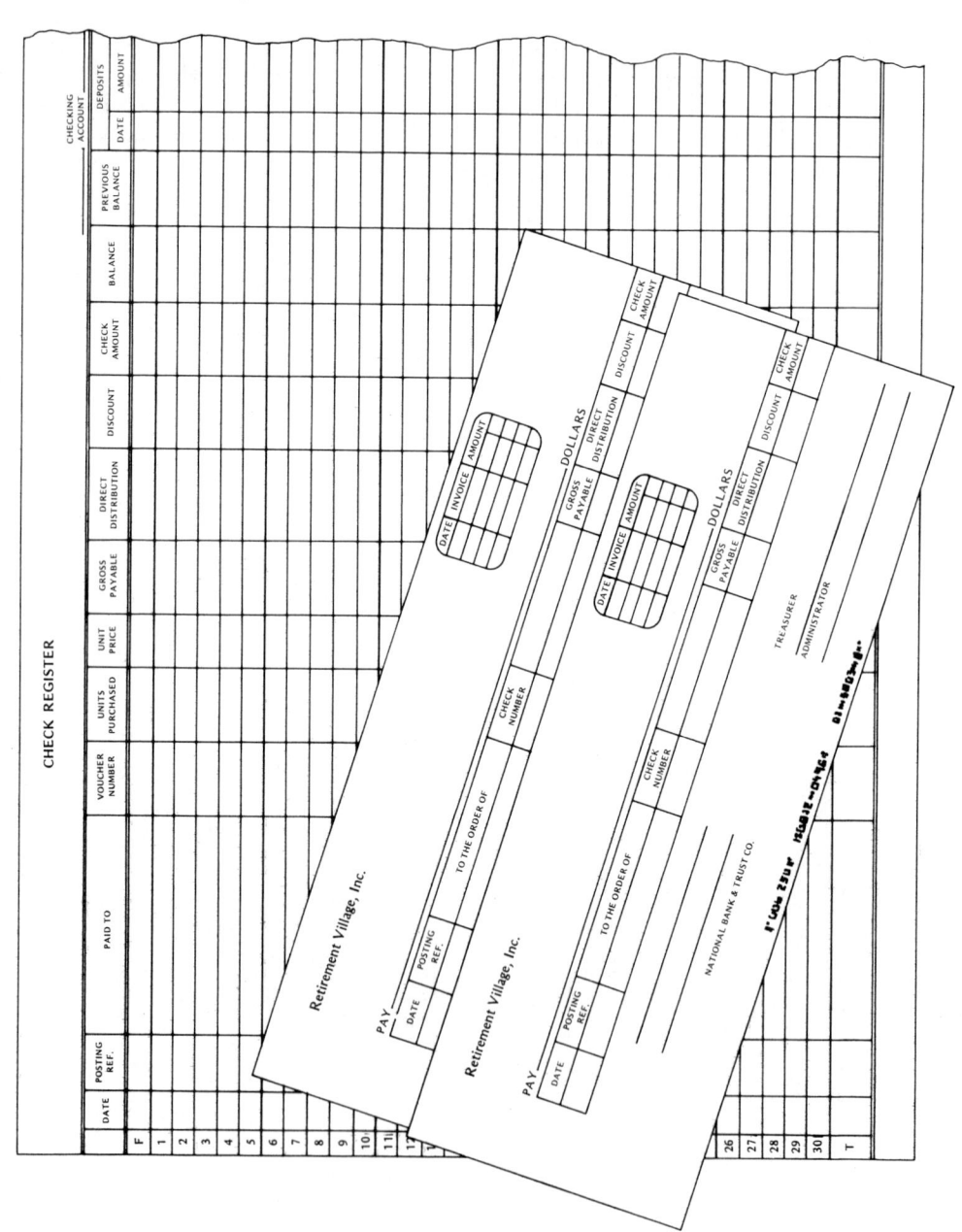

Exhibit 1-7 (cont.)

GENERAL JOURNAL

The General Journal is a book of original entry which records exceptional items that are not repetitive during an accounting period and do not warrant a specific purpose journal. Examples of these items are:

1. End of month entries
2. Adjusting entries
3. Correcting entries

Each entry in the General Journal is made up of debits and an equal amount in credits. As in the other journals the debits must always be equal to the credits. Also, there should always be clarifying explanation of the entry. There should be no doubt as to the reason for the entry.

In the other journals the summary totals are transcribed to the ledger, but in the General Journal each separate debit and credit is transcribed to the ledger. Many of the General Journal entries are repeated once every month. A set of *standard* General Journal entries helps significantly in the management of the General Ledger. Each month, the Journal Entry number is checked off so that nothing is overlooked. More than half the balancing problems of accountants are problems of omission—forgetting to record transactions completely.

Some typical General Journal entries which will be posted in the General Ledger in a normal situation are shown in Exhibit 1-8.

GENERAL LEDGER

The General Ledger is the book of *final entry*. All the other journals and registers, are books of *original entry*. All the summary accounting data accumulated in the journals and the General Journal are posted to the appropriate accounts in the General Ledger.

There is a separate page for each account listed in the Chart of Accounts. All accounts are numbered. There are accounts for Assets, Liabilities and Capital, Income, and Expenses. In tax-exempt nursing homes there are additional sections of the Chart of Accounts relating to Fund Accounting.

The General Ledger is arranged in the sequence in which it will be used in preparing financial statements. Monthly financial statements are prepared from the balances in the General Ledger accounts after they are closed and balanced. The first step in closing the General Ledger, after the journals are posted, is to list all the balances in a Trial Balance to be sure the General Ledger is in balance.

TRIAL BALANCE

Before monthly financial statements can be prepared from the balances in the General Ledger accounts, a Trial Balance should be drawn up.

A Trial Balance (Exhibit 1-9) is a list of the DEBIT and CREDIT balances of all the General Ledger Accounts. In keeping with the primary principle of accounting, the sum of all DEBIT balances should equal the sum of all the CREDIT balances. You cannot begin to prepare the financial statements until you have proven the totals to be equal.

Exhibit 1-8 General Journal

	A/C Number	Debit	Credit
1. Housekeeping—supplies		$2500	
Inventory—Housekeeping			$2500
To set up expense for supplies used during June.			
2. Accounts receivable—Patients		$ 83	
Cash—Operating Account			$ 83
To record a refund check.			
3. Provision for uncollectible receivables		$ 700	
Reserve for uncollectible receivables			$ 700
To set as an estimate of possible uncollectible accounts.			
4. Inventory—supplies		$2400	
Dietary expense—raw food			$1800
Laundry & Linen expense			200
Medical supplies			400
To adjust expense accounts for supplies on hand at the close of the period.			
5. Depreciation—movable equipment		$1000	
Accumulated depreciation—movable equipment			$1000

Just because the TOTALS of the DEBITS and CREDITS on the Trial Balance are determined to be equal, it should not be interpreted that the account balances themselves are correct. You should be aware that:

1. An incorrect amount may have been originally posted as a DEBIT or CREDIT.
2. A particular transaction may have been posted to the wrong account.
3. A transaction may have been omitted altogether.

Thus, it is important to use utmost precaution in posting the General Ledger Accounts and in recapping the balances of the accounts in the Trial Balance.

Note that the Trial Balance is divided into two parts:

1. The accounts that make up the Profit and Loss Statement
2. The accounts that make up the Balance Sheet

Also note that the grand TOTALS of DEBIT and CREDIT columns are equal.

PROFIT AND LOSS STATEMENT

After balancing the Trial Balance, you can prepare the Profit and Loss Statement, the components of which are described as follows:

1. The *Income* portion shows the billing of revenue for services rendered to patients.

Exhibit 1-9 Trial Balance

RETIREMENT VILLAGE, INC.

TRIAL BALANCE
5/31/80

Page 1

ACCOUNT NO.	DESCRIPTION	CURRENT PERIOD DEBIT AMOUNT	CURRENT PERIOD CREDIT AMOUNT	ENDING BALANCE DEBIT AMOUNT	ENDING BALANCE CREDIT AMOUNT
1000-0	ASSETS				
1000-1	CURRENT ASSETS				
1101-0	Cash In Bank - Operating	$183,578.35		$208,136.45	
1102-0	Cash In Bank - Building			$640.98	
1103-0	Cash In Bank - Gift Shop			$1,856.04	
1105-0	Cash In Bank - Trust Funds		$121.48	$15,772.91	
1108-0	Petty Cash Funds - Trust Fund			$250.00	
1109-0	Petty Cash Funds - Operating			$1,110.00	
1110-0	Imprest Payroll				$0.00
1111-0	Savings Account - Prudential			$3,911.33	
112-0	Savings Account - Building				
1113-0	Savings Account - Bonds		$10,336.17	$274,311.73	
1114-0	Savings Account - Chapel			$616.46	
1115-0	Investment - C.D.s			$153,300.00	
1116-0	Investment - Burial C.D.s			$7,000.00	
1117-0	Investment - Stocks			$2,650.00	

Acct #	Description			
1118-0	Investment – Bonds			$9,968.38
1119-0	Reserve For Bond Redemption	$1,856.25		$66,105.61
1121-0	Accts. Rec. —Private Patients	$24,022.16		$86,739.82
1122-0	Accts. Rec. —Medicaid	$8,588.96		$51,125.01
1123-0	Accts. Rec. —Medicaid Pending		$5,440.34	$2,440.50
1127-0	Accts. Rec. —Other			
1128-0	Hill-Burton Receivable			$8,194.00
1140-0	Real Estate Contracts Rec.		$48.92	$7,058.87
1141-0	Physician Fees – Clearing	$4,963.21		$40,238.48
1146-0	Accrued Interest Receivable			$927.50
1163-0	Unexpired Insurance			$1,779.75
400-0	CAPITAL ASSETS			
1405-0	Land			$96,017.50
1406-0	Land Improvements			$25,172.43
1411-0	Buildings – Original			$1,350,000.00
1412-0	Buildings – New			$1,230,842.33
1413-0	Buildings – Dycus			$916,911.13
1414-0	Buildings – Cottages			$769,634.15
1415-0	Buildings – Houses		$2,000.00	$107,044.35
1416-0	Buildings – Apartments			$395,909.49
1417-0	Buildings – House Trailer			$5,720.00
1418-0	Buildings—Wesley Ctr. —8 Bed			$6,600.23
1421-0	Building Improvements			$302,625.74
1431-0	Equip., Furniture & Fixtures	$178.00		$729,895.60
1432-0	Home and Cottage Furnishings			$45,065.53
1433-0	Apartment Furnishings			$61,235.00
1434-0	Office Equipment	$307.24		$13,027.27
1441-0	Transportation Equipment			$30,038.16
1506-0	Acc. Depr. —Land Improvements		$105.00	$4,487.30

Exhibit 1-9 (cont.)

RETIREMENT VILLAGE, INC.

TRIAL BALANCE
5/31/80

Page 9

ACCOUNT NO.	DESCRIPTION	CURRENT PERIOD DEBIT AMOUNT	CURRENT PERIOD CREDIT AMOUNT	ENDING BALANCE DEBIT AMOUNT	ENDING BALANCE CREDIT AMOUNT
1511-0	Acc. Depr. —Bldgs. —Original		$2,250.00		$389,250.00
1512-0	Acc. Depr. —Bldgs. —New		$2,052.00		$299,702.95
1513-0	Acc. Depr. —Bldgs. —Dycus		$1,528.00		$108,573.48
1514-0	Acc. Depr. —Cottages		$1,283.00		$77,752.17
1515-0	Acc. Depr. —Bldgs. —Houses		$199.00		$18,651.97
7963-0	Special Gifts—All Other		$44,208.95		$169,744.73
7964-0	Donated Oil Royalty Income		$578.17		$3,994.73
7965-0	Bake Sales & Bazaars				$618.60
7970-0	Rental Income – Beauty Shop		$100.00		$400.00
7981-0	Gain/Loss – Sale of Securities				
7991-0	Miscellaneous Income		$22.00		$311.54
		$800,622.02	$800,622.02	$9,775,485.63	$9,775,485.63

2. The *Expense* portion shows the expenditures of assets used in providing the services rendered to patients.
3. The *Net Profit* or *Net Loss* is the net increase or decrease in the nursing home's assets derived from services rendered to patients, that is, the difference between Income and Expense.

The Profit and Loss (P/L) Statement reflects the operating results for a specific period of time. Normally a P/L Statement is issued at the end of each month, showing the operating results for the month and year to date. The P/L Statement tells how the nursing home did financially for that particular month. If the actual results are compared to a budget, a better evaluation can be made as to whether the home is operating close to plan.

CLOSING THE INCOME AND EXPENSE ACCOUNTS

Once the Profit and Loss Statement has been completed for the fiscal year, the revenue and expense accounts in the General Ledger have served their purpose. They are annually "closed out" so that a new start can be made each year. Closing out the income and expense accounts is accomplished by one of two methods:

- *Method 1*—Record a closing entry for each individual revenue and expense account.
  a. *Debit* each separate account that has an ending credit balance.
  b. *Credit* each separate account that has an ending debit balance.
  c. *Debit or credit* the net difference (net profit is a credit; net loss is a debit) to the retained earnings account which represents the equity accumulation available for dividends.
- *Method 2*—Underscore each revenue and expense account as closed and record the net profit or loss figure in the retained earnings account. This keeps the books in balance and closes out the completed year.

BALANCE SHEET

After balancing the Trial Balance and preparing the Profit and Loss Statement, you can prepare the Balance Sheet, the components of which are described as follows:

1. The *Assets* are the resources of the nursing home consisting of personal and real properties owned (such as cash, buildings, and equipment).
2. The *Liabilities* are the creditors' claims against the Assets (such as accounts payable and mortgage payable).
3. The *Net Worth,* or *Capital,* or *Owners' Net Equity* is the equity of the owners in the Assets after deducting all liabilities. (In tax-exempt nursing homes, the term Fund Balance is used rather than Capital.)

The combined claims of creditors (Liabilities) and owners (Capital) must equal the value of the Assets.

The Balance Sheet is prepared monthly and reflects the financial status of the nursing home. For example:

Assets	$1,000,000
Less: Liabilities	800,000
Equals Capital	$ 200,000

THE JOURNAL SYSTEM

The advantages of the journal system for accounting are:

1. It summarizes details ultimately in one record, the General Ledger.
2. It permits two persons to work on the accounting records at the same time without interfering with the other.
3. It develops a control listing of all transactions and when they are due.
4. It segregates duties that might be vulnerable to embezzlement if not maintained by different persons.

CHAPTER 2
Accounting Control

How Accounting and Reporting Safeguard the Assets of the Nursing Home Business

In stating the objectives of accounting, we said that accounting is the arrangement of information pertaining to the conduct of a business entity in an appropriate manner that will enable the business manager to *control* assets and costs and establish prices and profit margins. Not only is this statement a truism, it is a fact. The business enterprise is basically intangible (not clearly in hand) until tangible (real, not vague or elusive) information is arranged and reported. To do this is not just the job of the bookkeeper or the accounting department. It *must be the result* of a defined, manageable system—system, meaning a way of doing the task, that is documented, understood, and used in the same manner each and every time. A simple example of a system is shown in Exhibit 2-1.

Even though this is simple and basic, it is imperative that the business manager understand that the systematic method is the heart of controlling the business enterprise. In this example, which is the heart of controlling the most valuable asset, cash, the purpose is to establish a focal point for arranging the information (check book) in an appropriate manner. Once this is accomplished, the intangible becomes real because it can be supported by canceled checks and deposit slips. Then the business manager (administrator) can *control cash* by comparing the canceled checks and deposit slips to the records. In accounting jargon this technique is called internal control; or in more literal terms "how to cover your assets."

In order that all assets are controlled, defined, manageable systems must be established for each category of business activity. The following paragraphs provide you with the basics of internal control that you can use to establish the system. The refinements and improvements will be your job as you understand it better by using it.

The organization of the system (and subsystems) of internal control must start at the top. So you first need an organization chart that specifies what the tangible

Exhibit 2-1

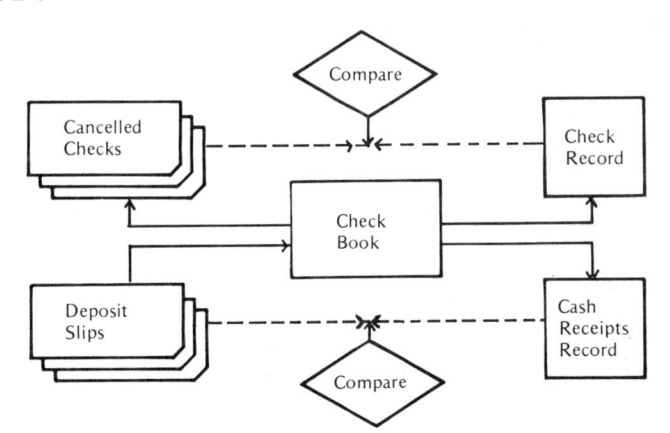

(real) responsibilities of each subsystem are. For an example, see Exhibit 2–2. We will now go through the functions and tasks and set down the basics of internal control for each.

MEDICAL

FUNCTION: MEDICAL/TASK: CHARGE SLIPS

Charge slips normally are created only for ancillary services, legend drugs, and major medical supplies. The charge to the patient for the room will be controlled through the patient census. The focal point for charge slip control is the record of charge slips issued to the departments.

The exercise of tracking charge slips (Exhibit 2-3) is worthwhile, for each charge slip lost is revenue lost. With a little extra effort better control over assets is accomplished.

Exhibit 2-2 Organization Chart for Internal Control

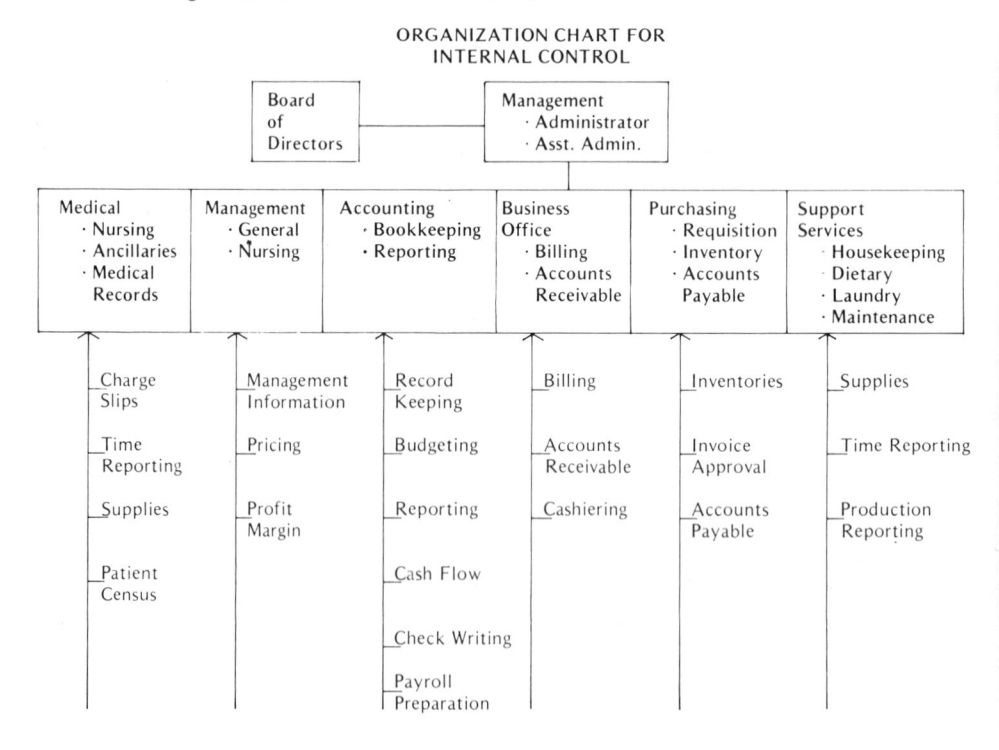

ORGANIZATION CHART FOR
INTERNAL CONTROL

Medical	Management	Accounting	Business Office	Purchasing	Support Services
· Nursing · Ancillaries · Medical Records	· General · Nursing	· Bookkeeping · Reporting	· Billing · Accounts Receivable	· Requisition · Inventory · Accounts Payable	· Housekeeping · Dietary · Laundry · Maintenance

Board of Directors — Management: · Administrator · Asst. Admin.

Charge Slips	Management Information	Record Keeping	Billing	Inventories	Supplies
Time Reporting	Pricing	Budgeting	Accounts Receivable	Invoice Approval	Time Reporting
Supplies	Profit Margin	Reporting	Cashiering	Accounts Payable	Production Reporting
Patient Census		Cash Flow			
		Check Writing			
		Payroll Preparation			

The responsibilities of each function (Medical, Administration, Accounting, Business Office, Purchasing and Support Services) relate to the specific tasks listed beneath the function. The responsibilities are to:
1. Protect the assets of the Business
2. Promote more efficient use of the assets of the Business
3. Help plan the use of the assets in the Business
4. Compare the actual use of assets to the original plan

FUNCTION: MEDICAL/TASK: TIME REPORTING

Time reporting should start with a time card that indicates the date, employee number, clock time in, clock time out, total hours, and estimated split of time for different levels of care. The focal point for the control of time reporting is the time cards and the payroll journal. The journal is a summary of the time cards, and it must agree with the staffing plan and the canceled checks. This establishes control over payroll expenditures as well as time reporting.

The exercise diagrammed in Exhibit 2-4 is worthwhile because each hour worked that is not in accordance with the staffing plan represents higher costs than expected and lower profit margins than were anticipated in establishing prices.

FUNCTION: MEDICAL/TASK: SUPPLIES

The supplies needed at the nursing stations should be requisitioned from a central storage area and charged to the patient as used. If the item is considered to be routine and included in the room rate, a patient charge slip will not be created, but a usage slip would be filled out and recorded. The focal point for the control of supplies is the Central Store's record and the floor record of receipts and requisitions, which indicate the actual usage of inventory.

This method of control (see Exhibit 2-5) is usually used only for the major supply items, but is worthwhile because it requires approved usage by formal requisitions and discourages waste or pilferage.

FUNCTION: MEDICAL/TASK: PATIENT CENSUS

The patient census is the most important task that nursing provides in the internal control scheme. The census determines present revenue levels, provides management with the major production unit, and allows management to plan out the best utilization of beds. The focal point of the patient census control is the bed

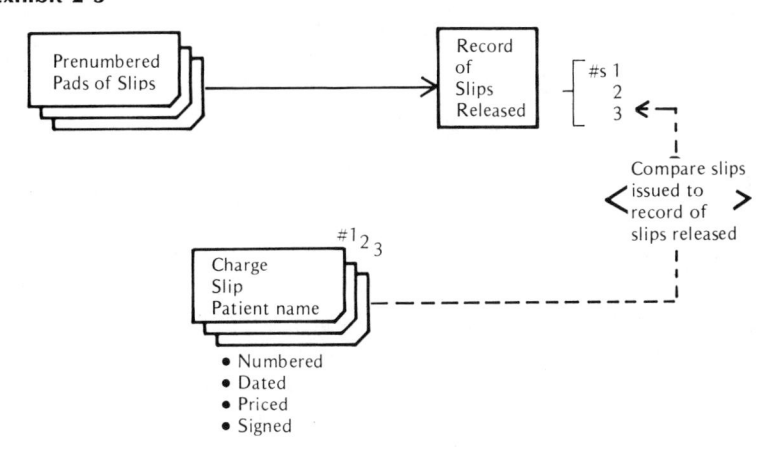

Exhibit 2-3

Exhibit 2-4

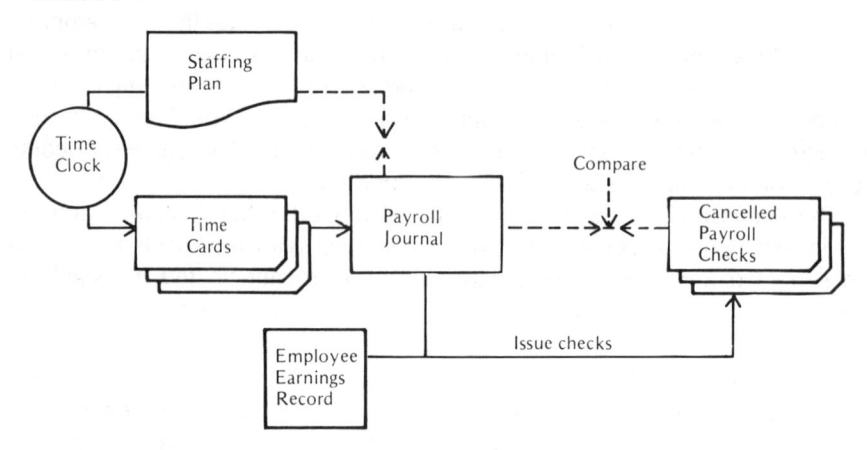

[Flowchart: Time Clock and Staffing Plan feed into Time Cards, which flow to Payroll Journal. Payroll Journal compares with Cancelled Payroll Checks. Employee Earnings Record issues checks.]

Exhibit 2-5

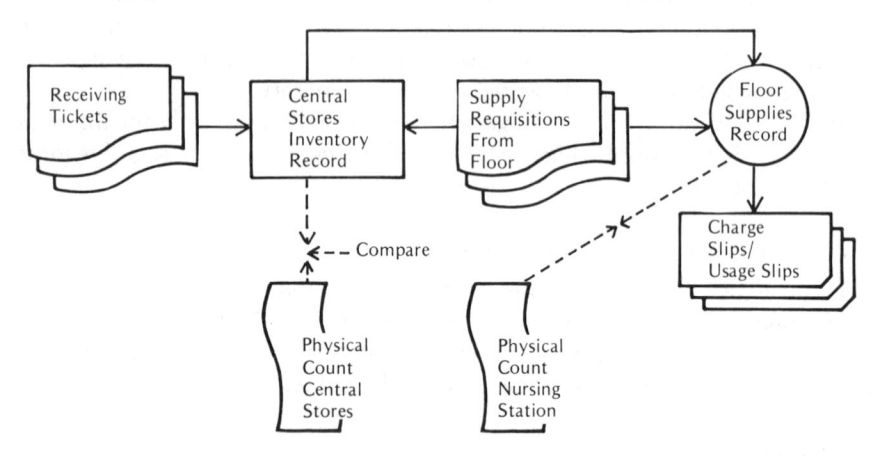

[Flowchart: Receiving Tickets flow to Central Stores Inventory Record. Supply Requisitions From Floor flow to Floor Supplies Record. Charge Slips/Usage Slips connect to Floor Supplies Record. Physical Count Central Stores compares with Central Stores Inventory Record. Physical Count Nursing Station connects to Floor Supplies Record.]

inventory listing. It is used for billing, placement of patients, and planning the staffing patterns. (See Exhibit 2-6.)

The patient-occupied bed is the primary indicator of utilized capacity. If accurate records are not kept, earned revenue can be lost.

ADMINISTRATION

FUNCTION: ADMINISTRATION/TASK: MANAGEMENT INFORMATION

The arrangement of information in a form that will allow management to anticipate needed actions accomplishes the objective of having reports. As the saying goes, "Being a domino or being an entrepreneur; the difference is in what you do and when you do it!" The focal points of the management information system are the production reports and the cost analysis report (see the Reporting Section for these forms).

Accounting Control

Exhibit 2-6

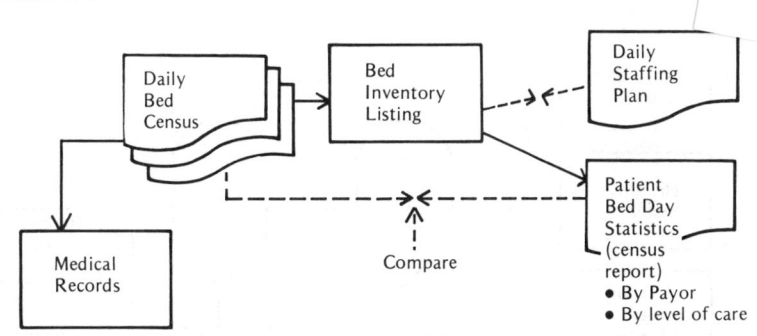

[Diagram: Daily Bed Census → Bed Inventory Listing; Daily Staffing Plan; Medical Records; Patient Bed Day Statistics (census report) • By Payor • By level of care; Compare]

If the management information system (MIS) provides this information to management on a timely basis, the business can be run like an enterprise. (See Exhibit 2-7.)

FUNCTION: ADMINISTRATION/TASK: PRICING

The establishment of adequate competitive prices is the lifeblood of a business. The nursing home is like any business; it needs adequate revenue to sustain itself. The problem the nursing home administration faces is the limited finances available to provide the quality care required by regulations (see Rate Setting section for the principles of pricing for nursing homes). The focal point for the pricing (which is the controlling factor over the long-range use of assets) task is the budget. (See Exhibit 2-8.)

FUNCTION: ADMINISTRATION/TASK: PROFIT MARGIN

The profit margin conceptually is defined as the difference between revenues and costs. It is the residual of the earned revenues and incurred costs, including economic costs for inflation and return on investment. The profit margin is fully

Exhibit 2-7

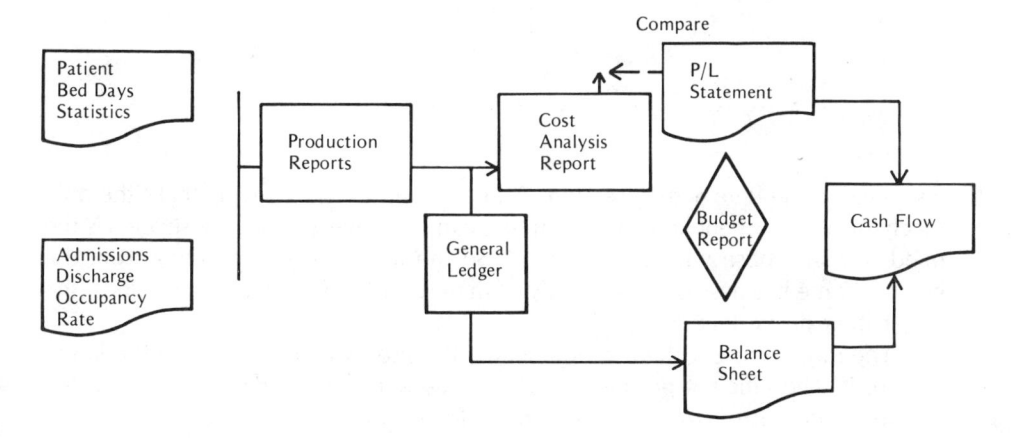

[Diagram: Patient Bed Days Statistics, Admissions Discharge Occupancy Rate → Production Reports → Cost Analysis Report, General Ledger; P/L Statement; Budget Report; Balance Sheet; Cash Flow; Compare]

Exhibit 2-8

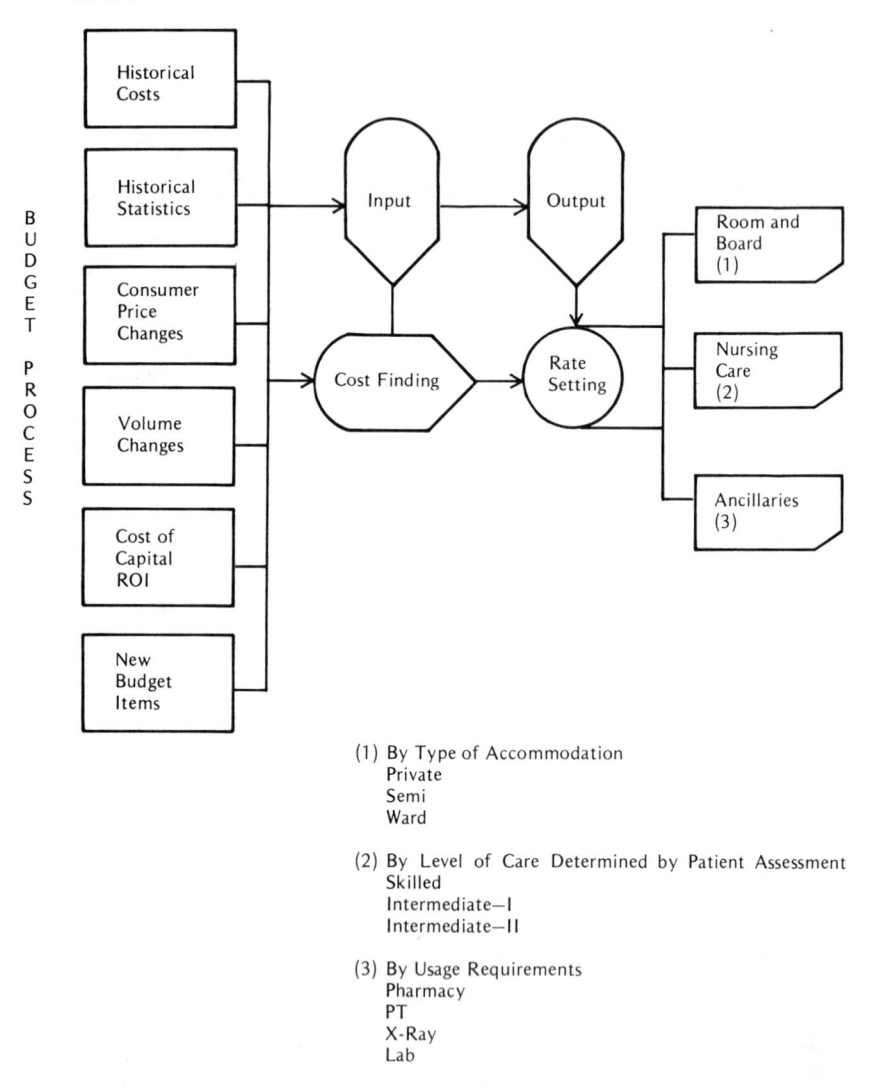

```
                    ┌──────────────┐
                    │ Historical   │
                    │ Costs        │
                    └──────────────┘
                    ┌──────────────┐                                      ┌──────────────┐
   B                │ Historical   │      ┌─────────┐     ┌─────────┐     │ Room and     │
   U                │ Statistics   │ ───> │  Input  │ ──> │ Output  │     │ Board        │
   D                └──────────────┘      └─────────┘     └─────────┘     │ (1)          │
   G                                           │              │           └──────────────┘
   E                ┌──────────────┐           ▼              ▼           ┌──────────────┐
   T                │ Consumer     │      ┌─────────┐     ┌─────────┐     │ Nursing      │
                    │ Price        │ ───> │  Cost   │ ──> │  Rate   │ ──> │ Care         │
   P                │ Changes      │      │ Finding │     │ Setting │     │ (2)          │
   R                └──────────────┘      └─────────┘     └─────────┘     └──────────────┘
   O                ┌──────────────┐                                      ┌──────────────┐
   C                │ Volume       │                                      │ Ancillaries  │
   E                │ Changes      │                                      │ (3)          │
   S                └──────────────┘                                      └──────────────┘
   S
                    ┌──────────────┐
                    │ Cost of      │
                    │ Capital      │
                    │ ROI          │
                    └──────────────┘
                    ┌──────────────┐
                    │ New          │
                    │ Budget       │
                    │ Items        │
                    └──────────────┘
```

(1) By Type of Accommodation
    Private
    Semi
    Ward

(2) By Level of Care Determined by Patient Assessment
    Skilled
    Intermediate—I
    Intermediate—II

(3) By Usage Requirements
    Pharmacy
    PT
    X-Ray
    Lab

discussed in the Rate Setting section. That section begins by saying that "the only mechanical instrument known to man that can conceive and believe success is the mind of man; those who use it profit." So the focal point of profiting from the nursing home business is the ingenuity of management. The better their minds, the better their profit. (See Exhibit 2-9.)

The more efficient the use of assets in the production of revenue, the larger the profit. The efficient production of revenue and the avoidance of loss in the business enterprise *is the way to manage for results.*

ACCOUNTING

FUNCTION: ACCOUNTING/TASK: RECORD KEEPING

The keeping of good records is on everyone's agenda but not on everyone's epitaph. In other words, good intentions and good records are separated by effort. If the effort is made to maintain good records and they are used for other tasks, such as management information systems, the potential for success is improved.

The focal point for good recordkeeping is the General Ledger. It sets the scene for cost accounting, financial analysis, and profit planning. (See Exhibit 2-10.)

FUNCTION: ACCOUNTING/TASK: BUDGETING

Budgeting is planning of a course of action that encompasses all facets of the business enterprise. If you were to drive to Clarksville without a map and got lost what would you do? Would you then take the time to plan the trip so you could

Exhibit 2-9

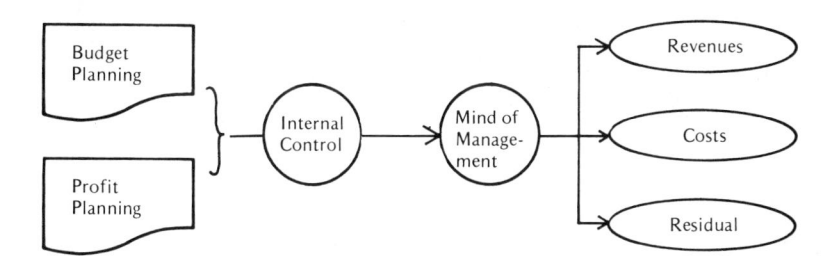

Exhibit 2-10

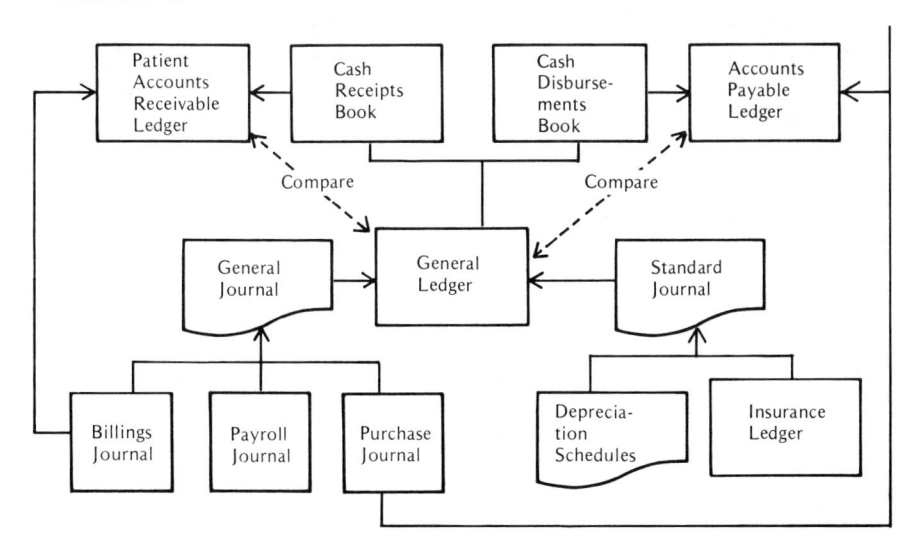

get to your destination? Of course you would! Then you would probably be a habitual map reader before setting out on the next trip. The same is true of budgeting; many businesses must get lost before they turn to planning. Once they are planners, they are always planners. It is too bad that some businesses become aware of the realities too late. The focal point of the budget (map to cost control and profit planning) is the forecast of production. See the Budgeting section for a full discussion of budgeting.

The budget then becomes the course of action. If the course can be maintained, the results will be as planned. If circumstances arise that cause a deviation from that course, alternate routes can be selected. Ultimately, the chances of getting to the desired results are far better with this approach (see Exhibit 2-11).

FUNCTION: ACCOUNTING/TASK: REPORTING

In the Reporting section we will discuss the uses of and usefulness of financial statements. Financial reporting is the focal point for controlling the finances of the business enterprise, but like a good book, they are not good until read and used. So it is important that they are readable and accurate, and fit into a comprehensive management information system which includes financial management reports and people management reports (see Exhibit 2-12). By this method good management is *in* the minds, not just on the minds, of all that receive the reports.

Exhibit 2-11

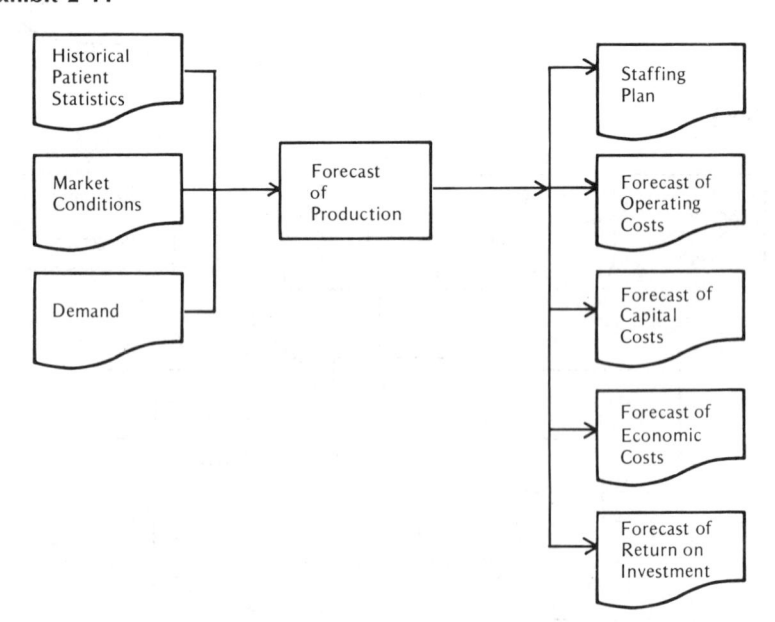

```
Historical
Patient         ─┐                              ┌─► Staffing Plan
Statistics       │                              │
                 │      Forecast                │
Market          ─┼─►    of          ──────────┬─► Forecast of Operating Costs
Conditions       │      Production            │
                 │                            ├─► Forecast of Capital Costs
Demand          ─┘                            │
                                              ├─► Forecast of Economic Costs
                                              │
                                              └─► Forecast of Return on Investment
```

FUNCTION: ACCOUNTING/TASK: CASH FLOW

The cash position of the business enterprise is the most important day-to-day concern of the accounting function. It is also the most demanding, as the industry comes under tighter regulatory control. The focal point for controlling the cash flow of the nursing home is the daily cash report, which should also report accounts receivable totals. (See Exhibit 2-13.)

Since the cost of doing business is paid for prior to the collection of earned revenue, every dollar in Accounts Receivable requires another dollar in capital. Since capital costs money, it is imperative to manage Accounts Receivable to reduce costs and improve profitability.

Exhibit 2-12

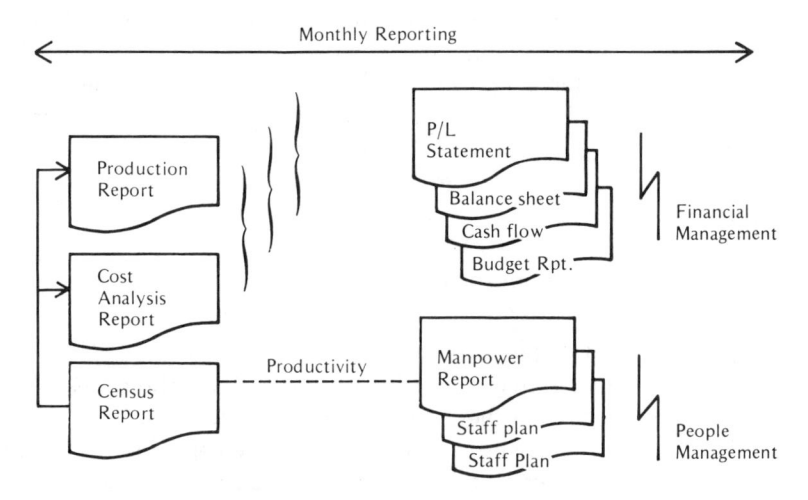

Exhibit 2-13

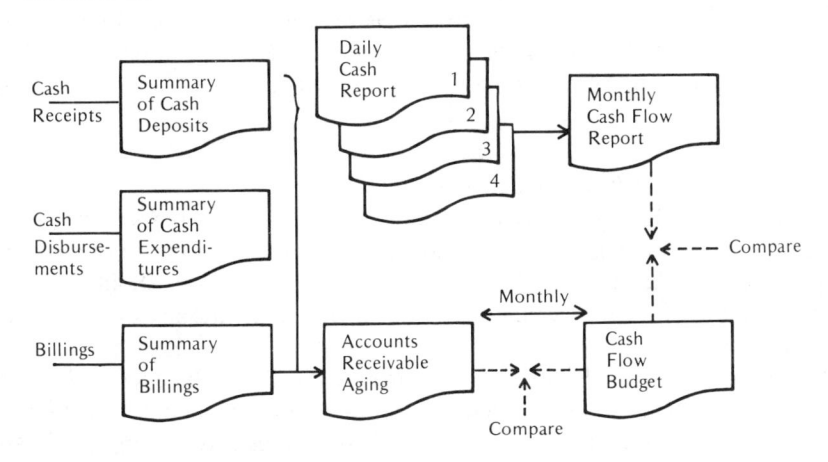

FUNCTION: ACCOUNTING/TASK: CHECK WRITING

The expenditure of cash must be controlled by a system of checks and balances so that duplicate payments are not issued or checks are not issued for unauthorized purchases. The focal point for this control is the Cash Disbursements Journal (check register).

Establishing control over cash expenditures with a small staff is like squeezing a balloon. The more you squeeze the more likely it is that something will happen. At best, the issuance of checks and the reconciling of the bank account should be done by different people. See Exhibit 2-14.

FUNCTION: ACCOUNTING/TASK: PAYROLL PREPARATION

The payroll preparation is a product of the time reporting received from each department and the withholding and fringe benefit authorizations on file. The focal point for the control payroll expenditures is the Payroll Journal.

Since payroll expenditures represent 50 percent of the expenses and 85 percent of the controllable expenses of a nursing home, it pays to establish adequate internal control over the payroll preparation (see Exhibit 2-15).

BUSINESS OFFICE

FUNCTION: BUSINESS OFFICE/TASK: BILLING AND ACCOUNTS RECEIVABLE

Nothing is deposited in the bank account of a nursing home for services rendered until a bill is prepared and submitted to the patient. The sooner the bill is prepared and sent, the sooner the bill will be paid. Therefore to improve cash flow and reduce the cost of having to maintain excessive capital in the business, billing should take priority over all other duties of the business office. This is the backbone of controlling finances. The focal point for the billing control is the patient's Accounts Receivable Ledger (see Exhibit 2-16).

The critical stage of the billing process is preparation of the Medicare and Medicaid billing. If the bills and patient open balance statements are slow in being mailed, the working capital requirements will be high as will be the cost of capital (interest).

FUNCTION: BUSINESS OFFICE/TASK: CASHIERING

As stated in the billing control procedures, fast turnaround in accounts receivable is imperative. Efficiency is also needed in the receipt and deposit of cash into the Operating Bank Account. At the same time, strong precautions should be taken to protect the business' most valuable asset—cash. The focal point of this control is the deposit slip.

As can be seen from Exhibit 2-17, control by check and balance is the focal point of true control. One person checking another by using balancing techniques is the best form of accounting control. If possible the duties of receiving checks and

Exhibit 2-14

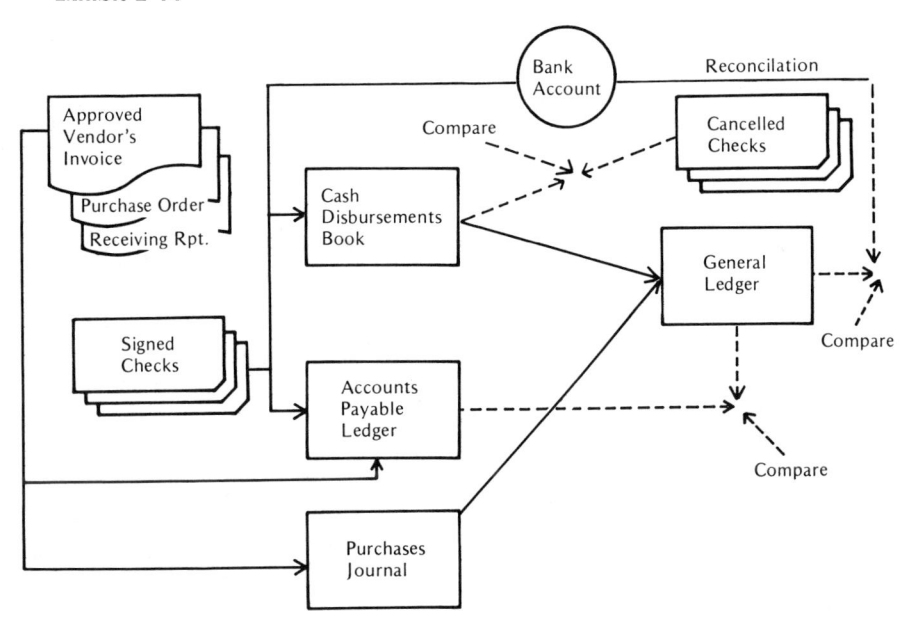

Exhibit 2-15

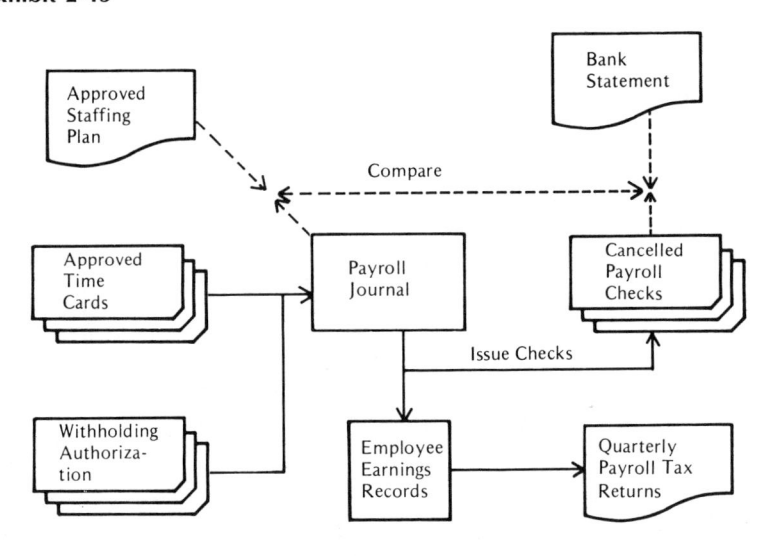

posting to accounts receivable should be handled by different employees. However, if this cannot be done because of a small staff, someone independent of cashiering should compare the deposit slip to the total of the checks received before the deposit is made and the records posted.

Exhibit 2-16

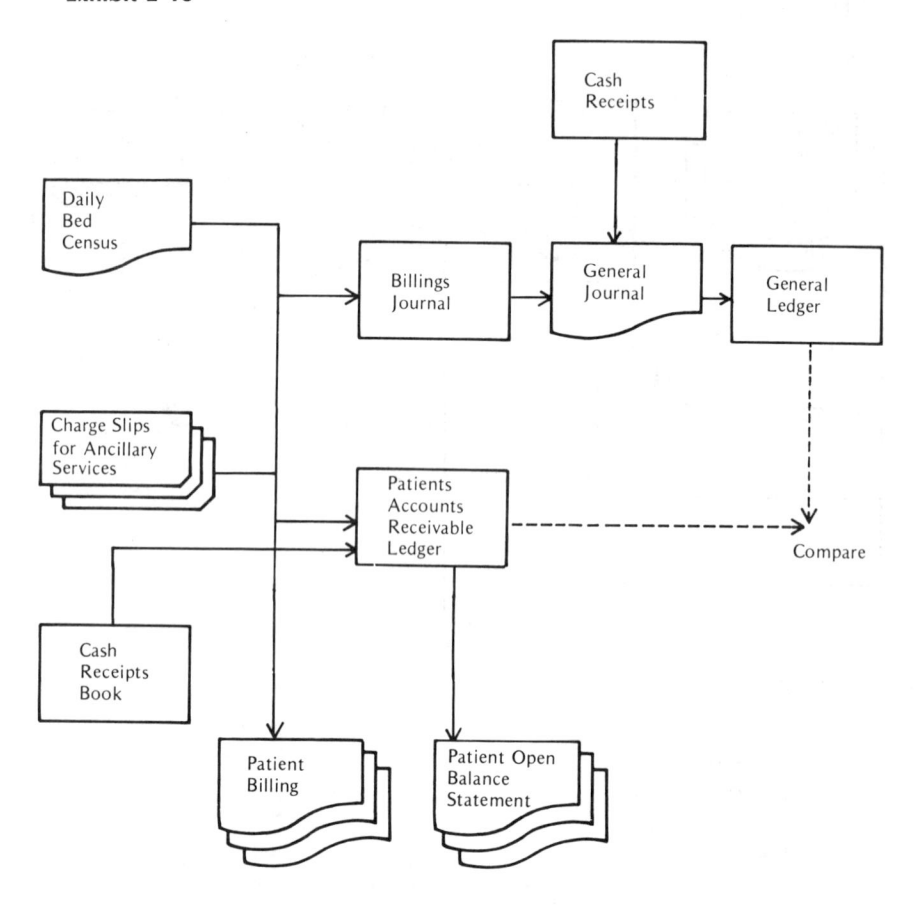

Exhibit 2-17

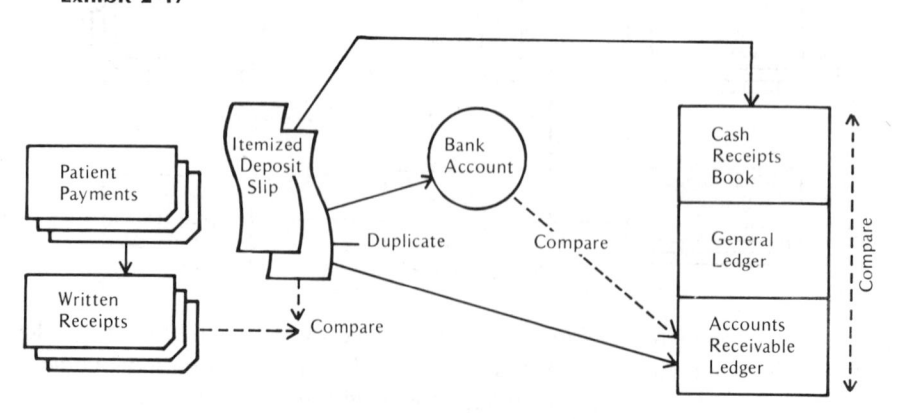

PURCHASING

FUNCTION: PURCHASING/TASK: INVENTORIES

The control over inventories of medical supplies, drugs, food, and of housekeeping, maintenance, and laundry supplies, after ordering and prior to requisition, is the responsibility of the purchasing agent (or the Administrator if that is his duty). The focal point of that control is a locked central storage area.

If proper reporting is done for the major inventory items, the General Ledger balance for those same items can represent a continuous record of current inventory. The balances in the accounts can then be verified by physical count and pricing once a year. See Exhibit 2-18.

FUNCTION: PURCHASING/TASK: INVOICE APPROVAL

Prior to the payment, all vendor's invoices should be checked, compared to the purchase order and receiving report, and then approved for payment. The focal point of this control is the invoice itself. See Exhibit 2-19.

No check should be drawn without approval by someone independent of Purchasing.

Exhibit 2-18

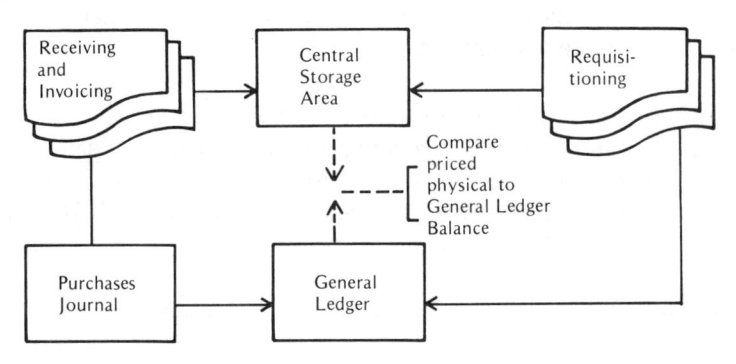

Exhibit 2-19

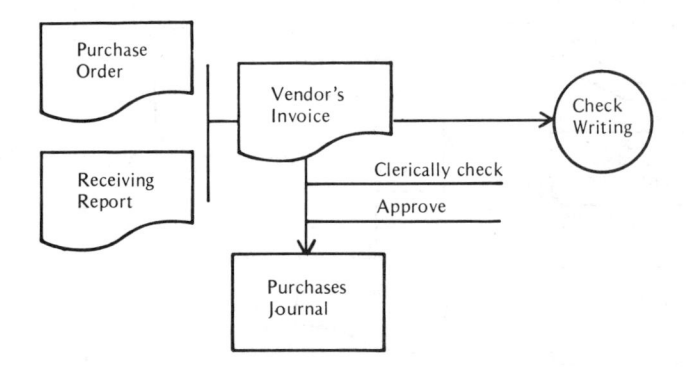

FUNCTION: PURCHASING/TASK: ACCOUNTS PAYABLE

To pay or not to pay and when are the questions that are asked when the cash position is weak. In nursing homes the practice of creative debtmanship may keep the float afloat. Creative debtmanship is paying only those invoices that must be paid. The focal point for this procedure and the control it establishes over cash expenditures is the Accounts Payable Ledger or file, if payables are on an open invoice file. An Accounts Payable Ledger and Purchase Journal are recommended if bills are not paid monthly. To do otherwise is to cause accounting havoc.

The purchasing function can be responsible for maintaining the Accounts Payable Ledger, and the Purchase Journal so long as the checks are signed by an independent party, who looks at approved invoices before signing. See Exhibit 2-20.

SUPPORT SERVICES

FUNCTION: SUPPORT SERVICES/TASK: SUPPLIES

The supplies used by the support services departments (housekeeping, dietary, laundry, and maintenance) should be requisitioned from a central storage area and charged to the user department. The focal point for the control of supplies is the Central Store's record of receipts, requisitions, and inventory.

This method of control (Exhibit 2-21) is usually used for only major supply items. It is worthwhile because it requires approved usage by requisitions, which should discourage waste and pilferage.

FUNCTION: SUPPORT SERVICES/TASK: TIME REPORTING

Time reporting should start with a time card that indicates the date, employee number, clock time in, clock time out, and total hours. The focal point for the control of time reporting is the time cards and the Payroll Journal. The journal is

Exhibit 2-20

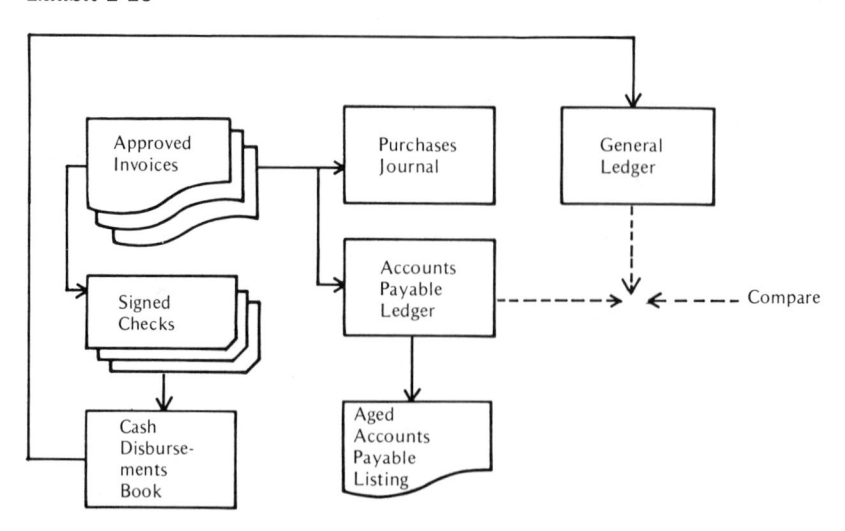

Exhibit 2-21

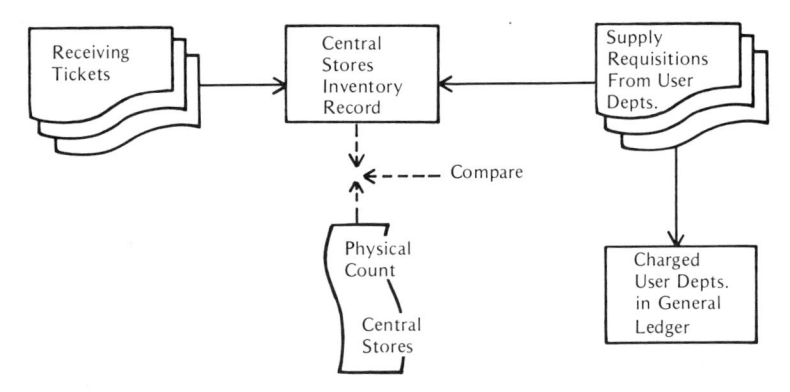

```
[Receiving Tickets] ───→ [Central Stores Inventory Record] ←─── [Supply Requisitions From User Depts.]
                               ↕ ←---- Compare                         │
                          [Physical Count                               ↓
                           Central Stores]                       [Charged User Depts.
                                                                  in General Ledger]
```

a summary of the time cards and it must agree with the staffing plan and the canceled checks. This establishes control over payroll expenditures as well as time reporting.

The exercise shown in Exhibit 2-22 is worthwhile because each hour worked that is not in accordance with the staffing plan represents higher costs than expected and lower profit margins.

FUNCTION: SUPPORT SERVICES/TASK: PRODUCTION REPORTING

The only indicator of indirect labor productivity that the nursing home business has are the statistics maintained by the support services department:

Department	Productivity Statistics
Housekeeping	Hours worked (by location)
Dietary	Meals served (by type)
Laundry	Pounds of laundry (by department)
Maintenance	Hours worked (by location)

If systematically gathered and recorded, these statistics provide management information for purposes of staffing. The only means of controlling productivity in the support services departments is to properly plan and control staffing requirements. The focal point of this control is the productivity log.

Exhibit 2-22

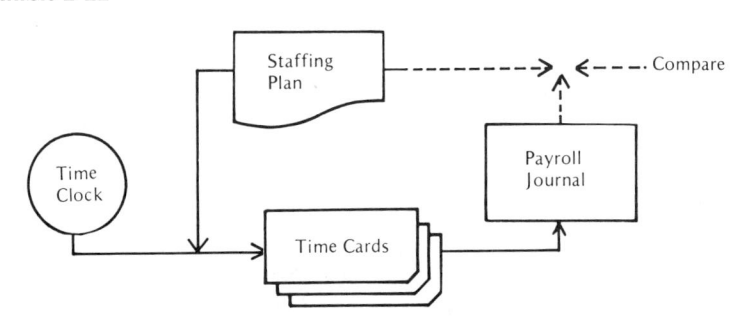

```
                    [Staffing Plan] --------→ ←---- Compare
                         │                    ↑
[Time Clock] ────────────┤                    │
                         │              [Payroll Journal]
                         ↓                    ↑
                    [Time Cards] ─────────────┘
```

As indicated earlier, payroll cost is at least 50 percent of the total expense and about 85 percent of the controllable expenses of a nursing home. If those costs are productive, the business can be termed efficient and improves its opportunity for a profit. See Exhibit 2-23.

Exhibit 2-23

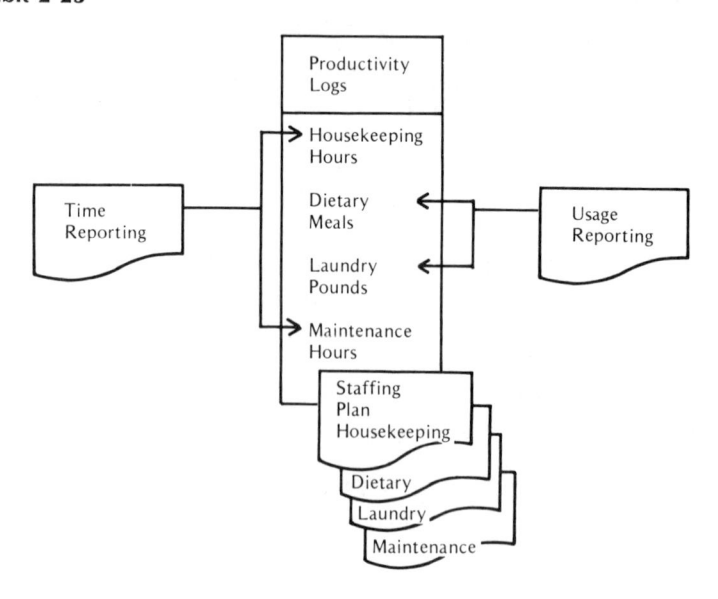

CHAPTER 3
Accounting Principles for Nursing Homes

Nursing homes require good accounting procedures and accounting principles to arrange information pertaining to the conduct of the business, so the business manager (administrator) may control assets and costs and establish prices and profit margins. The accounting principles that are uniformly used across an entire industry are called generally accepted accounting principles (GAAP). The uniformity that GAAP establishes is important because it establishes comparability between individual business units so such people as investors, bankers, and consumers can make comparisons for investment or purchase decisions.

The accounting principles in the nursing home industry are not necessarily unique from most small- to medium-sized service businesses, but they are not necessarily the same either. In the following pages we will discuss GAAP in general as they apply to nursing homes, with added emphasis on those areas of nursing home GAAP that are unique.

We will concentrate on the following accounting components, concepts, and terms in studying accounting for nursing homes:

Cash flow

Billings and accounts receivable

Contractual discounts (Medicaid and Medicare accounting) and third-party cost reconciliation settlements

Allowance for bad debts

Purchases, accounts payable, and inventories

Prepaid expenses and deferred charges

Current assets, liquidity, and long-term assets

Capital assets, depreciation, and construction in progress

Contingent assets

Accrued expenses

Unpaid income taxes

Current liabilities, liquidity, and long-term debt

Notes and mortgages payable

Deferred liabilities and deferred credits

Capital (or contributions for tax-exempt organizations)

Retained earnings (fund balance for tax-exempt organizations)

Contingent liabilities

Revenues

Capital costs (depreciation and interest) and lease expense

Patient funds

In the process of outlining GAAP, we will use examples and exercises to gain an understanding of accounting entries, accounting terminology, and accounting records. The goal is to provide you with an understanding of sound, uniform, and systematic accounting procedures. Just remember that generally accepted accounting principles are nothing more than a good recipe. If you put in the right ingredients, you will have an opportunity for good results; however you must watch very carefully, so that the results you get are those you expected.

Is Cash Position Still Important?

What you see in Exhibit 3-1 is a graphic example of what happens in a nursing home in terms of cash flow. As you can see, the expenditures for supplies, materials, labor, and overhead costs such as laundry expenses, dietary expenses, and administrative expenses are expended first. These expenses are incurred for purposes of caring for the patient. As a result a charge is assessed to the patient. In the case of a private patient you are generally collecting in advance. This is a very positive cash flow position because you are collecting the revenue before you incur the expense.

Exhibit 3-1 Cash Flow

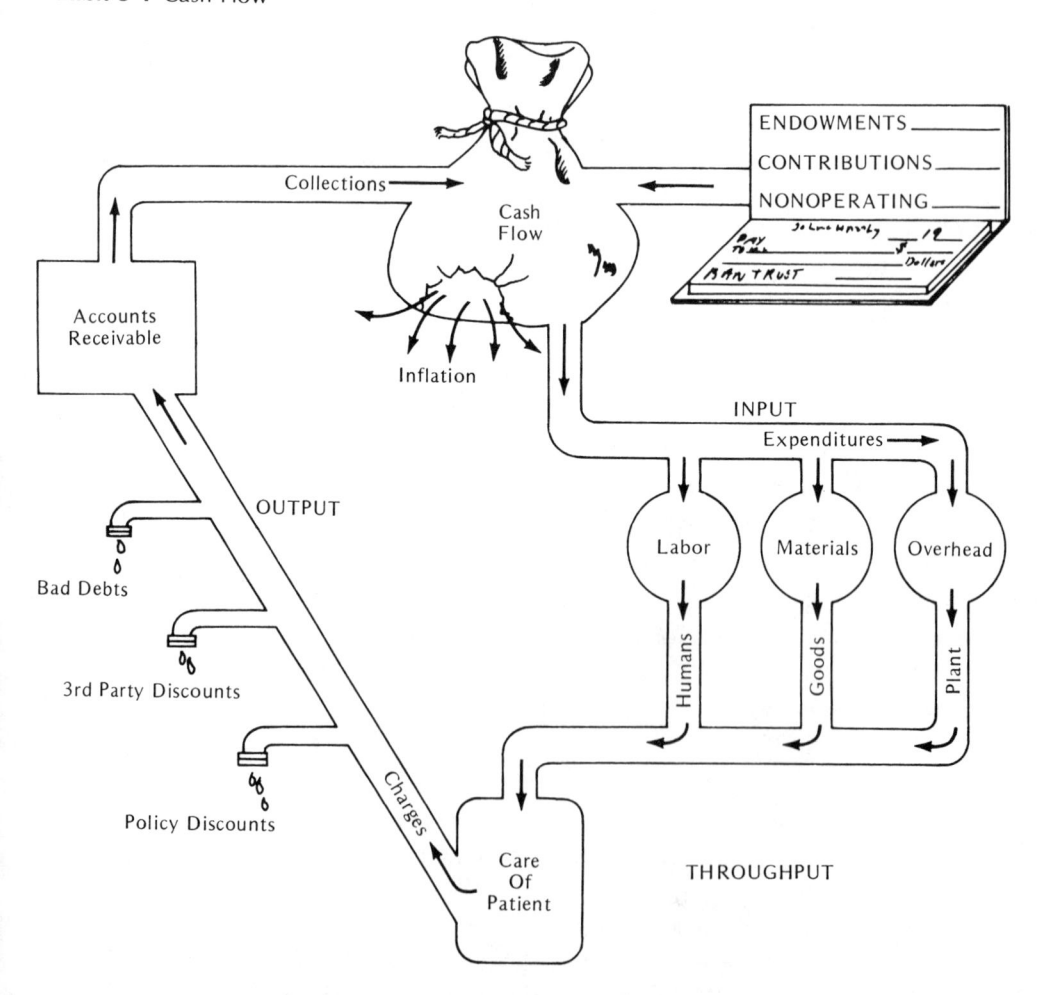

However, with third-party payers (which are becoming more and more predominant) the services are provided, the bill is prepared and submitted to the payers, and they pay, maybe. In this case, your cash flow is always in a negative position because you have already incurred the cost, expended the cash, and must wait for collection. This is why you need working capital. Working capital is needed to finance your business until the Medicare/Medicaid system processes a payment for you. (See Appendix 2 for an explanation of government health programs.) After billing there is a significant time lag before they process the payment. Eventually this payment will be deposited in the bank account, but meanwhile you must attempt to balance the cash cycle. In addition, a degenerating problem exists with the third-party payer system because of cost reimbursement (discount of customary charges to a level that the payer defines as cost). Discounting is your most negative cash flow factor because, if you were to deal with private pay patients rather than Medicare or Medicaid, the charge would result in full cash collections in advance. (Not only is the payment delayed from cost reimbursers, but there are discounts that reduce the potential cash flow.) Unfortunately, in the real world, nursing homes do not have the luxury of always collecting full customary charges; but on the other hand, the third-party payer programs enable nursing homes to serve all patients needing long-term care.

As can be seen in Exhibit 3–1, the sooner you can collect the money the more stable is your cash position. The longer it takes you to price the bill, submit the bill, and collect the bill, the more unstable your cash position will be, the higher your working capital requirements will be, and the lower your return on investment (ROI) will be. The reason your ROI is less is because the invested capital requirement is higher and profits are unchanged. As working capital needs increase, the cost of capital increases and the profit and return on investment become lower. And remember, for each dollar of capital invested and used to operate the business, a corresponding dollar of profit must be earned to replenish the capital if investors are to be paid a return and if services are to be expanded. For example:

Current Assets	$100,000
Current Liabilities	150,000
Working capital deficiency	$(50,000)
Invested capital	50,000
Capital available for dividends or expansion of services	$0
Source of capital is—	
Investor's capital	$ 50,000
Use of capital is—	
To pay operating expenses	50,000
Capital available for dividends or expansion of services	$0

In this example the investor's capital must be replaced by current operating profits before it can be used to pay dividends or improve future profit margins. What this shows is that capital borrowed or invested to cover a working capital deficiency must be replenished or it becomes just another cost of operations. Unfortunately many businesses do not recognize this phenomenon and do not include the cost of capital in their prices. The ultimate result is underpricing of the services and inadequate profit margins. Without profits there are no dividends and no internal financing of replacement of assets and expansion of the business.

This is why it is said that cash flow must be good or the return on investment is only a paper dream. And if the investment is only a paper dream, the day of awakening is a disaster. So cash flow is important. It takes cash to pay bills, to pay employees, and to pay investors. If you can manage the cash flow, you are managing the finances of the business.

Billings and Accounts Receivable

As each patient is billed, the detail is entered in the Billings Journal. (The Billings Journal is explained in detail in Chapter 1.) The revenue is broken down by type in the Billings Journal. The monthly totals for the billings are posted (credited) to the accounting records. This method is called accrual accounting because the revenue is recognized in the accounting records as billed (earned). So that the records balance, the other side of the revenue entries is a debit to Accounts Receivable. This is the technique used in double entry bookkeeping that allows the accountant to balance all entries made in the accounting records. For example, consider the following T accounts:

Revenue—Private Skilled		Revenue—Private Intermediate	
Debit	Credit	Debit	Credit
	$10,000 billing (1)		$10,000 billing (1)

Revenue—Medicare SNF		Revenue—Medicaid Skilled	
Debit	Credit	Debit	Credit
	$20,000 billing (1)		$40,000 billing (1)

Revenue—Medicaid Intermediate		Medicaid and Medicare Discounts	
Debit	Credit	Debit	Credit
	$20,000 billing (1)	$10,000 (2)	

Accounts Receivable Private		Accounts Receivable Medicare		Accounts Receivable Medicaid	
Debit	Credit	Debit	Credit	Debit	Credit
billings $20,000 (1)		billings $20,000 (1)	$3,000 (2)	billings $60,000 (1)	$7,000 (2)
		Bal. $17,000		Bal. $53,000	

(1) Billings for one month
(2) Discount of Medicaid and Medicare billings to cost

Accounting Principles for Nursing Homes

These T account illustrations of double entry bookkeeping allow the nonaccountant to get the feel for the balancing technique that is used in all double entry accounting systems.

The T accounts balance is as follows:

Debit		Credit	
Accounts Receivable—Private	$ 20,000	Rev. Private Skilled	$ 10,000
Accounts Receivable—Medicare	20,000	Rev. Private Intermediate	10,000
Accounts Receivable—Medicaid	60,000	Rev. Medicare SNF	20,000
Medicaid and Medicare Discounts	10,000	Rev. Medicaid Skilled	40,000
		Rev. Medicaid Intermediate	20,000
			$100,000
		Accounts Receivable—Medicaid	7,000
		Accounts Receivable—Medicare	3,000
	$110,000		$110,000

As the individual accounts receivable are collected, the payments are recorded in the cash receipts book as a debit to Cash and a credit to Accounts Receivable in the accounting records. The T account again depicts this procedure.

Cash		Accounts Receivable—Private	
Debit	Credit	Debit	Credit
Cash		Billings $20,000	$2,000 payments
Deposits $10,000		(2)	(1)
(1)		Balance $18,000	

Accounts Receivable—Medicaid		Accounts Receivable—Medicare	
Debit	Credit	Debit	Credit
Billings $20,000	$7,000 payments	Billings $60,000	$1,000 payments
(2)	(1)	(2)	(1)
Balance $13,000		Bal. $59,000	

(1) The bank deposit itemizes all the checks and the cash receipts book totals all deposits for a month and creates the double entries that are posted above.
(2) Billings for the month from billings journal.

The detail of each patient's balance is recorded in a record called the Patient Subsidiary Accounts Receivable Ledger. In that ledger, each patient has an account in which their individual billings and cash payments are recorded. Exhibit 3-2 depicts that record for a Medicare or Medicaid patient.

As can be seen, if a patient is billed in one month and the payment is received the next month, an accounts receivable for that patient exists. If all the individual

Exhibit 3-2 Medicare/Medicaid Patient Subsidiary Accounts Receivable Ledger

John Doe Patient #12345

Date	Charges (Billings)				Payments		Balance
	Room	PT	Drugs	Other	Date	Amount	
Aug.	$600	$50	$50	$10			$710.00
Sept.	600	50	50	10	Sept.	$710.00	710.00
Oct.	600	50	50	10	Oct.	710.00	710.00

accounts are totaled at month's end they must agree with the total in the accounting records. This comparison is done as follows:

Balance per accounting records at January 31, 198___	$31,000
Plus: Charges for February (billings journal)	30,000
Less: Collection in February (cash receipts book)	(27,000)
Balance per books at February 28, 198___	$34,000
Total of patients subsidiary accounts receivable accounts at February 28, 198___	$34,000

These amounts must agree!

Contractual Discounts (Medicare and Medicaid Accounting)

Besides billings and payments on account, Accounts Receivable are also affected by cost reimbursement formulas that are in effect for federal (Medicare) and state (Medicaid) health care programs. Basically, the customary billing to a private paying patient is more than the amount paid by the reimbursement formulas. If the Billings Journal is properly structured, *all* billings will be at the private paying rate and the difference of discount will be recorded as a deduction from gross revenue and a reduction of the Accounts Receivable balance. The reason for making this "paper" entry is to allow management to ascertain the impact on their operation of the cost-related health care programs.

As shown in the T account illustration of recording billings, the impact of discounting is as follows:

Gross Accounts Receivable	
Medicaid	$60,000
Medicare	20,000
	$80,000
Contractual Discounts	
Medicaid	$7,000
Medicare	3,000
	$10,000
Net Accounts Receivable	$70,000

The $10,000 represents the amount that the private paying patient pays in excess of the amounts received from cost reimbursers. Following is a complete example of the accounting procedures for recording contractual discounts.

THIRD-PARTY COST RECONCILIATION SETTLEMENTS

Exhibit 3-3 on Medicaid and Medicare accounting refers, in Entry 6, to Medicare Cost Report Settlement. This means that on a retroactive basis the Medicare Health Insurance Program (Part A) compares the actual reasonable-allowable costs incurred by the provider (participating skilled nursing facility) to the estimates paid to the provider during the fiscal year. This is referred to as a reconciliation between estimated costs and actual reported costs. The difference is called a settlement and is paid by the provider to a government intermediary, in a pay-back situation, or collected from the intermediary in an underpayment situation.

For example, consider the cost reimbursement formula in very general terms:

Costs per accounting records	$1,000,000
Nonallowable and unreasonable costs	(100,000)
Allowable reimbursable costs	$900,000
Amounts collected from program during year	850,000
Due from Medicare program	$50,000

Since the accounting records have been recording all billings and collections, with the Medicare program, on an estimated basis during the year, the $50,000 must be recorded to correct the estimates. The entry would be:

	Debit	Credit
Due from Medicare Program	$50,000	
Contractual Discounts		$50,000

This entry does not affect revenue or receivables if the billings are recorded properly, that is, if a discount for each bill is put in the billings journal (as you go), as depicted in the example.

The Medicaid programs are not necessarily on the same reimbursement system as Medicare. Medicare has a uniform method for all skilled nursing facilities certified to provide Medicare services. Each state has the option, so long as the system is cost related, to devise its own Medicaid reimbursement method or use the Medicare system. However, if the amount collected from the Medicaid program is less than the customary private paying patient rate, and the private pay rate is the customary rate that is needed to operate profitably, the accounting for the discount will be the same as it is for Medicare.

Allowance for Bad Debts

Bad accounts receivable are not a significant item for nursing homes. Generally bad accounts arise when patients do not pay deductibles and coinsurance amounts for Medicare stays or claims that are rejected by the Medicaid or Medicare programs. The bad accounts are not a factor for private paying patients because they are expected to pay for room and board in advance. Occasionally

Exhibit 3-3 Medicaid and Medicare Accounting

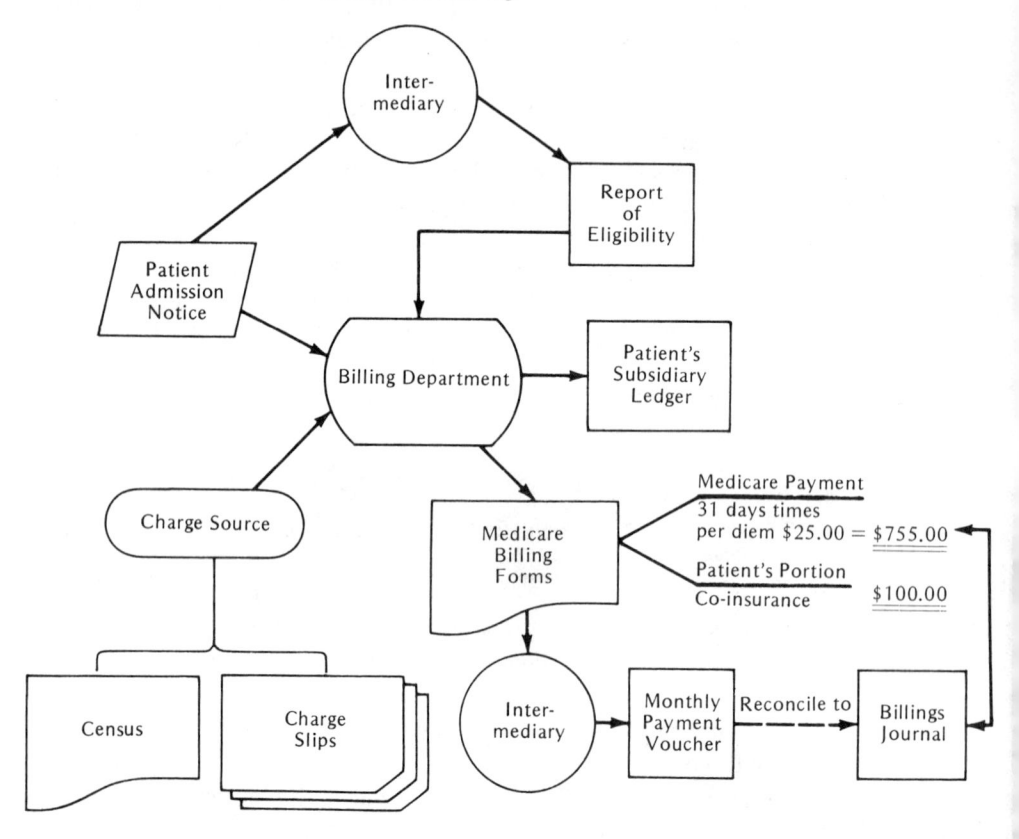

Accounting Entries—for Medicare Patients
(1) Record monthly charges
(2) Record payment per diem from Medicare billing form
(3) Record allowance (discount) from information taken from Medicare billing form
(4) Record monthly Medicare payment through cash receipts book
(5) Record, by journal entry, from year end Medicare cost report to book settlement
(6) Medicare cost report settlement made

*Accounting Entries—for Medicaid Patients on Retrospective Cost Reimbursement**
For Medicaid charges the flow through would be basically the same as for Medicare with the exception of deductibles and varying per diems (there would be no patient balance subsequent to Medicaid's remittance since no coinsurance nor deductible is normally involved). For accounting entries 1-4, substitute "Medicaid" for "Medicare" and disregard entries 5 and 6 unless the final cost report settlement is applicable.

*Under prospective reimbursement arrangements there may be no discount involved if incentive factors are included.

Exhibit 3-3 (cont.)

PATIENT'S SUBSIDIARY LEDGER								
	Charges					Debits		Credits	
Date	Routine Service	Pharmacy	PT	Other Service	Discount	Accounts Receivable	Description	Payments	Balance
1/31	$750.00	$90.00	$110.00			$950.00			$950.00
					$75.00		Med. Payment	$775.00	

```
   Patient's Accounts Receivable              Routine Service — Revenue
   (1) $950.00  | (2) $775.00                              | (1) $750.00
                | (3)    75.00
   Balance      | $100.00                         Pharmacy — Revenue
                                                           | (1) $90.00
      Medicare Control Account                  Physical Therapy — Revenue
   (2) $  775.00 | (4) $  775.00                           | (1) $110.00

      $65,000.00 | $65,000.00
                                                 Contractual Discount
                                                 (3) $  75.00
               Cash
   (4) $  775.00 |                               $ 1,000.00 | (5) $ 1,500.00
                                                 Balance $ 10,000.00
        $6,500.00
   (6)   1,500.00
        $9,000.00                                  Medicare Settlement
                                                 (5) $  500.00 | (6) $1,500.00
```

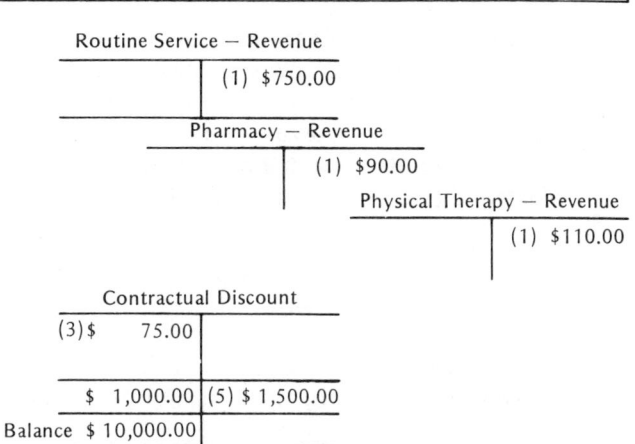

a private patient may not be able to pay for other services, but those amounts are usually minor.

Considering this, bad debts should be accounted for on a direct write-off method of accounting. In essence, the bad debt is not estimated but is written off to expense when it is evident that a specific amount will not be collected. The entry in the accounting records is as follows:

	Debit	Credit
Bad debt expense	$700.00	
Accounts receivable		$700.00

This method contrasts with the accrual method which requires that the bad debt expense be estimated on current revenue and recorded as follows:

	Debit	Credit
Bad debt expense	$1,000.00	
Estimated bad debts		$1,000.00

Then when a specific account becomes uncollectible the entry is:

	Debit	Credit
Estimated bad debts	$700.00	
Accounts receivable		$700.00

The difference in the two methods is purely in the timing of the expense. Under the accrual method bad debt expenses are recorded earlier, in an attempt to match the expense with the applicable revenue, rather than waiting for the bad debt to be confirmed, which may be in a later accounting period.

Under the direct write-off method, if the previously written-off bad debt is collected, the following entry is made:

	Debit	Credit
Cash	$450	
Recovery of a bad debt (an income account)		$450

Bad debts should be recorded as an expense of the administrative cost center. The recoveries should be offset against the expense.

Prepaid Expenses and Deferred Charges

Generally prepaid expenses in nursing homes are nominal; except for prepaid insurance. Prepaid insurance arises when a three-year premium is paid (or a contract signed to pay on the installment basis) in advance.

For example:

Premium for fire and extended coverage
January 1, 1976 to December 31, 1978 $15,000
Expense applicable to:
1976 $5,000
1977   5,000
1978   5,000
         $15,000

If a three-year contract payable is signed the entry would be:

	Debit	Credit
Prepaid insurance	$15,000	
Contract payable		$15,000
Contract payable	$5,000	
Cash (first year payment)		$5,000
Insurance expense	$5,000	
Prepaid insurance		$5,000

In the balance sheet of the nursing home at the end of the first year there would be the following accounts:

Prepaid insurance	$10,000
Contracts payable	$10,000
Insurance expense	$5,000
Cash paid for insurance	$5,000

The basic principle for prepaid expense is the same as inventory; if the expense applies to a future period, defer it until the expense is incurred. See the illustrative Schedule of Prepaid Insurance (Exhibit 3–4) which develops the accounting entries for recording expense.

Deferred charges generally consist of expenses that apply to a future period because that is when the benefits of the expenditure are experienced. A good example of this for nursing homes is rent paid in advance, such as a security deposit or escrow accounts for real estate taxes and insurance. At the time the expense becomes a benefit to the production of revenue, it must be removed from the deferral account and put into expense.

Deferred Rent	Cash	Rent Expense
(1) $1,000 | (2) $1,000	| $1,000 (1)	(2) $1,000 |

(1) Payment of rent in advance
(2) Recognition of expense when it becomes a benefit to the production of revenue

In some circumstances, income taxes or reimbursement amounts must be paid in advance due to a difference in method of recognizing the revenue or expense. These are referred to as timing differences or interperiod tax allocations. The best example of a timing difference is depreciation. This condition normally results in a deferred credit, because the depreciation taken for tax purposes is more than the depreciation recorded in the accounting records. Effectively the difference for each accounting period is due to the way the depreciation is calculated and not how much depreciation is taken in total. It is merely taken earlier for tax or cost reporting purposes. Thus enters the term *timing* difference. If the depreciation per the accounting records exceeds that on the tax return, you may have a deferred charge. If there is enough assurance that the difference is in fact an asset, which means it must be ultimately converted to cash, then it may be recorded as an asset. If it is not reasonably predictable that the taxable income will exist to allow for the use of the additional depreciation in later periods, no asset exists and none can be recorded.

Exhibit 3-4 Schedule of Prepaid Insurance

Insurer	Coverage	From	To	Premium	Prepaid at 12/31/74	Additions 1975	Expense 1975	Prepaid at 12/31/75	
Milwaukee Insurance (Examples)	#12-C-00263 Blanket	7/1/74	7/1/75		$1,342	—	$1,342	—	
XYZ Co.	#12345	1/1/75	2/1/75	$1,000		$1,000		$1,000	Paid 1/1/75 check #4000
Monthly entry	January	1/1/75	2/1/75				550	(550)	
Balance at 12/31/75					$1,342	$1,000	$1,892	$ 450	
					+	+	− =	$Prepaid	

(Reminder:

See the section on Deferred Revenue for the full accounting treatment for deferrals.

Purchases, Accounts Payable, and Inventories

The major purchases for nursing homes are for food, linens, medical supplies, and pharmaceuticals, with minor expenditures for support service supplies (housekeeping, laundry, maintenance, and office). The accounting should be on the accrual basis, which records the purchases as costs when the merchandise is received, not when it is paid for. The accounting method may vary, but the principles of recording costs in the period to which they apply hold. For example:

August food purchases received	$10,000
August food usage	8,000
Increase in food inventory	$2,000
Food inventory at first of August	2,000
Food inventory at end of August	$4,000

If the $2,000 in unused purchases of food during August were not put into the inventory account, which defers the cost until the food is used, the costs for August would have been $2,000 too high and profit $2,000 too low.

So generally speaking, *any* purchase (supplies, equipment, and so on) that is received in one accounting period but used in another period must be deferred and only put into cost when used. This exercise usually is accomplished through the Purchase Journal or the General Journal. (The Purchase Journal is explained in detail in Chapter 1.)

Current Assets, Liquidity, and Noncurrent Assets

The classification of assets as current or noncurrent is a technique used by all businesses to specify those assets that will or will not be converted to cash during the ordinary business cycle (normally one year). The placement of the assets in coding the accounting records and preparing the balance sheet are according to liquidity. The faster an asset is convertible to cash the more current it is. The following is the usual sequence of assets, normally called a chart of accounts:

Account Number

	Current Assets
100	Cash
110	Certificates of deposit
120	Marketable securities
130	Accounts receivable
140	Inventory
150	Prepaid expense

	Noncurrent Assets
170	Deposits
180	Cash surrender value of insurance
190	Deferred charges
	Fixed Assets
195	Land
196	Plant
197	Equipment

The relevance of liquidity is in the determination of working capital. The designation of an asset as current is an indication that it will be converted into cash during the operating cycle (usually one year) for the purpose of paying bills (current liabilities). The concept of working capital is covered more fully in Chapter 7.

The noncurrent assets usually represent assets that take longer than one year to convert to cash. In the case of fixed assets, the asset usually is not an expendable asset and does not become cash except in the course of producing revenue. In other words, the nursing home plant and equipment help produce revenue, that becomes accounts receivable, that becomes cash; but are considered fixed because they do not convert to liquid assets. That is why they are called fixed assets. The concept of deterioration and depreciation will be covered in the next section.

Capital (Depreciable) Assets and Construction-in-Progress

Depreciable assets consist of the plant and equipment costs and any other asset that is used in the production of revenue and lasts longer than two business cycles. To attribute the acquisition cost of the asset to more than one business cycle a rational and systematic method for depreciating the asset must be selected. Depreciation, therefore, is the systematic and rational recognition of cost over the life cycle of the capital asset. This amounts to a selection of the useful life of the asset and a method for calculating the cost for each period. For example:

Building cost	$1,000,000
Useful life	40 years
Cost per year	$25,000
using a straight-line method	
(same each year)	

See illustrative Depreciation Schedule (Exhibit 3–5) which develops the entries to expense.

The entry to record the depreciation each month in the accounting records would be:

	Debit	Credit
Depreciation expense	$1250	
Reserve for depreciation		$1250

This is a paper entry but it has an effect on profit or loss and has an influence on cash flow. For example, if the asset being depreciated is financed, the difference between the depreciation expense and the principal payment represents the amount of cash that must be paid from owner's capital.

Exhibit 3-5 Depreciation Schedule

Nursing Wing—Depreciation Schedule

Description	Date Acquired	Life	Method of Depreciation	Cost	Accumulated Depreciation	Depreciation 9/30/73	Depreciation 9/30/74	Depreciation 9/30/75
Buildings:								
Example building	10/1/72	40 years	Straight-line	$600,000.00				
Depreciation @ 9/30/73					$ -0-	$15,000.00		
Accumulated depreciation @ 9/30/73					15,000.00	$15,000.00		
Depreciation @ 9/30/74					$15,000.00		$15,000.00	
Accumulated depreciation @ 9/30/74					15,000.00		$15,000.00	
Depreciation @ 9/30/75					$30,000.00			$15,000.00
Accumulated depreciation @ 9/30/75					15,000.00			$15,000.00
					$45,000.00			
Equipment:								
4 beds (4 @ $250.00)	10/1/73	10 years	Straight-line	$ 1,000.00			$ 100.00	$ 100.00
Television—RCA (SN. 0493)	4/1/74	10 years	Straight-line	500.00			½ 25.00	50.00
Air conditioner (Fedder)	4/1/74	10 years	Straight-line	2,500.00			½ 125.00	250.00
				$ 4,000.00	$ -0-			
Depreciation @ 9/30/74					250.00		$ 250.00	
Accumulated depreciation @ 9/30/74					$ 250.00			
Depreciation @ 9/30/75					400.00			$ 400.00
Accumulated depreciation 9/30/75					$ 650.00			

Cost of plant	$1,000,000
Useful life	40 years
Mortgage	$800,000
Mortgage term	20 years
Depreciation expense	$25,000
Principal payment on mortgage	40,000
Amount to be paid by owner's capital	$15,000

In this situation unless the nursing home revenues exceed expenses by at least $15,000, the owner receives no replenishment of the capital expended until the mortgage is paid. The $15,000 does not represent profit; it is a replenishment of capital. By the time the plant needs to be replaced, due primarily to inflation, the $200,000 capital that is available, unless it has been supplemented by profits in excess of the inflation rate, will not be adequate to finance rebuilding.

BASIS OF VALUATION

Property, plant, and equipment must be valued on the basis of cost. Cost is defined as acquisition cost or the fair market value of donated property, plant, and equipment at the date of donation.

Historical cost is the cost incurred by the present owner in acquiring the asset and preparing it for use. Generally such cost includes costs that would be capitalized under GAAP.

Historical cost for lease-purchase assets for which a purchase option has been exercised is the sum of the lease payments and other acquisition costs less amounts allowed as rent. Some lease agreements are essentially the same as installment purchases of facilities or equipment. The existence of the following conditions will generally establish that a lease is essentially a purchase:

1. The rental charge exceeds rental charges of comparable facilities or equipment in the area.
2. The term of the lease is less than the useful life of the facilities or equipment.
3. The facility has the option to renew the lease at a significantly reduced rental, or has the right to purchase the facilities or equipment at a price significantly less than fair market value.

If the lease is essentially a purchase, the rental charge is cost only to the extent that it would have been included in expense if legal title were held to the asset. The cost of ownership, such as straight-line depreciation, taxes, insurance, and interest, therefore represents cost rather than rent. The difference between the amount of rent paid and the amount recognized as rental expense is capitalized as part of the historical cost of the asset. If the asset is returned to the lessor without passing title, the difference is expensed in the year the asset is returned.

CAPITALIZATION OF DEPRECIABLE ASSETS

If a depreciable asset has an estimated useful life of at least two years and a cost of say $200, or, if it is acquired in quantity and the cost of the quantity is, say, $500, its cost must be capitalized and written off ratably over the estimated useful life of the asset. If a depreciable asset has a historical cost of less than $200, or, if it is acquired in quantity and the cost of the quantity is less than $500, or if the asset has a useful life of less than two years, its costs are expensed in the year acquired. Alterations and improvements which extend the life or increase the productivity of an asset should be capitalized and depreciated over the remaining useful life of the asset to which they are fixed. Repair and maintenance costs that do not extend the life or productivity are expensed in the current accounting period.

USEFUL LIFE OF DEPRECIABLE ASSETS

The estimated useful life of a depreciable asset is its normal operating or service life to the facility. The factors to be considered in determining useful life include normal wear and tear, obsolescence due to normal economic and technological advances, climatic and other local conditions, and the facility's policy for repairs and replacement. In selecting a proper useful life for computing depreciation, facilities should utilize the useful life guidelines published by the Internal Revenue Service.

USEFUL LIFE OF LEASEHOLD IMPROVEMENTS

The costs of improvements that are the responsibility of the facility under the terms of a lease will be amortized over the useful life of the improvement or the remaining term of the lease, whichever is shorter. The term of the lease includes any period for which the lease may be extended.

CONSTRUCTION-IN-PROGRESS

Construction-in-progress represents the expenditures made towards an expansion of the present facility or the stages of completion of a new facility. According to good accounting principles the costs incurred in constructing a capital asset must be accumulated in a long-term asset category and systematically assigned to each operating cycle, in a rational manner. The book definition of depreciation is: "the systematic and rational recognition of cost over the life cycle of the capital asset."

This process starts when the asset is put into production, for example, the date the beds are available for patients. This is the date that the construction-in-progress becomes a depreciable capital asset. The following are the accounting T accounts to demonstrate the accounting treatment:

Construction-In-Progress	Building	Movable Equipment
(1) $1,000,000 | (2) $500,000	(2) $400,000 |	(2) $50,000 |

Fixed Equipment	Cash	Notes Payable
(2) $50,000 |	| (1) $500,000	| (1) $500,000

(1) Expenditures for construction bills and financing for debt capital:

	Debit	Credit
Construction-in-progress	$1,000,000	
Cash		$500,000
Notes payable		500,000
	$1,000,000	$1,000,000

(2) Completed portion of building opened for admission of patients:

	Debit	Credit
Building	$400,000	
Movable equipment	50,000	
Fixed equipment	50,000	
Construction-in-progress		$500,000
	$500,000	$500,000

The depreciation would start at this point.

Contingent Assets

Contingent assets are those items that may materialize but there is not sufficient documentation to assure an outsider that the potential asset has value. For example:

Description	Reasoning
• Net operating loss tax purposes	• Not an asset until a future year produces taxable income.
• Carryover of Medicare settlement amounts for lower of cost or charges	• Not an asset until a future year allows the settlement amount to be recovered.
• Lawsuits for past due accounts that have been previously written off as uncollectible	• Not an asset until the account is collected.

The accounting theory states that assets do not become assets until there is reasonable assurance that the item will be converted to cash in the next operating cycle. Recording transactions that are not reasonably expected to become a cash receipt within a year are called "window dressing the balance sheet" because they do not represent real assets; they are merely potential assets. The rule is anything you cannot eventually spend or anything you have not eventually paid cash for is not an asset.

Accrued Expenses

Recall that the definition of accrual accounting specified that incurred expenses, those that are incurred in the operation of the nursing home, must be recorded at the time they become payable. For example, drug purchases that have been received and are either on hand as inventory or are being administered to patients but have not been paid for are accrued expenses. They accrued in the accounting category of accounts payable. The T accounts depict the accounting principle:

Drug Inventory		Accounts Payable	
(1) $1,000	(3) $750	(2) $500	(1) $1,000
Balance $250			$500 Balance

Drug Expense		Cash	
(3) $750			(2) $500

(1) Purchase of drug inventory

	Debit	Credit
Inventory	$1,000	
Accounts Payable		$1,000
	$1,000	$1,000

(2) Payment of an account payable for a supplier's inventory.

(3) Use of drugs for patient care. The cost of the drugs is taken out of inventory as they are used and put into expense.

This example shows the cycle of a drug purchase. The principle also applies to any supply purchase, including raw food.

Lists of other accrued expenses are presented as follows:

Description
- Accrued Payroll

Source of Information
- The payroll register, for the pay period (or a part of a pay period that has expired but is not completed) that has not been paid to the employee.

Pay periods normally end according to calendar weeks. Consequently during a month four pay periods can end:

S	M	T	W	T	F	S
		1	2	3	④	5
6	7	8	9	10	⑪	12
13	14	15	16	17	⑱	19
20	21	22	23	24	㉕	26
27	28	29	30			

or five pay periods can end:

S	M	T	W	T	F	S
				1	②	3
4	5	6	7	8	⑨	10
11	12	13	14	15	⑰	17
18	19	20	21	22	㉓	24
25	26	27	28	29	㉚	

If the payrolls were recorded in the accounting period that they are paid, as shown by the preceding example, some months would have four payrolls and some would have five. To make sure that thirty or thirty-one days of payroll expense are recorded in each month, payrolls are accrued. In the example the first month would have an accrual for four days (27, 28, 29, and 30) and the second month there would be no accrual unless the payroll checks were not released until the following month.

Some other accrued expenses are:

Description	Source of Information
• Accrued payroll taxes	• The payroll register, for the taxes that have not been paid to the bank or to the State or Federal agency.
• Accrued real estate taxes	• Prior years' tax payments.
• Accrued interest	• The mortgage payment book for interest that is due but not paid. At the end of the accounting period if the mortgage payment is not due, a certain amount of interest is *accrued* based on the number of days since the last mortgage payment. This accrual of interest expense is accomplished by a General Journal entry.

An expense that is attributable to a specific accounting period must be recorded in that period. If a check has not been drawn for that expense an accounting entry must be made. Normally, the accounting entry comes from the General Journal as a part of the regular accounting system.

Unpaid Income Taxes

Income taxes are an expense of doing business. They are assessed according to a tax return filed after the close of the accounting year. The expense accrues as income is earned. This occurs monthly. Also, if the tax is of a certain amount, quarterly payments are payable as estimated tax payments. Therefore, the tax on this income must be estimated and recorded monthly. If it is not recorded, the profit that is shown by the accounting records is overstated.

The estimate is determined as follows:

Profit for the month	$20,000
Federal tax rate	48%
	$9,600
Surtax exemption ($14,000 for entire year × ¹⁄₁₂ for one month)	1,166
Federal tax for month	$8,434
State tax for month	1,566
Total tax expense for month	$10,000
Profit for the month	$20,000
Tax expense	10,000
Net profit for month	$10,000

The accounting entry would be:

Accrued Taxes		Tax Expense		Cash	
(2) $30,000	(1) $10,000	(1) $10,000	(3) $4,000		(2) $30,000
	(1) 10,000	(1) 10,000			
	(1) 10,000	(1) 10,000			
(2) $30,000	(1) 10,000	(1) 10,000			
	(1) 10,000	(1) 10,000			
	(1) 10,000	$120,000			
		(4,000)			
		Balance $116,000			

(1) This entry would be originated from the General Journal and recorded monthly until the end of the year.
(2) If a quarterly payment is due it would be paid and recorded as a reduction of the accrual.
(3) After the tax return is prepared and the final taxes determined, an adjustment may be required to reflect the actual amount due at the end of the year.

In the example the total tax expense for the year would be $116,000. The accrual at the end of the year would be the amount of the monthly accrual less the quarterly payments adjusted to the tax due as shown on the tax return:

Accrual	$120,000
Quarterly payments	(90,000)
Accrual at end of year	$30,000
Adjustment to actual taxes	(4,000)
Actual taxes per the return	$26,000

Current Liabilities, Liquidity, and Long-Term Debt

The classification of liabilities as current and long-term is a technique used by all businesses to specify those liabilities that will or will not be paid in cash during the ordinary business cycle (normally one year). The placement of the liabilities in coding the accounting records and preparing the balance sheet are according to liquidity. The sooner a liability is required to be paid the more current it is. The liabilities are deemed to be due in accordance with the terms of the underlying agreement.

For example, liabilities that are secured with collateral and due within one year, such as the mortgage payments, take creditor precedence over unsecured debt, such as accounts payable. Therefore the mortgage payments due the next year are more current than accounts payable. The following is the sequence of liabilities:

Account Number

	Current Liabilities
200	Notes payable, secured
210	Current portion of mortgage debt
220	Accounts payable

230	Notes payable, unsecured
240	Accrued expenses
250	Accrued taxes
	Long-Term Debt
270	Mortgage notes payable
280	Notes payable
290	Bond indentures payable

The relevance of liquidity, as with current assets, is for matching the assets available during the operating cycle to pay bills due during the operating cycle. The longer it takes to liquidate a debt, the longer the business has to produce profits to make the payments. Therefore current liabilities are matched with current assets and long-term debt payments are compared to cash available from profits to pay principal payments on long-term obligations.

NOTES AND MORTGAGES PAYABLE

The debt capital to finance the business is normally obtained on a long-term basis. The portion that is due annually is a current liability and the portion due beyond one year is long-term debt. The interest expense that accrues with the principal payment that is due is recorded as it becomes due. It is accrued until paid.

Any finance costs related to the debt that are included in the mortgage are normally recorded at the same time as the related asset. If the finance costs relate to the purchase of a building but the debt repayment period is different than the depreciable life of the asset, the cost is amortized over the repayment term of the debt.

An exception to this general rule is the treatment of interest expense incurred during the construction period. For example, assume that $1,000,000 is borrowed to pay construction bills as the nursing home building is being built. Assume that the mortgage covering the debt financing starts when the building is complete. In other words, the interest expense incurred during the construction period relates to temporary financing not the long-term debt. The question is, what should the accounting treatment be? Should the expense be a cost of that short period or should it be included in the cost of the building and depreciated over the life of the assets?

Accounting principles stipulate three alternatives under the appropriate circumstances. The alternatives are:

1. Expense the full amount in the period incurred.
2. Include incurred amount in the cost of the building.
3. Expense the amount incurred and include an imputed amount in the cost of the building that represents the cost of capital at its present value if invested for the life of the asset.

The impact on the profit and loss statement of each alternative can be substantial. In the example the difference would be:

	Alternatives		
	One	Two	Three
Interest incurred at 9%	$90,000	$90,000	$90,000
Expense			
Interest	$90,000	$ –	$90,000
Depreciation (40-year life)	–	2,500	–
Capital cost	–	–	$10,000
Total expense charged against profit	$90,000	$2,500	$100,000

As you can see, the difference is substantial. A further complication is that the Medicare and Medicaid regulations require that this type of interest expense must be included in the cost of the building and spread over the life as a part of depreciation. The Securities and Exchange Commission (SEC) requires registered companies to expense construction interest in the period incurred. And the IRS specifies that the treatment will normally be that interest during construction be spread over the life of the asset, unless otherwise justified.

Realistically and logically the construction interest cost applies to a very specific period of time: the time it takes to construct the building. The debt capital it takes to finance the building to cover its construction costs normally arises when the mortgage becomes effective for the operating plant. Then the interest paid on the debt capital represents the debt capital costs for each succeeding period. The cost of the building then only includes construction costs of the capital asset and the annual depreciation represents the cost of the capital asset over its life cycle.

The cash has been expended. The cost applies to a specific period of construction. The cost must be recovered now through profits if the cash outflow is to be covered. Therefore, in the nursing home industry, the first alternative seems to be the most appropriate from an accounting standpoint.

However, if this method is selected the treatment for reimbursement and taxes will require extensive dual accounting. This so called "timing difference" and interperiod tax accounting will be discussed extensively in the section on deferred credits.

Deferred Income, Liabilities, and Credits

Deferred amounts, in accounting circles, are a means of matching revenue with expenses. So when an item applies to a future period it must be deferred. For example, if a private patient pays room and board charges in advance of the month that it applies, the revenue must be delayed until the month when the service is provided. This is called deferred income. Following is the accounting treatment for deferred income and the recognition of prepaid taxes (i.e., deferred charge):

	Per Books	Per Tax Return
Room and Board Paid in Advance		
Income	—	$100,000*
Deferred income	$100,000	—
Taxable income	—	100,000
Tax effect	—	$48,000

*Tax ruling is that prepaid revenue is taxed as collected regardless of when earned.

The accounting entries would be:

Tax Expense		Tax Liability
(1) $100,000		(1) $100,000
		(2) 48,000
		Bal $148,000

Deferred Charge
(2) $48,000

(1) Record tax expense on book income which is lower than taxable income because the revenue collected in advance is deferred.

(2) Record the increase to the actual amount due on the tax return. The difference of $48,000 is the deferred (prepaid) tax that will not be an expense per books until the revenue is recognized as earned.

Deferred liabilities are items that represent an expense of the current business cycle but will not be paid for some time. A good example is pension funding, in which the pension agreement requires a funding method that attributes pension costs to current wage levels but does not require that all of the costs be paid in cash immediately. In other words, the cost is related to current period salaries and is a cost of doing business for the current period and must be recorded. However cash funding of the pension cost may be at a different time. Therefore a deferred liability must be established so the cost and commitment can be recorded as it is incurred as an expense.

Deferred Pension Liability		Pension Expense
(2) $10,000	(1) $15,000	(1) $15,000
	Balance $5,000	

Cash
(2) $10,000

(1) Record pension expense that relates to the current period.
(2) Record payment of pension funding.

Deferred credits generally consist of revenue that is not earned until a future period. The example that is most common is deferred income taxes. As pointed out in the discussion of deferred charges, amounts that arise because of a difference in the manner an item is earned must be accounted for. The timing of the accounting treatment usually depends on the method selected to determine the amount. In the case of income taxes, if a method of calculating the amount of revenue on prepaid room and board charges is different for tax purposes than it is for book purposes, we have a timing difference. This is calculated as follows:

	Per Books	Per Tax Return	Timing Difference
Straight-line depreciation	$100,000	$100,000	$ —
Accelerated depreciation	—	50,000	50,000
	$100,000	$150,000	$50,000
Tax effect at 46%	$46,000	$69,000	$23,000

This means that the tax paid with the tax return will be $24,000 less than the tax would be on book income because more depreciation is currently taken on the tax return. In later years the situation will "reverse" itself as the accelerated depreciation is less than straight-line. Remember that over the life of the asset the total depreciation will be the same. Only the timing of the expense is different. The accounting entries would be:

Tax Expense		Tax Liability	
(1) $100,000		(2) $23,000	(1) $100,000
			Balance $77,000

Deferred Credit (taxes)
(2) $23,000

(1) Record tax expense on book income which is higher than taxable income because of lower depreciation.
(2) Record the reduction of the tax liability account to the $77,000 actually due to the government. The difference is the deferred taxes that will be used up in later years as the process (timing) reverses itself.

In tax accounting you should also be aware that differences in taxable income and book income that are due to nondeductible expenses are "Permanent Differences" that are due to regulations not method. These differences do not reverse themselves and therefore do not lead to deferred credits. In these cases the tax on the tax return is the amount recorded in the accounting records. A good example of this would be nondeductible travel and entertainment expenses. The expense is in the books and records and not in the expenses for tax purposes, hence the permanent difference.

The timing difference theory also holds true for Medicare and Medicaid reimbursement. If the difference is due to timing and will reverse itself, the difference should be recorded as a deferred item. If it is due to unallowable costs it is not a deferred item; it is a charge or credit to the current period's profit or loss.

Capital Stock, Contributions, and Retained Earnings

The invested capital, often referred to as equity capital, consists of the following:

Description	Source
• Capital stock (all classes) less repurchased stock for treasury (treasury stock)	• Investment of cash or donation of productive assets to the business including the capital paid-in in excess of par value. Any stock redeemed for cash or assets reduces the invested capital stock amount.

Description	Source
• Contributions	• Donation of cash or assets to a tax exempt organization is a form of capital. It is not redeemable to an investor but is all-essential in the provision of capital to the business.
• Retained earnings less dividends	• The excess of revenue over expense, net income, is retained by the business for working capital, replacement and expansion capital, and dividends. As the investors are paid a return—cash or stock dividends—on their investment, the dividends must be met out of retained earnings or they represent a return of investment not dividends.
• Fund Balance	• The excess of revenue over expense accumulated by a tax-exempt organization is for working capital and replacement and expansion capital.

The Capital section of the accounting records and balance sheet represents the performance record of the nursing home from inception. It must somehow be accounted for at a level that represents the excess of spendable assets over payable liabilities. If shown any differently, it is distorting the financial position of the nursing home. Therefore the creation of capital by recording intangible assets that will not result in cash benefits or the overlooking of liabilities that eventually must be paid is called "window dressing." This practice must be avoided because it is not only misleading to investors and bankers but also to all who hope to benefit from the nursing home business.

The Capital section is the basis for determining a number of financial ratios:

- Return on capital
- Return on investment
- Debt to equity ratio

These will be discussed in Chapter 7.

Contingent Liabilities (Loss Contingency)

The Financial Accounting Standards Board (FASB) in their Statement of Financial Accounting Standards No. 5, Accounting for Contingencies, defines a contingency as an existing condition, situation, or set of circumstances involving uncertainty as to possible gain (gain contingency) or loss (loss contingency) that will be resolved in the future. Contingencies are limited, in an accounting sense, to those events that cannot be reasonably estimated and valued, until they are resolved.

When a loss contingency exists, the likelihood that the future event will result in a loss ranges from probable to remote:
- *Probable*—The event is likely to occur.
- *Reasonably possible*—The chance the event will occur is possible.
- *Remote*—The chance the event will occur is remote.

These terms are important in deciding whether the contingencies are predictable enough to record. If they are predictable in value and probable in occurrence, they should be recorded in the period that it arises.

According to Statement No. 5:

> An estimated loss from a loss contingency shall be accrued by a charge to income if both of the following conditions are met:
> a. Information available prior to issuance of the financial statements indicates that it is probable that an asset had been impared or a liability had been incurred at the date of the financial statements. It is implicit in this condition that it must be probable that one or more future events will occur confirming the fact of the loss.
> b. The amount of loss can be reasonably estimated.

Examples of loss contingencies include:
- Collectibility of receivables
- Obligations related to product warranties and product defects
- Risk of loss or damage of property by fire, explosion or hazards
- Threat of expropriation of assets
- Pending or threatened litigation
- Actual or possible claims and assessments
- Risk or loss from catastrophes
- Guarantees of indebtedness of others
- Obligations of banks for letters of credit
- Agreements to repurchase receivables or real property

If the loss contingency is probable and can be valued it should be recorded as follows:

Loss Due to Malpractice Settlement	Malpractice Settlement
$10,000 (1)	$10,000 (1)

(1) This condition can only exist if the claim is asserted and is likely to be settled for the amount recorded. If doubt of the outcome is beyond the estimation of probability, the event should be disclosed in a footnote to the statements. For further guidance you should seek guidance from FASB Statement 5 and the American Institute of Certified Public Accountants.

Revenues

Revenues in a nursing home consist of room and board charges, nursing care, and numerous add-on charges for rehabilitative services. The revenue should be recognized on the accrual basis (as earned) which is normally earned as follows:

Payer	Earned Revenue Value	Timing of Collection
Self-Pay (Private)	Customary charge	At beginning of month
Medicare	Reasonable cost	Monthly on an estimated basis reconciled at end of year. There is usually a 30-day lag between billing date and collection date.
Medicaid	Cost-Related Contracted Price	Monthly on a contracted basis. In some states an annual reconciliation is required. The monthly payment usually lags for 30 days after billing.

The method of determining the value of the gross earned revenue and the net earned revenue depends on who is purchasing the services. The private paying patient will pay the list price for services and it will be recorded as follows:

```
      Private Pay                            Private Pay
  Accounts Receivable                 Room and Board Revenue
  $600.00  (1) | $600.00 (2)                   | $300.00 (1)
   200.00  (3) |
   800.00      |
  Bal. $200.00 | $200.00 (4)
```

```
                                            Private Pay
                                  Standard Nursing Care Revenue
                                              | $300.00 (1)

                                            Private Pay
           Cash                              Drugs Revenue
  $600.00 (2) |                               | $50.00 (3)
   200.00 (4) |
                                            Private Pay
                                    Physical Therapy Revenue
                                              | $100.00 (3)

                                            Private Pay
                                    Medical Supplies Revenue
                                              | $50.00 (3)
```

(1) This assumes that the patient is billed for room and board and standard nursing care on the first day of the month.

(2) Private patient pays shortly after being billed.

(3) The patient is billed in the first two or three days of the following month for the actual usage of add-on services.

(4) The $200.00 accounts receivable for add-ons is then paid in the following month. If it is not paid it could become a bad debt.

The Medicare patient has a slightly different method because the Medicare program pays a discounted rate based on reasonable cost (which includes a return on net equity for proprietary providers) as determined by a prescribed formula. A discount normally is required to recognize the elimination of the mark-up from the list price the private patient pays.

To account for the amount of the discount for an operating period, the customary private pay rate is recorded for Medicare patients and a contractual discount recorded when Medicare makes a payment. The payments for individual accounts are reconciled at the end of the accounting year to the total costs for providing services to all Medicare beneficiaries.

Discounting is used by management to determine the optimum utilization of beds. It is also required by the Medicare regulations because *Medicare charges* at customary prices are used in the Medicare cost reimbursement formula as follows:

	Customary Charges				
	All Patients	Medicare Patients	% Utilization	Total Cost	Medicare Cost
Room and board and nursing care	$120,000	$30,000	25%	$100,000	$25,000
Ancillary services	30,000	20,000	66	25,000	16,666
Total settlement	$150,000	$50,000		$125,000	$41,666

This method of reimbursement is known as the Ratio of Charges to Charges as Applied to Costs (RCCAC). It was initially used for all providers. It became an optional method before being replaced by a method called the combination method. The combination method used a per diem approach for room and board and nursing (routine services) and an RCCAC approach for ancillaries.

In the example, if the total patient days were 6,000 and the Medicare days 2,000 the Medicare cost would be:

	Total Cost	Patient Days	Cost Per Day	Medicare Days	Medicare Cost
Room and board and nursing	$100,000	6,000	$16.66	1,700	$28,322
Ancillary services					16,666
Total reimbursable cost					$44,988

The Medicare cost is then compared to the amount paid for each Medicare patient during the accounting year and the reconciliation is settled, dollar for dollar, with the Medicare program. If the combination method is used the settlement would be as follows:

Total reimbursable cost	$44,988
Amount paid by patient for deductibles and coinsurance	$5,500
Less deductibles and coinsurance considered to be uncollectible	500
	$5,000
Amount to be paid by Medicare	$39,988
Total amount paid or to be paid by Medicare during year	38,555
Amount owed to nursing home by Medicare	$1,433

Under these circumstances the revenue and discount would be recorded in the accounting records as follows:

Medicare Accounts Receivable		Medicare Room and Board and Nursing Care Revenue
$50,000 (1)	$38,555 (2)	$30,000 (1)
	5,000 (3)	
	6,445 (4)	
	$50,000	

Cash		Medicare Ancillary Services Revenue
$38,555 (2)		$20,000 (1)
1,433 (5)		
$39,988		
5,000 (3)		
$44,988		

Medicare Contractual Discount	
$6,445 (4)	$1,433 (5)
Balance $5,012	

(1) A bill for each Medicare patient is created and recorded as an accounts receivable.

(2) The payment is received from the Medicare paying agent (Intermediary) monthly on an estimated amount per patient day. The example shows the total for the year but in reality it is paid monthly.

(3) The amount the patient pays for deductibles and coinsurance.

(4) The payment from Medicare in final settlement of the annual cost reconciliation.

The discounting procedure was primarily developed for retrospective cost reimbursements plans. The Medicaid Program did not become cost related until July 1, 1976. Many of the state plans are similar or identical to the Medicare Principles of Reimbursement. In those cases the accounting would be the same as Medicare. However, many of the plans are going to be using negotiated prospective reimbursement contracts that do not pay costs that are specifically attributed to each facility. The accounting for discount in these situations may have to take a different form.

For example if a target price, independent of each facility and including a factor for profit, is less than the private pay rate, a discount may not exist. This negotiated price with Medicaid is probably the best price available for the bed and there is no intent to charge more. To assume that a discount is being given, when the bed would be empty otherwise, is not appropriate. In these circumstances the negotiated price would be the customary rate that is recorded as revenue and no discount would be recognized. In most cases, if a discount were recorded it more than likely would not be realistic because the customary private pay rate is subsidizing the lower Medicaid price. Therefore the difference between the Medicaid price and the regular price is not a discount; it is merely the difference of prices because of market conditions.

When it is decided that the discounting procedure is not appropriate, the revenue recordkeeping for Medicaid is the same as private pay. If the Medicaid reimbursement is retrospective the revenue recordkeeping would be the same as Medicare.

See the Billing and Accounts Receivable section for more specific guidance on Medicare and Medicaid accounting.

Capital Costs

The definition of capital and the cost of capital is covered in the Glossary. Basically it asks what the costs are of having investors commit their dollars to the business. The accounting principles for capital costs require that the costs be based on incurred costs. Those incurred costs consist of:

- *Depreciation expense*—The systematic and rational assignment of the acquisition cost of plant and equipment to each accounting period during the useful life of the asset.
- *Interest expense*—The interest paid or accrued on debt incurred for financing the plant and equipment.
- *Real estate taxes*—Taxes that relate to the cost of the property (not to the cost of operations) and can be viewed as cost of the capital asset. Building insurance has also been categorized as capital cost.
- *Rent expense*—Rent incurred for leasing the plant and/or equipment (versus depreciation and interest for owned capital assets). The rent for each accounting period is a ratable measurement of capital cost.

If the plant and equipment are leased with ownership conditions, it may, in reality, be an installment purchase. According to authoritative GAAP originally promulgated by the American Institute of Certified Public Accountants (AICPA) Accounting Principles Board:

> The determination that lease payments result in the creation of an equity in the property obviously requires a careful evaluation of the facts and probabilities surrounding a given case. Unless it is clear that no material equity in the property will result from the lease, the existence, . . . of one or more circumstances such as those shown below tend to indicate that the lease arrangement is in substance a purchase and should be accounted for as such.
>
> a. The property was acquired by the lessor to meet the special needs of the lessee and will probably be usable only for that purpose and only by the lessee.
> b. The term of the lease corresponds substantially to the estimated life of the property, and the lessee is obligated to pay costs such as taxes, insurance, and maintenance, which are usually considered incidental to ownership.
> c. The lessee has guaranteed the obligations of the lessor with respect to the property leased.
> d. The lessee has treated the lease as a purchase for tax purposes.

Whenever it is determined that the lease is in fact a purchase, the leased asset must be recorded as an owned depreciable asset and the debt for principle lease payments must also be recorded. The costs for interest and for real estate taxes and insurance, if applicable, must be valued and recorded with each lease payment or amortized as a cost of capital.

Total rent payments	$2,000,000
Value of Property	$100,000
Plant	700,000
Equipment	200,000
	$1,000,000
Interest	1,000,000
Total cost	$2,000,000
Capital cost (prorated to each accounting period)	
Depreciation	$1,000,000
Interest	1,000,000
	$2,000,000

Depreciation

A number of methods can be used in computing depreciation. Under the straight-line method the annual allowance is determined by dividing the cost of the asset (less any estimated salvage value) by the years of useful life. This method produces a uniform allowance each year. Under accelerated methods the amount of depreciation is more in the early years of the useful life, and less in later years.

The nursing home should establish a policy as to the amount of depreciation to be taken in the year of acquisition. Acceptable policies are:

1. Computing first year depreciation based on the portion of time the asset is in use during the year. That is, if a depreciable asset is received and in use in the first eight months of the year of acquisition, two-thirds of a full year's depreciation expense is recognized in that first year.
2. Recording one half of the yearly depreciation expense in the year of acquisition and year of disposal, regardless of the date of acquisition.
3. Recording a full year's depreciation expense if the asset is acquired in the first half of the year. If the asset is acquired in the last half of the year, no depreciation expense is recognized.

The theory underlying accelerated depreciation is related to economics as well as physical deterioration. In the earlier example, where the useful life was forty years and the mortgage term was twenty years, the difference between the cash required to pay the principal and the cash provided by depreciation could be reduced by using an accelerated method of depreciation. For example:

Cost of plant	$1,000,000
Useful life	40 years
Depreciation method	Double the straight-line method times the net book value of the plant

Mortgage	$800,000
Mortgage term	20 years
Depreciation using accelerated method	$50,000
Principal payment	40,000
Amount to put into retained earnings for replenishment of capital	$10,000

This forces management to include a higher amount of depreciation in its pricing structure to cover the cash flow requirements of the principal payments. If this is accomplished, the bottom-line amounts are available for dividends or capital funding of replacement. The impact of inflation also is minimized because the capital is replenished at a faster rate if the retained earnings are invested in income producing investments.

Patient Funds

Accounting for patients' funds began as a way to safeguard patient valuables. The accountability only required that the patients' property be placed in envelopes bearing their names. Giving receipts for the valuables and accounting for the funds were performed informally, if at all. With the advent of the Supplementary Security Income (SSI) law in 1972, the quantity of the patients' funds and the accountability requirements have increased. To make matters worse, when SSI was passed, little attention was paid to the administration of the funding and many states permit the patients to retain more than the minimum.

In those instances where the family members receive funds on behalf of the patient there are problems in insuring the use of the funds for the patient's immediate benefit. Where the patient receives the funds directly, there are problems with the patient's competence to spend the funds in a meaningful manner. Where the facility is the named recipient, additional administrative burdens are encountered in cashing funds and disbursing the funds between personal use and care billings.

The facility's receipt of a patient's funds needs to be documented by a legal document establishing a trustee relationship between the patient and the facility. This document may be a clause in the facility's admission agreement or a court order decreeing the facility custodian for the patient. Once the trustee relationship is established, the facility can properly take custody of the patient's funds.

The patient funds accounting should establish individual patient accounts to record the cash transactions. Patient fund receipts should be deposited in a separate bank account, termed Patient Trust Fund Account, distinct from all other bank accounts of the facility, and entered in the individual patient accounts showing date, amount, and from whom received. Only minimal amounts should be kept on hand to meet the day-to-day needs.

The documentation of disbursing patient funds is very important. The disbursement system must also accommodate patients who are senile. There must be documentation that the disbursements are clearly shown to be for the personal wants of the patient. At discharge, the patient or other responsible party can be given a check made payable to the patient representing the balance in the account. At the death of a patient, the payee must be determined.

At least quarterly, a statement of the patient's receipts and disbursements should be given to each patient or designated guardian. On a monthly basis, the individual patient fund accounts should reconcile to the cash on hand and in the bank. Annually the patient fund transactions should be filed with the appropriate state agency together with a certification by the facility that the designated purpose of patient funds have been met.

Recording and reporting the fiduciary responsibility for patient funds as an asset and liability of the facility is not appropriate. The responsibility is separate from the operating statements of the facility. The best alternative is to record the patient funds in a separate report following the facility's financial information.

The patient funds can best be depicted as follows:

Patient Trust Fund Account		Trust Fund Liability
(1) $25		(1) $25

Patient Account	
Receipt	Disbursement
$25	$25

(Separate Accounting Report)

Trust Fund Account	$25
Trust Fund Liability	$25

(1) These amounts should agree.

Life Care Contracts: An Accounting Nightmare

Life care contracts represent a form of life insurance policy. They originally were not conceived to be such, but based on inadvertent overzealousness to raise money, the life care concept got distorted to the point where it became a tool for raising front end capital to build retirement centers. The theory behind the life care prepayment was that it would enable a tax exempt organization to raise capital for purposes of building retirement centers and nursing homes. The benefit to be derived by the purchasers of the life care contract was that they would be assured of a place to live and be cared for, for the rest of their lives. But like many good ideas, this idea was only good for a few short years.

In the beginning, there was very little, if any, borrowing to finance the construction of brick and mortar. The deep-seated problem which arose was related to the fact the seller of the life care contract was trying to establish a mini-insurance company with a limited population. This meant the actuarial experience was not statistically sound, and one or two major exceptions to the rule could spell disaster. Unfortunately, the capital usually was spent in building the capital assets as it was expected that the operation would carry itself, enabling the organization to put aside future prepayments to provide life care to "living" residents. In reality, the prepayment was normally inadequate to cover the added costs of care resulting from higher quality standards and inflation. The only way the organization could make ends meet was to negotiate long term borrowing, using the property as collateral, or by pyramiding the number of units to be sold so the capital kept flowing in.

There are a number of reasons why this concept was not financially sound. In addition to the increase in quality standards and inflation, the residents, under "no stress" conditions, began to live longer than expected. Statistically, the 1958 life expectancy tables, used to determine the amount of prepayment, were not representative of the life expectancy of the elderly in a fraternal type of organization such as a not-for-profit retirement centers. This meant that the residents were living longer and using more services, which reduced the opportunities for the facility to accumulate any capital.

Accountants did not help in this process, because they really did not understand how to establish values which reflected the total commitment to the life care contract holders. It was their assumption that the prepayments were deferred income, with prepayment of the life fee to be amortized over a determinable period. This step in accounting theory was a step up from what was originally practiced, which was to record all collections as revenue when collected. The amortization method required that the prepayment be recognized as revenue using:

1. A contractual period of time
2. Life expectancy tables

This method of accounting did not really work because it was assuming that the prepayment was going to be adequate to cover the life care costs of the resident. Unfortunately, the prepayments were not actuarially determined, but were determined based purely upon circumstances. Many of the life care contract holders paid in their life savings and were told this would buy them long-term care services for life. But if the prepaid life care fee were $20,000 and the cost of care goes up 15 percent, it would mean within approximately six and one half years, the initial prepayment would be worth one-half of what it was originally. Therefore, there was no feasible way for the prepayment to cover the services required by the resident, unless the resident lived for less than their life expectancy. What actually happens in practice is that the people under life care contracts tend to live longer because of the responsibilities assumed for them. (In many of the institutions which have life care, there is literally no worry on the part of the resident as to where the money is coming from.) As a result, these residents live longer than expected, and utilize more services than expected.

It does help somewhat to look at insurance accounting when you are dealing with life care. Many of the reserve requirements, which are standard operating procedure in insurance companies, also have applicability to the life care concept. For example, when a resident is admitted under a life care contract, and it is actuarially determined that the resident will incur more costs over their remaining life than their prepayment covers, less any payments they have made towards their care, an insurance reserve should be established and funded. Ideally, this insurance reserve should be funded with cash. The insurance reserve represents the present value of the life commitment, based upon actuarially determined life expectancy, less any payments the resident will make towards their own care. Following is the step-by-step formula and the accounting for the life care commitment:

1. Statistical information regarding the resident must be gathered, for example: date of admission, age at admission, placement in the facility, current monthly

rate, currently monthly payment on behalf of the resident, age at date of computation, expected remaining life (based upon life expectancy tables, plus a percentage factor—a percentage factor must be added because of the deviation from the normal life expectancy statistics), a copy of the contract.

2. The current cost of care, which can be the amount charged to the resident for their services, less the mark-up, is the basis for determining the long-term care commitment. In other words, if a resident is sixty-eight when he is admitted, and seventy-eight in 1980 and expected to live four more years, then the commitment will be the monthly cost times the number of months that the resident is expected to live. This will be reduced by the amount of revenue the resident is contractually required to pay towards the cost of care. This present value of the commitment must be recorded on the books of the facility.

You might ask, "Why should the liability be recorded before it is due?" We must point out that the day the life care contract is signed, there is an obligation on the part of the facility to provide lifelong care. To be able to determine if the prepayment is adequate, the life care commitment should be valued and it should be compared to the amount of revenue expected to be collected from the resident over their remaining life. Ideally, this calculation should be done prior to the signing of the contract to make sure there is adequate front-end money to do the job, or some provision in the contract which will allow the facility to receive a monthly maintenance cost, or an alternative, whereby the facility can seek other resources for payment (i.e., Medicaid and Medicare). If the front-end payment is not going to be adequate to cover the life care commitment and it is signed by both parties, even though ignorant of the facts, the organization is contractually obligated to provide life care, and the value of the commitment should be recorded at the date of executing the contract. If it is deferred or not recorded at all, then the period of time in which the resident is still in the facility, with very little or no cash income, becomes a financial nightmare for management (for example, Pacific Homes in California). But if management diligently records the total commitment, compares it to expected receipts, and the net amount of the obligation for life care contracts is reflected in the balance sheet, then the financial position of the institution is properly stated. To understand the calculation, please review the schedule shown in Exhibit 3-6, which is a sample listing of life care contracts for a 320-unit retirement campus. The accounting entries for recording life care contracts, after the mechanics are worked out, are not very difficult. The front-end prepayment is a debit to cash and a credit to deferred income. The deferred income should be amortized independently, using the current charge for care. (See Exhibit 3-7.)

The actuarial value of the life care commitment, less any payments which are expected to be received from the resident over their lifetime, represents the life care commitment. The initial accounting entry for the commitment is a credit to life care commitment and a debit to a valuation reserve account in the capital section of the balance sheet. The effect on the current operating year is the fluctuation of the valuation reserve due to fluctuations in cost of care, deaths, and new contracts. Any

Exhibit 3-6 Sample Life Care Commitment Accounts

Residential Sheltered Care	Birth Date and Date of Entry	Age at Entry	Age at 12-31-78	Life Expectancy (Plus 15%)	Monthly Rate Residential Nursing	
Tom Baker	08-08-1898 08-21-1978	80 (1)	80	6.73	$ 495.00 975.00	$495
Wayne Franklin	01-11-1903 11-29-1969	66 (1)	75	8.98	450.00 975.00	
Jerry Rhoads	07-23-1895 12-20-1978	83 (1)	83	5.62	495.00 975.00	$185.80
Mary Kaiser	02-26-1896 10-07-1969	73 (1)	82	5.97	495.00 975.00	$450
Marie Holcomb	12-18-1890 09-03-1976	85 (1)	88	4.08	495.00 975.00	$450
Janet Huette	03-14-1897 03-31-1971	74 (1)	81	6.34	495.00 975.00	$510
Jane Jensen	04-15-1911 11-26-1974	63 (1)	67	13.49	450.00 975.00	$184.50
Sally Miller	08-23-1889 08-04-1977	87 (1)	89	3.81	495.00 975.00	$200
Pat Donnelly	03-07-1901 01-11-1978	76 (1)	77	8.03	495.00 975.00	$157.40
Erma Opperman	05-08-1900 12-01-1966	66 (1)	78	7.58	495.00 975.00	$460
Keith Poshard	02-07-1890 10-02-1978	88 (1)	88	4.08	495.00 975.00	$326
John Spitzer	08-24-1895 10-03-1973	78 (1)	83	5.62	495.00 975.00	$410
William Wrigley	08-18-1903 11-19-1975	72 (1)	75	8.98	495.00 975.00	$250

Exhibit 3-6 (cont.)

Contract Amount Payable	Liability Difference × ½ Life Expect.	Age at 12-31-79	Life Expectancy (Plus 15%)	Monthly Rate Residential Nursing	Contract Amount Payable
295.00 but Public Aid	$ 8,090.00 —	81	6.34	$ 560.00 1,110.00	$295.00 495 but P.A.
165.00 165.00	15,355.00 43,640.00	76	8.50	560.00 1,110.00	165.00 165.00
170.10 but Pub. Aid	10,955.00 —	84	5.29	560.00 1,110.00	185.80 185.80 P.A.
283.00 but Public Aid	7,605.00 —	83	5.62	560.00 1,110.00	450.00 450 but P.A.
350.00 but Public Aid	3,550.00 —	89	3.81	560.00 1,110.00	450.00 450 but P.A.
460.00 but Public Aid	1,330.00 —	82	5.97	560.00 1,110.00	495.00 510 but P.A.
166.20 but Pub. Aid	22,990.00 —	68	12.85	510.00 1,110.00	184.50 184.50 P.A.
200.00 but Public Aid	6,760.00 —	90	3.52	560.00 1,110.00	200.00 200 but P.A.
142.90 but Pub. Aid	2,515.00 —	78	7.58	560.00 1,110.00	157.40 157.40 P.A.
395.00 but Public Aid	4,548.00 —	79	7.14	560.00 1,110.00	460.00 460 but P.A.
326.00 but Public Aid	7,980.00 —	89	3.81	560.00 1,110.00	326.00 326 but P.A.
395.00 but Public Aid	3,372.00 —	84	5.29	560.00 1,110.00	410.00 410 but P.A.
250.00 but Public Aid	13,200.00 —	76	8.50	560.00 1,110.00	250.00 250 but P.A.

Exhibit 3-6 (cont.)

Liability Difference ½ Life Expect.	Deferred Entrance Fee 12-31-78	12-31-79	Cash %/Fee % or Payment Limit	Village Liability 12-31-78	12-31-79
$10,080.00 –	$14,613.50	$12,018.50	$495.00	$ 14,613.50	$ 12,018.50
20,145.00 48,195.00	8,475.58	4,725.58	165.00	58,995.00	68,340.00
11,880.00 –	3,912.60	–	185.80	10,955.00	11,880.00
3,710.00 –	7,148.69	5,245.69	450.00	7,605.00	5,245.69
2,515.00 –	12,111.24	10,476.24	450.00	12,111.24	10,476.24
2,330.00 –	7,621.82	7,281.82	510.00	7,621.82	7,281.82
25,095.00 –	37.01	–	184.50	22,990.00	25,095.00
7,605.00 –	10,267.88	6,532.88	200.00	10,267.88	7,605.00
18,310.00 –	10,686.01	5,422.81	157.40	10,686.01	18,310.00
4,285.00 –	5,008.23	5,072.88	460.00	5,008.23	5,072.88
5,350.00 –	14,493.00	12,270.00	326.00	14,493.00	12,270.00
4,760.00 –	2,010.92	660.92	410.00	3,372.00	4,760.00
15,810.00 –	12,971.96	9,742.46	250.00	13,200.00	15,810.00
			Sub Total	$191,918.68	$204,165.13

Exhibit 3-7 Life Care "T" Accounts

Cash		Life Care Commitments	
(1) $50,000		(2) $5,000	(1) $50,000
			(3) 10,000
			(4) 60,000
			(5) 55,000

Resident Revenue	
	(2) $5,000

Provision for Valuation Reserve		Valuation Reserve Fund Balance	
(3) $5,000		(3) $5,000	

(1) Prepayment
(2) Amortization of current charges for service to revenue
(3) Life care valuation reserve—to restate the life care commitment based on actuarilly determined liability commitment, for current and prior periods
(4) Life care commitment
(5) Reassessed valuation, ending balance—

Prepayment (1)		(1)	50,000
Current amortization		(2)	(5,000)
			45,000
Valuation reserve			
Prior		(3)	5,000
Current		(4)	5,000
Life care commitment		(5)	55,000

residents who forfeit a portion of their life care prepayment, due to death or departure from the facility, shall be removed from the life care commitment and recorded through the valuation reserve.

The balance sheet and income statement (see Exhibits 3-8, 3-9) portray the reporting of the life care contracts. In addition to the basic financial statements, there should also be a footnote explaining the life care concept, the number of residents with contracts, a summary of the provisions of those contracts, and a description of the accounting principles to be applied. Note a sample of that footnote as shown in Exhibit 3-10.

Exhibit 3-8

Retirement Village, Inc.
Balance Sheet
December 31, 1979

ASSETS

		December 31, 1979
Current Assets:		
Cash		$ 54,965
Investments:		
Marketable equity securities (at cost)	$ 4,075	
Savings accounts, government bonds, certificates of deposit	86,496	
Unexpended bond proceeds and escrow account	307,141	397,712
Accounts receivable:		
Residents	98,818	
Hill-Burton grant	8,194	
Real estate contracts	88,706	195,718
Accrued interest receivable		928
Deferred charges - bond program		54,143
Patient deposits		26,075
Unexpired insurance		2,373
Total current assets		731,914
Capital Assets (at cost and appraisal):		
Land		96,017
Land improvements	25,172	
Buildings:		
Nursing care	3,806,929	
Apartments, houses, cottages	1,280,308	
Equipment:		
Nursing care	736,474	
Residential	102,944	
Transportation	31,093	
	5,982,920	
Less accumulated depreciation	1,428,825	4,554,095
Construction in progress		74,308
Total capital assets		4,724,420
Total assets		$5,456,334

Exhibit 3-8 (cont.)

LIABILITIES AND CAPITAL

		December 31, 1979
Current Liabilities:		
Notes payable to banks and savings and loans		$ 274,500
Current installments-mortgage payable		51,125
Accounts payable		63,523
Salaries and wages payable		29,561
Accrued liabilities:		
Payroll taxes	$ 7,740	
Interest	49,598	57,338
Liability residents:		
Deposits	17,075	
Burial funds	9,000	
Annuities	68,802	94,877
Total current liabilities		570,924
Long-term debt, net of current installments:		
Bonds payable		753,750
Mortgage payable		691,229
Total long-term debt		1,444,979
Unfunded life care commitments (see note)		2,167,796
Capital:		
Fund balance, before restatement		2,609,011
Valuation life care commitments, December 31, 1978, resulting from a prior period correction of fund balance for errors in infunded liability		(652,439)
Fund balance, as restated		1,956,572
Reserve for valuation of unfunded life care commitments, resulting from an excess of life care commitment over related revenues		(745,175)
Net income for the period		61,238
Total capital		1,272,635
Total liabilities and capital		$5,456,334

Exhibit 3-9

Retirement Village, Inc.
Statement of Income
The Year Ended December 31, 1979

	December 31, 1979
Revenue:	
Membership fees	$1,632,550
Recognized revenue life care commitments, being amortized on the life expectancy method (see note)	347,351
	1,979,901
Provision for 1979 valuation of life care commitments (see note)	92,736
Total revenue	1,887,165
Operating Expense:	
Salaries	1,093,080
Employee benefits	115,090
Insurance	49,393
Consultants	38,549
Utilities	163,067
Supplies	243,549
Medical	82,020
Other	76,661
Total operating expense	1,861,409
Capital Expense:	
Interest	170,314
Depreciation	176,907
Total capital expense	347,221
Total expense	2,208,630
Operating loss	(321,465)
Other Income:	
Interest	31,291
Houses	34,250
Contributions	206,509
Gain from sale of stock and property	97,214
Miscellaneous	13,439
Total other income	382,703
Net income for the year	61,238
Non-cash Items:	
Depreciation	176,907
Recognized revenue life care commitments	(347,351)
Cost adjustment life care commitments	92,736
Cash flow	$ (16,470)

Exhibit 3-10

RETIREMENT VILLAGE, INC.
NOTES TO FINANCIAL STATEMENTS
December 31, 1979

Accounting Principles - Life Care Commitments

Life Expectancy

1. 1958 Commissioner's Standard Ordinary Mortality Table, plus 15% for changes in life expectancy due to improved longevity at the Village (no differences have been reflected for males vs. females).

2. In residential apartments and cottages, the life expectancy is assumed to be spread 1/2 in residential and 1/2 in nursing center.

3. In nursing center the entire life expectancy is assumed to be in the nursing center.

Contractual Obligation

1. For residents, where the life expectancy commitment (unfunded liability) exceeds the unamortized prepaid entrance fee, the life expectancy calculation is used as the liability.

2. For residents, where the life expectancy commitment is less than the unamortized prepaid entrance fee, the unamortized entrance fee is used as the liability. This is necessary because most of the contracts provide for a payment by the residents only after their prepayment is fully amortized.

Contractual Arrangements

1. Most of the 300 plus contracts provide for some payment after the prepayment is fully amortized. If the resident is unable to pay, the Village is normally able to obtain Medicaid (Public Aid) funds to cover their commitment.

2. Some contracts call for a set monthly payment, after their prepayment is fully amortized. After the prepayment is fully amortized, a nominal monthly payment is received. This payment reduces the life expectancy commitment.

3. Where a resident qualifies for Medicaid, after their prepayment is fully amortized they are considered to be full pay. So the unfunded life care commitment for them is the unamortized prepayment.

4. Burial fees and medical expenses contractually assumed by the Village are ignored in the calculations.

# of Residents	Unfunded Life Care Commitment	1978	1979	Decrease in Commitment
141	Apartments & cottages	$1,881,981.32	$1,813,995.94	$ (67,985.38)
50	Wesley I	212,370.03	136,032.19	(76,337.84)
59	Wesley II	189,575.73	118,396.53	(71,179.20)
60	Dycus	97,189.91	58,077.37	(39,112.54)
10	Various residencies	41,293.50	41,293.50	-0-
320		$2,422,410.49	$2,167,795.53	$(254,614.96)

CHAPTER 4
Operating Budget

Business Failures

Business failures are often blamed on lack of capital or a poor ma*real* reason too often rests with faulty top management. The prime reasons for business failures are:

1. Faulty accounting records.
2. Management of finances by chance rather than by plan.
3. Failure to plan strategy.

FAULTY ACCOUNTING RECORDS

Inaccurate, late, or misleading accounting and production records can create crisis after crisis. Failure-prone business managers often compound their problems by hiring incompetent people, to save money, or by trying to keep the records themselves. Ironically failure-prone business managers short cut what will help them the most—good accounting records.

At a minimum these records should consist of:

- Cash expenditure record
- Payroll record
- Cash received record
- Billings record
- Purchases record
- Inventory record
- Depreciation record
- Insurance record
- Double entry set of books
- Accounts receivable record
- Accounts payable record

They should be maintained on a daily basis and summarized monthly for the preparation of the following reports:

1. *Balance sheet*—a summary of assets, liabilities, and capital.
2. *P/L statement*—a summary of revenues, expenses, and taxes.
3. *Cash flow statement*—a summary of cash in and cash out.

If you are not receiving the above information for every month by the fifteenth of the following month, you are not managing your resources; they are managing you.

MANAGEMENT OF FINANCES BY CHANCE RATHER THAN BY PLAN

Failure-prone business managers too often are lured into expansion and capital improvements in the hope that this will pick up the business. Meanwhile they become short of critically needed cash. Cash and cash alone pays bills and meets unexpected expenses.

It is important to keep adequate cash reserves at all times. How much can be determined by consulting your accountant and banker? If your cash reserves are low try the following:
- Move to more of a cash-only basis with customers or give discounts to those paying cash.
- Pay bills on time. Take advantage of discounts and do not fall into the habit of paying late. This indicates poor management.
- Collect past due accounts. Hire an independent collection agency if you cannot do it yourself.
- Learn to *plan* cash requirements six months in advance.

FAILURE TO PLAN STRATEGY

Failure-prone business managers tend to get so engrossed in the day-to-day operations they fail to think creatively about the future and plan their actions accordingly. Strategic planning means asking such critical questions as:
- What sort of business will mine be in two years?
- What are my competitors' biggest handicaps and how can I capitalize on them over the next two years?
- What shape is my industry in now and where will it be in two years?

A recent study of businesses actually using strategic planning indicated such planning does help the business manager to influence the future. The critical factors of successful planning are top management commitment, involvement of key subordinates in the creation of the plan, a timetable for attaining the goals established in the plan, and a willingness to revise the plan as reality sets in.

Peter Drucker, the renowned author and father of Management by Objectives, has been quoted as saying, "The responsibility of business managers is to avoid loss." The theory is that in the avoidance of failure the business will profit and attain success. This book is intended to help the business manager avoid failure. The reader must understand and work towards the achievement of the following objectives to avoid business failure:

1. To develop an understanding of the uses of accounting information.
2. To develop an understanding of how the accounting information is gathered.
3. To demonstrate how the accounting system can be used to control the business transactions.
4. To illustrate the basic accounting records needed by a nursing home.
5. To develop an understanding of the uses of budget information.
6. To develop an understanding of how budget information is gathered.
7. To demonstrate how the accounting information and budget information can be used to control the business enterprise.

The objectives are attainable for readers with a minimal amount of accounting training. However, it is not a bookkeeping course. It is assumed that bookkeepers, accountants, and public accountants will be resources available to the average nursing home.

The underlying objective is therefore the improvement of management awareness and capability through the use of accounting and budgeting. We encourage you to take advantage of this opportunity to better prepare yourself because "the difference between being a domino or an entrepreneur is in what you do and when you do it!"

Budgeting

DEFINITION OF BUDGETING

Budgeting is the planning of a course of action that encompasses all facets of the business enterprise. It is not simply "projecting" the current plan for next year. True planning means starting without preconceptions. It means not to be intimidated by what has happened in the past. It means ignoring the dictates and biases of previous plans and keeping an open mind with respect to alternative courses of action. Nothing is firm or sacred even after the alternatives are selected. It requires the planner to justify the plan—component by component—and to evaluate the alternatives for achieving the business' objectives in the most efficient and effective manner.

OBJECTIVES OF BUDGETING

Every element of the business must be viewed with a fresh look. Management can then analyze alternatives, make "tradeoffs," and set priorities in a systematic manner. This is the most effective decision-making method known to modern-day business. So, in essence, the objective of budgeting is to provide management with a fresh look at what is planned for the business for the next year. Then if alternatives (tradeoffs) are necessary they can be decided on intelligently. This is the decision-making process that weighs alternatives. As it becomes a part of management's procedures it becomes as indispensable as a flight plan is to a pilot. No sound decision can be made without it.

PURPOSE OF BUDGETING

At one time a budget of any kind was considered optional. It was only done if you had the time and the personnel available to do it. The problem was, who ever has the time until they make time? No one! And who ever has the people to do it? Everyone is busy with his present tasks. Just ask!

Well, the day has come when everyone must take the time and find the people to prepare the "flight plan" (realistic budgets) and follow it. Why now? Several factors now require that each facility take the budgeting task seriously. A budget is no longer a luxury, but a tool for survival. In a crisis, the quality of management procedures must improve. In today's volatile economy, those who do not carefully plan and keep their thumb on the pulse of their business transactions are lost. With costs increasing, as they have been, it becomes a day-to-day struggle to stay afloat.

A good budgeting system will provide management with current financial information and enable it to act on current conditions after weighing all possible alternatives. Some of these alternatives are:
- Should we raise prices?
- Should we borrow more capital?
- Can we cut costs?
- Should we change the quality of our service?
- Can we hold out under these conditions if none of the above alternatives are possible?
- Should we sell the business?

Questions like these are being asked daily in the nursing home industry. The facilities that have a flight plan are able to respond to them. They are able to look at current conditions, in relation to their plan, and alter their course. The facilities that do not have a flight plan fly in circles until they crash. The facility with good management can survive the crisis. The facility with a good budget has provided management with the instrument that will help them weather the storm.

Budgeting is a necessity to proper and adequate cost-related reimbursement from Medicaid and Medicare. With the enactment of the 1972 Social Security amendments (Public Law 92-603) the role of government control was expanded. It became evident that the biggest buyer (state and federal government) wants the highest quality of care at the lowest possible price. To accomplish this, regulations are slowly being implemented to encourage planning and budgeting. It is called prospective reimbursement. Eventually, this concept will replace the retrospective method now used by Medicare and most states in purchasing nursing home care.

To attain cost control, the system must include the following basic steps, at all levels:

1. List and rank operating objectives in order of importance. The steps should relate to the use of all available resources: capital, people, plant, equipment, and materials.
2. Examine the revenue and cost components in relation to the stated operating objectives.
3. Form "decision packages" consisting of the revenue and cost components of the various alternative courses of action. Rank them in order of acceptability.
4. Compare the results to be produced by each alternative course of action and select the "package" that is most compatible with the stated operating objectives.
5. Review the "tradeoffs" (alternatives) with top management and get their approval.
6. Execute the plan and watch it very carefully.

HOW A BUDGET PLAN IS PREPARED

An effective budget is a collection of the carefully conceived financial plans for all departments. The basic steps are:

1. *Establish goals and objectives* for the facility and for each department. To have impact the budget must be able to guide the behavior of the organization. An operating philosophy must be adopted by the owners, the administrator, and the staff before the budget can be prepared. Formulating an operating philosophy is primarily the function of the owners and the administrator. The operating philosophy must be communicated in writing to the entire staff or the budget exercise will not be totally effective.
2. *Prepare budget package plan* to establish individual responsibilities. It is a plan that must be supplemented by organization charts, information gathering procedures, and forms. Usually the system exists in an established facility. If not, it must be set up. Then management must establish a timetable for preparation of the budget and designate the period of time to be covered by the budget. This is basically called getting organized. The budget (decision package) to be constructed by each department should include alternative courses of action if there is any question on the direction that department will be taking. It is then management's responsibility to select the acceptable alternative.
3. *Prepare a staffing plan* by department for all personnel.
4. *Forecast production units* by department.
5. *Budget departmental operating costs* by general ledger expense categories and perform cost accounting.
6. *Determine profit margin* and return on investment.
7. *Determine prices* including profit mark-up.
8. *Budget revenues* by type of service based on forecasted production units and price per unit of service.
9. *Determine contractual discounts* (Medicare and Medicaid loss) using budget revenues and operating costs.
10. *Develop reports* that compare budget to actual financial data. To accomplish this, realistic and controllable goals are set in the budget for each department. Responsibility reports are the key to financial control; they advise a department head how well the department is doing in relation to its goals.
11. *Compare actual results to budgeted amounts* and explain variations. In responsibility reporting, current operating revenues and expenses are reported and compared with the budgeted amounts by department. The difference between them, or variance, is also reported. If actual performance improves on the budget (i.e., higher revenues or lower cost), the variance is called a favorable variance. If actual results are lower than the budgeted amounts (i.e., lower revenues or higher costs), the variance is termed unfavorable. For detailed information on the analysis of variances you should inquire about the training materials on standard costing.
12. *Take prompt action on variances,* which are signals for action. Each department head must determine the cause of the variance he or she is responsible

for and decide on appropriate action. That action must be directed towards influencing the department's activities in the future. Timely reporting makes prompt action possible and can prevent further setbacks.

13. *Revise the budget,* if necessary, in light of the variances. If the forecasts were too optimistic or unforeseen changes occur, the budget should be revised to establish more realistic goals.

In summary, preparation of a budget can be reduced to its simplest elements by remembering the italicized words used in the preceding list:

- Establish goals and objectives
- Prepare budget package plan
- Prepare a staffing plan
- Forecast production units
- Budget departmental operating costs
- Determine profit margin
- Determine prices
- Budget revenues
- Determine contractual discounts
- Develop reports
- Compare actual results to budgeted amounts
- Take prompt action on variances
- Revise the budget

HOW A BUDGET IS CONTROLLED

The control of the business operation is the primary purpose of budgeting. If the budget plan is to be used properly the business operation must be organized so responsibilities are assigned to the people in a chain of command (pecking order). It is like the military; you tell the troops in the trenches what their job is, train them to do it, check to see if they are doing it, then reward them for doing it or replace them if they do not. Somewhere in the process discipline must be established. You will find that a good organization has some form of discipline in its pecking order. See Exhibit 4-1 for a simplified example of an organization chart.

The organization chart is very much like the line-up of a baseball team. Each team member is given a position based on demonstrated talents and with that position go certain duties. They keep their position in the line-up only if they perform. See Exhibit 4-2 for an example of how the general responsibilities of preparing a budget are doled out.

As you can see from the line-up, each team member must fill his position adequately to enable administration to construct the budget package for the Board of Directors' approval. Once done in this manner, the budget becomes "everyone's" budget because the team participated in putting it together. This is the essence of participative management and responsibility accountability—involving

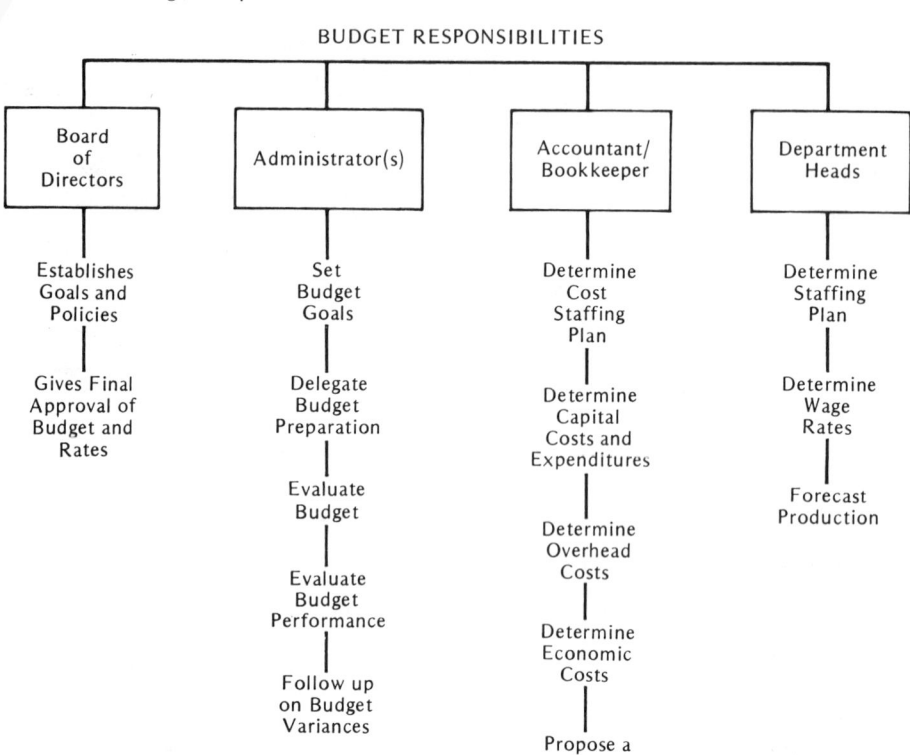

Exhibit 4-2 Budget Responsibilities

BUDGET RESPONSIBILITIES

Board of Directors	Administrator(s)	Accountant/ Bookkeeper	Department Heads
Establishes Goals and Policies	Set Budget Goals	Determine Cost Staffing Plan	Determine Staffing Plan
Gives Final Approval of Budget and Rates	Delegate Budget Preparation	Determine Capital Costs and Expenditures	Determine Wage Rates
	Evaluate Budget	Determine Overhead Costs	Forecast Production
	Evaluate Budget Performance	Determine Economic Costs	
	Follow up on Budget Variances	Propose a Rate Structure Using Budgeted Costs	

positions is the first step in a good *written* game plan. The only way to know the positions is to define them in writing so there is no doubt in anyone's mind about what is required to get the job done.

The following work program and assignment of responsibilities will cover the organization chart for:

- Board of Directors
- Administrators
- Accounting
- Department Heads

Annual Operating Budget

THE BOARD OF DIRECTORS' WORK PROGRAM

The objective of the work program is to construct a budget for the next operating cycle (fiscal year), then use it for controlling the actual operations. To achieve this objective, use the following procedures:

1. Create a written expression of operating goals in order of importance. The goals should relate to the use of all available resources: capital, people, plant, equipment, and materials.
2. Review the budgeted revenue and cost components in relation to the stated operating goals.
3. Review "decision packages" consisting of the budgeted revenue and cost components of the various alternative courses of action. Rank them in order of acceptability. (In many cases there may be only one obvious course of action and only one obvious decision possible. The thought that goes into this type of decision should be the same as would go into one with multiple alternatives because it is the review of the obvious that promotes new ideas.)
4. Compare the results to be produced by each alternative course of action and select the package that is most compatible with the stated operating goals.
5. Review the tradeoffs (alternatives) and make the decision on courses of action and communicate the decisions to administration.
6. Review the execution of the budget plan monthly and determine if the plan needs revision or if alternative decisions must be made.

THE ADMINISTRATOR'S WORK PROGRAM

The objective of the operating budget work program is to gather information regarding the expected results of operations for the coming fiscal year. The estimates of staffing levels, patient load (production), and controllable expenses will become the guidelines to the department heads for the next fiscal year.

To achieve this objective, use these general procedures:
1. Create a written expression of each department's staffing, production, and operating plans for next fiscal year.
2. Attribute costs to the written plans.
3. Evaluate the results to be attained from the written plans.
4. Resubmit to department heads for revision, if necessary.
5. Submit the final budget package to the board of directors for approval.
6. Execute the plan and watch it very carefully.

The following table lists specific procedures:

Procedure	Target Date	Responsible Person
1. Develop a budget package (forms, goals, etc.) and meet with accounting and department heads to answer questions and set target dates.		Administrators

Procedure	Target Date	Responsible Person
2. Accumulate controllable costs individually for nursing, ancillary, and standard services, including: 　Staffing plan by month 　Wage rates for each position 　Total supplies required 　new equipment required and when required		Dept. Heads
3. Accumulate semifixed expenses for: 　Utilities 　Insurance 　Fringe Benefits 　Consulting fees 　Administration		Accounting
4. Accumulate fixed expenses for: 　Depreciation or rent 　Interest 　Real estate taxes 　Other taxes		Accounting
5. Assemble budgeted operating costs by department. Revise if information is not realistic.		Accounting
6. Group costs by department for cost finding. The support service (overhead) departments should be allocated (assigned) to the nursing and ancillary (production) departments.		Accounting
7. Determine the amount of cost Medicare and Medicaid will pay and the amount they will not pay. This represents the contracual discount (loss) incurred in dealing with cost reimbursers.		Accounting
8. Determine the amount of profit required to meet the Board of Directors' operating goals.		Administration
9. Establish a pricing structure that will produce revenue adequate to meet the budgeted operating costs plus an adequate profit margin, at the expected level of production (patient load).		Accounting
10. Calculate the estimated cash flow that will result using the budgeted operating results. The payment of budgeted revenues and expenses must be determined from past experience. Also the amount of expenditures for inventory and equipment must be included.		Accounting
11. Submit budget package to the Board of Directors for review. If alternative courses of action are proposed for the board's decision they should be shown as alternative budgets.		Administrator
12. Revise budget if the board needs clarification for its decisions.		Administrator
13. After the budget is approved each department head should be advised of the decisions for their department. They should also be reminded of their responsibilities and how they will be reviewed and rewarded.		Administrator

14. Send monthly budget report to department head showing actual figures compared to budget for: Accounting
   Staffing hours
   Salary costs by job classification
   Wage rates
   Supply costs
15. Review departmental responses to budget variances. Follow up necessary decisions.   Administrator
16. Review the monthly accounting reports of actual production for each department. The reports should cover: Administrator

Production	Cost/Income
Census	Total costs per day
Staff hours	Variable costs per day
Therapy hours	Revenue per patient-day
Prescriptions	Net income per patient-day

17. Review monthly accounting report of actual revenue, semifixed, and fixed expenses in total compared to budget.   Administrator
18. Advise board on progress towards operating goals by presenting them with a monthly management summary on production and cost and income analysis.   Accounting to prepare Administrator to prepare

Nursing Services Budget

DIRECTOR OF NURSING RESPONSIBILITY PROGRAM

The objective of the nursing services responsibility program is to gather information on estimated patient load, staffing plan, wage rates, and supply and equipment needs for the next fiscal year.

To accomplish this objective, these general procedures should be followed:

1. Assemble production information on patient days and staffing hours by patient care areas for the next year.
2. Determine wage rates to be paid each job classification for the next fiscal year.
3. Determine total medical supply and drug expense for the next fiscal year.
4. Determine the needs for new or replacement equipment for the next fiscal year.
5. Submit budget package to administrator for approval.
6. Execute the plan and watch it very carefully.
   See the following table for procedures that apply to each nursing station.

	Target	Responsible
Procedure	Date	Person
1. Summarize patient statistics by month for prior three years (patient days by level of care and by private, Medicare, Medicaid, and other category and nursing hours).		Dept. Head
2. Forecast monthly patient levels for the next fiscal year, in terms of historical statistics.		D.O.N.
3. Forecast staff hours by month based on expected patient load.		D.O.N.
4. Present productivity levels to department heads for their review.		D.O.N.
5. Calculate salary costs at the monthly productivity levels using staff hours and wage rates by job classification.		D.O.N.
6. Calculate supply and drug costs based on patient load levels.		D.O.N.
7. Present calculations to department heads for their review.		D.O.N.
8. Consolidate all nursing stations.		D.O.N.
9. Finalize the budget package and submit it to administration for approval.		D.O.N.
10. Compare monthly actual performance to budget for: Staffing hours Salary costs by job classification Wage rates Supply costs		D.O.N. and Dept. Heads
11. Respond to budget variances. Follow up on necessary actions		

Ancillary Services Budget

ASSISTANT ADMINISTRATOR RESPONSIBILITY PROGRAM

The objective of the ancillary services responsibility program is to gather information on estimated volume by department, staffing, wage rates, and supply and equipment needs for the next fiscal year.

To achieve this objective, these general procedures should be followed:

1. Assemble production information on physical therapy hours, rehabilitative procedures, prescriptions filled, and staffing hours for the next fiscal year.
2. Determine wage rates to be paid each job classification for the next fiscal year.
3. Determine the needs for supplies and new or replacement equipment for the next fiscal year.
4. Submit budget package to administrator for approval.
5. Execute the plan and watch it very carefully.

See the following table for procedures that apply to each ancillary department.

Procedure	Target Date	Responsible Person
1. Summarize usage statistics for prior three years.		Dept. Head
2. Forecast monthly usage statistics		Dept. Head
3. Forecast staff hours by month based on expected usage statistics.		Dept. Head
4. Calculate costs at the monthly productivity levels sing staff hours and wage rates by job classification.		Dept. Head
5. Calculate supply costs.		Dept. Head
6. Finalize the budget package and submit it to administration for approval.		Dept. Head
7. Compare monthly actual performance to budget for: Staffing hours Salary costs by job classification Wage rates Supply costs		Dept. Head
8. Respond to budget variances. Follow up on necessary actions.		Dept. Head

Support Services Budget

ASSISTANT ADMINISTRATOR RESPONSIBILITY PROGRAM

The objective of the support services (overhead) responsibility program is to gather information on estimated staffing hours, wage rates, and supply and equipment needs for the next fiscal year.

Follow these general procedures:
1. Assemble staffing hours for the fiscal year for:
    Housekeeping
    Maintenance
    Dietary
    Laundry
    Medical records
2. Determine wage rates to be paid each job classification for the next fiscal year.
3. Determine the needs for supplies and new or replacement equipment for the next fiscal year.
4. Submit budget package to administration for approval.
5. Execute the plan and watch it very carefully.

See the following table for specific procedures that apply to each overhead department:

Procedure	Target Date	Responsible Person
1. Forecast staff hours by month based on expected staffing plan.		Dept. Head
2. Calculate costs of the monthly staffing plan using expected wage rates by job classification.		Dept. Head
3. Calculate supply costs.		Dept. Head
4. Finalize the budget package and submit it to administration for approval.		Dept. Head
5. Compare monthly actual performance to budget for: Staffing hours Salary costs by job classification Wage rates Supply costs		Dept. Head
6. Respond to budget variances. Follow up on necessary actions.		

Administrative Budget

ACCOUNTING DEPARTMENT'S RESPONSIBILITY PROGRAM

The objective of the accounting department's responsibility program is to gather the budget packages from all departments and assemble the semifixed and fixed expenses (uncontrollables) portion of the budget.

The following procedures are used:

Procedure	Target Date	Responsible Person
1. Assemble the estimate of the uncontrollable expenses for the next fiscal year based on historical experience for: Utilities Insurance Fringe Benefits Consulting fees Administration Capital costs (interest and depreciation/rent) Real estate taxes Sales taxes Income taxes		Accounting
2. Submit budget packages to administrator for approval in the following segments: *Controllables* *Uncontrollables* Staffing Plant and capital costs Wage rates Taxes Supplies Administration		Accounting

3. Prepare monthly budget reports comparing actual controllable expenses to budget by responsibility department. — Accounting

4. Follow up on budget variances on noncontrollable expenses, if necessary.

COST FINDING AND RATE SETTING WORK PROGRAM

The objective of the cost finding and rate setting work program is to assign overhead costs to the nursing and ancillary services departments so costs per patient day and per production unit can be determined. After the costs per unit are known a mark-up can be applied and prices set for the next fiscal year.

The following procedures are used:

Procedure	Target Date	Responsible Person
1. List all budgeted operating costs by department. Assign the following expenses to room and board, nursing, or ancillary departments (using a simple step-down cost accounting method): Housekeeping—work hours; Maintenance—work hours; Dietary—patient and employee meals; Laundry—pounds; Depreciation/rent—square footage; Real estate taxes—square footage; Insurance—square footage; Administration—total direct expense		Accounting
2. Determine budgeted costs per patient day for room and board and nursing, and per production unit for ancillaries.		Accounting
3. Add a percentage factor for Medicare and Medicaid discounts and bad debts.		Accounting
4. Add a mark-up for profit using a return on investment formula applied to the current value of the equity and debt capital.		Accounting
5. Establish prices for nursing services and ancillary services adequate to meet operating goals and estimated productivity.		Accounting
6. Submit to administrator for approval.		Accounting
7. Revise, if necessary. Then determine cash flow that would result from the budgeted expenses and revenues.		Accounting
8. Advise administrator of the cash position that can be expected.		Accounting
9. Revise until cash flow is at an acceptable level.		Accounting
10. Prepare a monthly cash flow report comparing actual cash position with budgeted cash position and follow up accordingly.		

Sample Annual Operating Budget

Schedule 1
Nursing Center, Inc.
Consolidated Net Profit Goals
For Year Ended November 30, 1978

Basis of Net Profit Goals
1. Quality service.
2. Debt coverage— two times as much profit as the principal and interest payment.
3. Reasonable prices.
4. Funding of book depreciation and accumulation of capital to cover economic costs.
5. Return on investment (debt and equity) of 20% before capital costs and income taxes.

Debt Coverage
   Mortgage Payments (building corporation)

First Federal	$ 2,356	
City Bank	2,356	
State Bank	842	
	$ 5,558	
Number of payments	12	
	$ 66,709	
Debt coverage factor	2	
Debt coverage—profit	$133,418	
Rounded		$134,000
Building Corp. Budgeted Profit		
Rent from operating company	$140,500	
Interest	$ 36,000	
Depreciation	30,000	
Insurance	12,000	
Property taxes	24,000	
Directors	6,000	
Salaries	15,000	
Misc.	4,000	
	$127,000	
Net profit before income taxes	$ 13,500	
Add back interest expense	36,000	
Net profit excluding interest	$ 49,500	49,500
Net profit goal for operating company		$ 84,500

Schedule 1 (cont.)
Nursing Center, Inc.
Consolidated Net Profit Goals

Funding of Depreciation and Capital Costs (Return *of* investment)

Book depreciation		$ 30,000
Plant cost	$ 687,600	

Equipment cost	87,600	
	$ 775,200	
Inflation factor (10 years at 6% per year)	160%	
Current value	$1,240,300	
Depreciation rate	3.5%	43,400
Profit needed to cover economic depreciation costs		$ 13,400
Book interest		$ 36,000
Current value of investment	$1,240,300	
Return on asset rate	10%	124,000
Profit needed to cover economic capital costs		$ 88,000
Economic costs		
Depreciation		$ 13,400
Capital		88,000
Profit needed to reach economic breakeven		$101,400
Return on Investment		
Total capital investment		$775,200
Rate of return		20%
		$155,000
Less book costs for—		
Depreciation	$ 30,000	
Interest	36,000	66,000
Profit needed to generate a 20% ROI		$ 89,000

Schedule 1 (cont.)
Nursing Center, Inc.
Consolidated Net Profit Goals

Net Profit Goal (criteria for decision)	
Alternative 1	
Debt coverage requirement	$134,000
Alternative 2	
Economic breakeven requirement	$101,400
Return on investment requirement	89,000
	$190,400
	$324,400
Average of two	$162,200
Building corporation	49,500
Profit goal operating company	$112,700
Per patient day at 39,785 forecasted days	$ 2.83
Realistic profit per patient day at 94% occupancy rate	$ 2.40

Conclusion

Based on the two profit goal alternatives the final decision is to attempt to establish a pricing structure that will produce a profit, before income taxes, of $95,000 (39,785 × $2.40 per patient day) for the operating company. If this is not possible, the decision must be made as to what level of profitability is attainable and if it is acceptable.

Schedule 2
Nursing Center, Inc.
Forecast of Volume Based on
Historical Experience

Nine Months Actual Patient Load (274 Days)

Level of Care	Private	Welfare	Medicare	Total	Average Occupied Beds
Intermediate	7,181	5,204	—	12,385	45
Skilled					
200 wing	4,592	2,227	1,080	7,899	28
100–300 wings	6,887	3,341	—	10,228	38
Nine month totals	18,660	10,772	1,080	30,512	111.4
Nine month	÷274	÷274	÷274	÷274	
Annualized	24,880	14,362	1,440	40,682	111.4
Average Patients	68	39	3.9	111.4	
Budget	66	38	5	109	

Budgeted Patient Days for Year Ended November 30, 1978

	Total Licensed Beds	Assumed Occupied Beds	Occupancy Rate	Budgeted Patient Days (1)	%
ICF	46	44	95.6%	16,060	40.4%
SNF					
200 wing	28	26	92.8	9.490	23.8
100–300 wings	42	39	92.8	14,235	35.8
	116	109	94.0	39,785	100.0%
Private		66		24,090	
Public Welfare		38		13,870	
Medicare		5		1,825	
		109		39,785	

(1) Assumed occupied beds times 365 days in year

Schedule 3
Nursing Center, Inc.
Budgeted Staffing Costs—Aides
ICF Building (46 Beds—44 Average Occupied Beds)

Description	Total Staff	Clock Time	Hours Per Day	Total Hours
Days	1	7 AM–3 PM	8	8
	1	7 AM–12:30 PM	5	5
Afternoons	1	3 PM–11 PM	8	8
Nights	1	11 PM–7 AM	8	8
	Aide hours per day			29
	Number of days in year			×365
	Total aide hours			10,585

Expected average wage rate	$ 3.00
Total salary cost	$31,775
Rounded	$32,000
Average wage rate for aides	
Average rate per last payroll	$ 2.62
Increase	
Minimum wage (including ripple effect)	.38
Expected average wage rate	$ 3.00

Schedule 3 (cont.)
Nursing Center, Inc.
Budgeted Staffing Costs—Aides
SNF-ICF 100–300 Wings (42 Beds—39 Average Occupied Beds)

Description	Total Staff	Clock Time	Hours Per Day	Total Hours
Days	2	7 AM–3 PM	8	16
	3	7 AM–12 PM	5	15
Afternoons	2	3 PM–11 PM	8	16
	2	3 PM–8:30 PM	5	10
Nights	2	11 PM–7 AM	8	16
	Aide hours per day			73
Rehab. Aide	1	7 PM–3 PM	8	8
	Total aide hours per day			31
	Number of days in year			×365
	Total aide hours			25,915
	Expected average wage rate			$ 3.00
	Total salary cost			$77,745
	Rounded			$78,000

Schedule 3 (cont.)
Nursing Center, Inc.
Budgeted Staffing Costs—Aides
SNF 200 Wing (28 Beds—26 Average Occupied Beds)

Description	Total Staff	Clock Time	Hours Per Day	Total Hours
Days	2	7 AM–3 PM	8	16
	2	7 AM–12:30 PM	5	10
Afternoons	2	3 PM–11 PM	8	16
	1	3 PM–8:30 PM	5	5
Nights	1	11 PM–7 AM	8	8
Ward Clerk	1	8 AM–5 PM	8	8
	Aide hours per day			63
	Number of days in year			×365
	Total aide hours			25,915
	Expected average wage rate			$ 3.00
	Total salary cost			$77,745
	Rounded			$78,000

Schedule 3 (cont.)
Nursing Center, Inc.
Budgeted Staffing Costs—Licensed Personnel
ICF Building (46 Beds—44 Average Occupied Beds)

Description	Total Staff	Clock Time	Hours Per Day	Total Hours	Annual Hours
LPN Days	1	7 AM–3 PM	3*	3	1,095
LPN Afternoons	1	3 PM–11 PM	3*	3	1,095
LPN Nights	1	11 PM–7 AM	1*	1	365
		Licensed hours per day		7	
		Number of days in year		×365	
		Total licensed hours		2,555	2,555
		Expected average wage rate		$ 4.50	
		Total salary cost		$11,497	
		Rounded		$11,500	

*Floating staff time between ICF and SNF

Schedule 3 (cont.)
Nursing Center, Inc.
Budgeted Staffing Costs—Licensed Personnel
SNF-ICF 100–300 Wings (42 Beds—39 Average Occupied Beds)

Description	Total Staff	Clock Time	Hours Per Day	Total Hours	Annual Hours
LPN Days	1	7 AM–3 PM	5*	5	1,825
LPN Afternoons	1	3 PM–11 PM	5*	5	1,825
LPN Nights	1	11 PM–7 AM	3*	3	1,095
		Licensed hours per day		13	
		Number of days in year		×365	
		Total licensed hours		4,745	4,745
		Expected average wage rate		$ 4.50	
		Total salary cost		$21,352	
		Rounded		$21,500	

*Floating staff time between ICF and SNF

Schedule 3 (cont.)
Nursing Center, Inc.
Budgeted Staffing Costs—Licensed Personnel
SNF 200 Wing (28 Beds—26 Average Occupied Beds)

Description	Total Staff	Clock Time	Hours Per Day	Total Hours	Annual Hours
RN Days	1	7 AM–3 PM	8	8	2,920
RN Afternoons	1	3 PM–11 PM	8	8	2,920
					5,840
RN Nights	1	11 PM–7 AM	4*	4	1,460

109 Operating Budget

```
Licensed hours per day          20
Number of days in year        ×365
Total licensed hours          7,300      7,300
```

Classification	Salary Cost Present Rate	Raise Minimum	Merit	Budget	Total Cost	Rounded
RNs	$4.62	$.35	$.53	$5.50	$32,120	$32,200
LPNs	$3.74	$.35	$.41	$4.50	6,570	7,000
						$39,200

*½ time spent in 200 wing, ½ in ICF wings

Schedule 3 (cont.)
STAFFING PLAN SUPPORT SERVICES

DIETARY EMPLOYEES

Employees Dietary	Date Employed	Wages for December 1977	Hourly Increase	Wages for January 1978	Staff Hours	Budgeted Amount
Dietitian	5-4-67	$3.50	$.50	$4.00	1,950	$ 7,800
Head Cook	3-10-71	2.50	.25	2.75	1,950	5,362
Head Cook	9-16-75	2.30	.45	2.75	1,950	5,362
Cook's Helper	8-16-77	2.30	.35	2.65	1,950	5,168
Cook's Helper	11-14-77	2.30	.35	2.65	1,950	5,168
Asst. Dietitian	5-13-76	2.30	.45	2.75	1,950	5,168
Dishwasher	7-8-77	2.30	.35	2.65	1,950	5,168
Dishwasher	2-14-72	2.40	.35	2.75	1,950	5,362
Dishwasher	1-17-76	2.40	.35	2.75	1,950	5,362
Tray Girl	11-23-77	2.30	.35	2.65	1,950	5,168
Tray Girl	7-6-77	2.30	.35	2.65	1,950	5,168
					21,450	$60,256
Part-time Helpers	Various	2.30	.35	2.65	3,676	9,744
					25,126	$70,000

HOUSEKEEPING AND LAUNDRY EMPLOYEES

Employees Housekeeping						
Supervisor	6-5-68	$2.75	$.25	$3.00	2,080	$ 6,240
Housekeeper	11-21-77	2.30	.35	2.65	500	1,325
Housekeeper	4-10-75	2.40	.35	2.75	1,040	2,860
Housekeeper	1-13-76	2.30	.40	2.70	500	1,350
Housekeeper	10-22-74	2.50	.25	2.75	1,040	2,860
Housekeeper	9-8-77	2.30	.35	2.65	500	1,325
Housekeeper	8-23-76	2.30	.40	2.70	2,080	5,616
Housekeeper,	5-17-76	2.30	.40	2.70	—	—
Fill In	8-19-77	2.30	.35	2.65	159	424
					7,899	$22,000

HOUSEKEEPING AND LAUNDRY EMPLOYEES

Employees Laundry	Date Employed	Wages for December 1977	Hourly Increase	Wages for January 1978	Staff Hours	Budgeted Amount
Supervisor	10-8-73	$2.30	$.45	$2.75	1,950	$ 5,300
Laundry Helper	11-15-77	2.30	.35	2.65	500	1,300
Laundry Helper	4-10-77	2.30	.45	2.75	830	2,200
Laundry Helper	3-7-75	2.30	.45	2.65	1,200	3,200
					4,480	$12,000

MAINTENANCE EMPLOYEES

Supervisor	10-8-71	$3.50	$.25	$3.75	1,950	$ 7,300
Helper	10-1-77	2.65	—	2.65	1,018	2,700
					2,968	$10,000

ACTIVITIES EMPLOYEES

Director	8-3-69	$3.50	$.25	$3.75	1,950	$ 7,300
2 Assistants	Various	2.65	—	2.65	3,283	8,700
					5,233	$16,000

Schedule 4
Nursing Center, Inc.
Nursing Hours Per Patient Day

Area	Budgeted Patient Days	RNs	LPNs	Aides	Total	Budgeted Nursing Hours Per Day
SNF 200 wing	9,490	5,840	1,460	25,915	33,215	3.50
SNF-ICF 100–300 wings	14,235	—	4,745	29,565	34,310	2.41
ICF building	16,060	—	2,555	10,585	13,140	.82
	39,785	5,840	8,760	66,065	80,665	2.03
Director of nursing					2,080	.05
Total nursing hours					82,745	2.08
Total salary cost					$282,700	
Average cost per hour					$3.42	

Notes
1. Weekends covered by a regular aide around the clock in place of two rehab. aides.
2. Training hours and sick time hours are offset by cushion in aide hours.

Schedule 5
Nursing Center, Inc.
Budgeted Operating Costs
And Capital Costs

	9 Months Ended	12 Months Projected	Projection Inflation	Projection Other	Budgeted Costs	Per Patient Day
Administrative						
Salary	$ 15,767	$ 21,000	$ 1,100	$ —	$ 22,100	
Office salaries	18,238	24,300	2,800	—	27,100	
Office supplies	1,469	2,000	200	—	2,200	
Nursing admin.	—	—	—	Reclas. 11,050	11,050	
Travel	4,328	5,800	—	(3,400)	2,400	
Advertising/PR	4,281	5,700	—	(3,900)	1,800	
Licenses & dues	2,796	3,700	—	—	3,700	
Professional services	6,284	8,400	—	(400)	3,000	
Unemployment comp.	9,619	12,800	2,500	—	15,300	
Social Security taxes	19,376	25,800	2,000	—	27,800	
Insurance/group	5,383	7,200	—	(2,200)	5,000	
Sales taxes	3,668	4,900	200	—	5,100	
Misc.	299	400	100	—	500	
	$ 95,578	$122,000	$ 8,900	$ 1,150	$132,050	$3.32
Property (Capital costs)						
Interest	$ 291	$ 400	$ —	$ (100)	$ 300	
Rent—Bldg.	105,381	140,500	—	—	140,400	
Rent—Equip.	5,218	7,000	—	(2,400)	4,600	
Depreciation	4,650	6,200	—	—	6,200	
Dep.—Bldg. Imp.	513	700	—	—	700	
	$116,053	$154,800	$ —	$(2,500)	$152,300	3.83

Schedule 5 (cont.)
Nursing Center, Inc.
Budgeted Operating Costs and Capital Costs

	9 Months Ended	12 Months Projected	Projection Inflation	Projection Other	Budgeted Costs	Per Patient Day
Plant Operations						
Salaries	$ 6,786	$ 9,000	$ 1,000	—	$ 10,000	
Utilities—Elec.	14,045	18,700	1,500	—	20,200	
—Gas	8,211	10,900	900	—	11,800	
—Water	2,107	2,800	200	—	3,000	
Purchased services	2,224	2,900	200	—	3,100	
Repairs	9,225	12,300	—	—	12,300	
Supplies	894	1,200	100	—	1,300	
	$43,492	$57,800	$3,900	—	$61,700	1.55
Dietary						
Salaries	$49,247	$65,700	$4,300	—	$ 70,000	
Food	58,445	77,900	6,200	—	84,100	
Supplies	3,884	5,200	400	—	5,600	
	$111,576	$148,800	$10,900	—	$159,700	$ 4.01
Laundry						
Salaries	$ 8,333	$11,100	$ 900	—	$ 12,000	
Linen	1,409	1,900	100	—	2,000	
Supplies	1,634	2,200	100	—	2,300	
	$11,376	$15,200	$1,100	—	$ 16,300	.41
Housekeeping						
Salaries	$15,944	$21,300	$ 700	—	$ 22,000	
Supplies	2,352	3,100	200	—	3,300	
	$18,296	$24,400	$ 900	—	$ 25,300	.64

Pharmacy					
Salaries	$ 7,337	$ 9,800	$ 200	—	$ 10,000	
Medical supplies	8,369	11,200	900	—	12,100	
Drugs	22,545	30,100	2,400	—	32,500	
	$ 38,251	$ 51,100	$ 3,500	—	$ 54,600	1.37
Recreation						
Salaries	$ 11,811	$ 15,700	$ 300	—	$ 16,000	
Consultant	891	1,200	—	—	1,200	
Supplies	1,913	2,500	200	—	2,700	
Travel	103	100	—	—	100	
	$ 14,718	$ 19,500	$ 500	—	$ 20,000	.50
Physical Therapy						
Salaries	$ 9,785	$ 13,000	—	Reclas. $(10,100)	$ 2,900	
Lab	$ 848	$ 1,100	$ 100	$ —	$ 1,200	
Beauty/Barber Shop	5,519	7,400	200	—	7,600	
In-service—Salaries	5,857	7,800	—	Reclas. (7,800)	—	
—Misc.	809	1,100	—	Reclas. (1,100)	—	
Physician Services	270	400	—	—	400	
Medical Director	1,150	1,500	—	—	1,500	
U R Committee	700	900	100	—	1,000	
	$ 15,153	$ 20,200	$ 400	$ (8,900)	$ 11,700	$ .29
Nursing Costs—Schedule 6	474,278	$626,800	$30,100	$(20,350)	$636,550	$15.99
	175,004	233,300	29,050	20,350	282,700	7.11
	$649,282	$860,100	$59,150	—	$919,250	$23.10
Patient Days					39,785	
Average Cost Per Patient Day					$23.10	

Schedule 6
Nursing Center, Inc.
Budgeted Operating Costs by Level of Care

	Nursing Hours Per Day	Total Budgeted Hours	ICF Building	SNF 200 Wing	SNF 100–300 Wings	Total	Per Patient Day	Salary Cost Per Hour
Nursing Costs								
Aides	1.70	66,065	$ 32,000	$ 78,000	$ 89,000	$199,000	$ 5.01	$3.00
LPNs	.22	8,760	11,500	7,000	21,500	40,000	1.01	4.57
RNs	.15	5,840	—	32,200	—	32,200	.81	5.51
Totals	2.07	80,665	$ 43,500	$117,200	$110,500	$271,200	$ 6.82	$3.36
D.O.N.		2,080	4,400	2,800	4,300	11,500	.29	5.75
Nursing Costs		82,745	$ 47,900	$120,000	$114,800	$282,700	$ 7.11	$3.42
Support Service Costs (1)								
Plant Operations			$ 24,927	$ 14,685	$ 22,088	$ 61,700	$ 1.55	
Dietary			64,519	38,009	57,172	159,700	4.01	
Laundry			6,585	3,879	5,836	16,300	.41	
Housekeeping			10,221	6,021	9,058	25,300	.64	
Recreation			8,080	4,760	7,160	20,000	.50	
Medical Director			606	357	537	1,500	.03	
U R Committee			404	238	358	1,000	.03	
Support Costs			$115,342	$ 67,949	$102,209	$285,500	$ 7.17	
Administration (1)			$ 53,348	$ 31,428	$ 47,274	$132,050	$ 3.32	
Capital Costs (1)			$ 61,530	$ 36,247	$ 54,523	$152,300	$ 3.83	
Operating Costs			$278,120	$255,624	$318,806	$852,550	$21.43	
Patient Days			16,060	9,490	14,235	39,785		
Per Patient Day			$ 17.36	$ 26.94	$ 22.40	$ 21.43		

Ancillary Services
Pharmacy $ 54,600
Physical Therapy 2,900
Barber and Beauty 7,600
Lab 1,200
Physician Services 400
Ancillary Costs $ 66,700

(1) Detail of cost finding is on the second part of this schedule.

Schedule 6 (cont.)
Nursing Center, Inc.
Budgeted Operating Costs by Level of Care Cost Finding

Allocation Basis						SNF	
Patient Days	Percent	Cost Center	Total Budgeted Cost	ICF Building	200 Wing	100–300 Wings	
16,060	40.4	Plant Operations	$ 61,700	$ 24,927	$14,685	$ 22,088	
9,490	23.8						
14,235	35.8	Dietary	159,700	64,519	38,009	57,172	
29,785	100.0	Laundry	16,300	6,585	3,879	5,836	
		Housekeeping	25,300	10,221	6,021	9,058	
		Recreation	20,000	8,080	4,760	7,160	
		Medical Director	1,500	606	357	537	
		U R Committee	1,000	404	238	358	
		Total Support Costs	$285,500	$115,342	$67,949	$102,209	
		Administration	$132,050	$ 53,348	$31,428	$ 47,274	
		Capital Costs	$152,300	$ 61,530	$36,247	$ 54,523	
		Director of Nursing	$ 11,500	$ 4,400	$ 2,800	$ 4,300	

Schedule 7
Nursing Center, Inc.
Budgeted Revenues According to Goals

Payer	Budgeted Patient Days	Cost Rate	Private Rate (1)	Projected Revenue	Rounded
Medicare	1,825	$26.94		$ 49,200	$ 49,000
Medicaid					
ICF	6,658	$17.36		115,583	115,000
SNF	7,212	$22.40		161,549	161,500
	13,870			$ 326,332	$ 326,000
Private					
ICF	9,402		$20.00	$ 188,040	$ 188,000
SNF	14,688		$28.50	418,608	417,000
	24,090			$ 606,648	$ 605,000
Ancillaries				$ 84,000	$ 84,000
Total Revenue				$1,016,980	$1,015,000
Total Operating Cost					920,000
Profit Goal	39,785				$ 95,000

Schedule 7 (cont.)
Nursing Center, Inc.
Budgeted Revenues According to Goals

						Budget	
Private Rates (2)	Days	Cost Per Day	Total Cost	Mark-up	Total Revenue	Price Per Day	Rounded
ICF	9,402	$17.36	$163,200	$24,000	$187,200	$19.91	$20.00
SNF	14,688	24.79	364,100	53,700	417,800	28.44	28.50
	24,090		$527,300	$77,700	$605,000		
				14.7%			
		14.7%	77,700				
			$605,000				

(1) Management could not get the $28.50 rate for private skilled nor the $20.00 for Intermediate. See Schedule 8 for final determination of rates.

(2) The mark-up on private payers is determined as follows:

Budgeted cost	$ 920,000
Third party	(326,000)
Ancillaries	(66,700)
Total private cost	$ 527,300
ICF	(163,200)
SNF	$ 364,100
Budgeted cost	$ 920,000
Profit goal	95,000
Total revenue required	$1,015,000
Revenue from third-party payers	(326,000)
Revenue from ancillaries	(84,000)
Revenue required from private payers	$ 605,000
Operating cost	527,300
Required mark-up	$ 77,700
Percent of operating cost	14.7%

117

Schedule 8
Nursing Center, Inc.
Budgeted Revenues and Profit
According to Final Competitive Rates

Payer	Patient Days	Cost Rate	Annual Private Rate	Projected Revenue	Rounded	Monthly	Per Patient Day
Medicare	1,825	$26.94		$ 49,200	$ 49,000	$ 4,100	
Medicaid							
ICF	6,658	17.36		115,583	115,500	9,600	
SNF	7,212	22.40		161,549	161,500	13,500	
	13,870						
Total third-party payers	15,695			$326,332	$326,000	$27,200	$20.77
Private							
ICF	9,402		$18.00	$169,236	$170,000	$14,200	$18.00
SNF							
200 wing 40	5,875		28.00	164,500	164,500	13,700	28.00
100–300 wings 60	8,813		25.00	220,325	220,300	18,300	25.00
	14,688						
Total private payers	24,090			$554,061	$554,800	$46,200	$23.03
Total revenue routine services	39,785			$880,393	$880,800	$73,400	$22.14
Operating costs routine services					852,550	71,000	21.43
Net income routine services					$ 28,250	$ 2,400	.71
Ancillary services							
Revenue					$ 84,000	$ 7,000	
Cost					66,700	5,600	
Net income ancillary services					$ 17,300	$ 1,400	$ .44
Total profit at 109 beds occupied					$ 45,550	$ 3,800	$ 1.15

Notes:
Additional occupancy impact (3 beds per day = 112)
1 bed in 200 wing (365 × $25 per day) $ 9,125
2 beds in 100–300 wings (730 × $28 per day)   20,440
Less food costs (1,095 days × $2 food cost per day)   (2,450)
                                                         $ 27,115

Total profit at 112 beds occupied (including ancillaries) $ 72,665 $ 1.78
Total profit at 116 beds occupied (including ancillaries) $ 91,870 $ 2.17

Schedule 9
Nursing Center, Inc.
Potential Revenue and Profit
At Full Capacity

	Beds Available	Days	Private Rate		Projected Revenue
All beds at private rates					
ICF	46	16,790	$18.00		$302,220
200 wing	28	10,220	28.00		286,160
100–300 wings	42	15,330	25.00		383,250
	116	42,340			$971,630
			Cost	Private	
Discount for third party					
Medicare		1,825	$26.94	$28.00	$ (1,900)
Medicaid					
ICF		6,658	17.36	18.00	(4,300)
SNF		7,212	22.40	27.00	(33,200)
					$(39,400)
Total revenue for 116 beds					$932,230
Operating costs					852,550
Additional raw food costs (2,555 days @ $2.00 per day)					5,110
Total operating costs for 116 beds					$857,660
Net profit for 116 beds					$ 74,570
Ancillaries net profit					17,300
Total net profit for 116 beds					$ 91,870

Pertinent Profit Considerations:
Potential profit lost on third parties $ 39,400
Potential profit lost on 109 bed occupancy $ 46,320
Potential profit lost on 112 bed occupancy $ 19,205

Budget Analysis

Budget analysis is the comparison of actual operating results to forecasted sales and projected cost of sales and budgeted selling and administrative expenses. The total budget plan effectively is a form of management by objectives. The forecast of sales is the establishment of quotas and targets. The projection of expected cost is the production goal. The budget of administrative expenses is the guideline for spending. Each segment of the plan represents the objectives (goals) for the attainment of the profit margin.

The attainment of the goals is a day-by-day process that requires checks and balances. In other words, it is not just something that happens; it must be made to happen. (This reminds me of the remark made to me by a converted budget skeptic: "I never knew I could predict the future until I did a budget and made it happen!")

The easy part is doing the budget, the hard part is *making it happen!* Making it happen consists of the following:

- Good financial reports
- Timely financial reports
- Good and timely production reports
- Comparison of actual operating results and productivity to the plan
- Follow-up on the variances of actual results versus planned results
- Influencing the actions of people to keep them on the game plan
- Refinement of the plan if it is not reasonable

Budget analysis should normally be done by an accountant on a timely basis. A trained administrator can also analyze why the business is not "on" budget. The analysis consists of these two steps.

1. A comparison of the output production quotas (forecast) to the actual production should be made as often as possible and no less than monthly. It will tell the administrator whether the volume of patients being cared for (beds occupied) is adequate to meet the monthly budget quotas. It will also indicate if the number of Private Pay patients is adequate to subsidize the Medicare and Medicaid patient load. The analysis consists of:
   a. Volume
   b. Patient mix

This is called the output analysis which is illustrated in detail in Chapter 7. This analysis should be done separately for routine services exclusive of ancillaries. The ancillaries should be analyzed using hours of service or number of procedures.

2. The comparison of the forecasted input production units to the actual will tell the administrator whether the labor component is according to plan (staffing plan) and whether the labor production levels are producing adequate units to demonstrate efficiency. This consists of:
   a. Direct- and indirect-labor hours per patient day (by level of care)
   b. Number of nursing hours per patient day (by level of care)
   c. Number of nursing staff per patient day (by level of care)
   d. Meals served to patients and employees

e. Pounds of laundry processed

f. Housekeeping and maintenance hours per occupied bed

This analysis is indicative of the efficiency of the direct- and indirect-labor component.

Let's look at an example to put the revenue (output) budget analysis in perspective.

	Forecasted Quotas	Monthly Actual Productivity	(+) Favorable (−) Unfavorable Variance
Patient Days			
Skilled			
Private	500	450	(−) 50
Medicaid	1,000	1,050	(+) 50
Medicare	400	350	(−) 50
Veterans	100	100	−
	2,000	1,950	(−) 50
Intermediate			
Private	500	400	(−) 100
Medicaid	1,500	1,650	(+) 150
Veterans	−	50	(+) 50
	2,000	2,100	(+) 100
	4,000	4,050	(+) 50

This table shows that the home as a whole exceeded the forecasted production level by 50 days. This is a favorable variance because it adds potential output units to the facility's revenue. However, the further analysis of production levels indicates that the patient mix has shifted to the intermediate level and has reduced the private pay patient load by 150 days. The problem highlighted is that the overall revenue of the facility for the month will be under budget while the patient load productivity exceeds budget. Let's price it out to determine the impact:

	Variance	Price	Variance Impact
SNF			
Private	(−) 50	$40.00	(−) $2,000
Medicaid	(+) 50	22.00	(+) 1,100
Medicare	(−) 50	28.00	(−) 1,400
Veterans	−	−	−
	(−) 50		$(2,300)
ICF			
Private	(−) 100	29.00	(−) $2,900
Medicaid	(+) 150	18.00	(+) 2,900
Veterans	(+) 50	27.00	(+) 1,350
	(+) 100		(+) $1,350
	(+) 50		(−) $ (950)

122 Basic Accounting and Budgeting for Long-Term Care Facilities

If this same thing happens each month, and it can compound if a trend develops, the impact on the bottom line can be substantial. For example:

	Annualized 50 Days	½ Year 50 Days	¼ Year 50 Days	Total
January	$950			$950
February	950			950
March	950			950
April	950			950
May	950			950
June	950			950
July	950	$950		1,900
August	950	950		1,900
September	950	950		1,900
October	950	950	$950	2,850
November	950	950	950	2,850
December	950	950	950	2,850
	$11,400	$5,700	$2,850	$19,950

This presumes that patient days increased by 1,050 for the year but the mix changed to lower potential revenue by $19,950. Unless staffing levels and labor costs are adjusted downward by a corresponding amount, the bottom line can decrease up to $19,950. The reason for doing this analysis monthly is to determine whether the labor costs or prices are compensating for the patient mix. If they are not, a decision must be made to either revise the staffing plan or revise the prices.

The direct-labor (output) budget analysis we have just looked at analyzes the impact of variances on revenue. The input budget analysis will accomplish the same objective on the costs. Now let's look at an example of the impact of variances in input units on costs.

		Monthly Forecasted Quotas	Actual Productivity	(+) Favorable (−) Unfavorable Variance
Direct Labor				
Skilled Unit				
RNs	3	600	700	(−) 100
LPNs	4	800	900	(−) 100
Aides	20	4,000	3,800	(+) 200
	27	5,400	5,400	−
Intermediate				
RNs	−	−	100	(−) 100
LPNs	3	600	500	(+) 100
Aides	15	3,000	3,500	(−) 500
	18	3,600	4,100	(−) 500
		9,000	9,500	(−) 500

This indicates that direct-labor hours exceeded quotas by 500 which is an unfavorable variance because it increases labor costs. But let's see what effect this has on costs before we call it unfavorable.

	(+) Favorable (−) Unfavorable Variance	Actual Wage Rate Per Hour	Variance Impact
Skilled			
RNs	(−) 100	$6.00	(−) $ 600
LPNs	(−) 100	4.50	(−) 450
Aides	(+) 200	2.80	(+) 500
	—		(−) $ (550)
Intermediate			
RNs	(−) 100	6.00	(−) $ 600
LPNs	(+) 100	4.50	(+) 450
Aides	(−) 500	2.80	(−) (1,400)
	(−) 500		(−) $(1,550)
Net Direct-Labor Variance			(−) $(2,100)

These figures indicate that the salary costs increased by $2,100, and this is unfavorable. But do we have the whole story? What about the wage rate per hour and the level of productivity? These are variables that constitute the full explanation of why the labor costs increased and if the variance is favorable or unfavorable. The effect of wage rate on the variance is as follows:

	Budgeted Wage Rate	Actual Wage Rate	(+) Favorable (−) Unfavorable Variance
RNs	$6.25	$6.00	(+) $.25
LPNs	4.75	4.50	(+) .25
Aides	2.70	2.80	(+) .10

Impact on cost is as follows:

	Variance	Forecasted Hours	(+) Favorable (−) Unfavorable Variance Impact
RNs	(+) $.25	600	(+) $150
LPNs	(+) .25	1,400	(+) 350
Aides	(+) .10	7,000	(+) 700
			(+) $1,200

The actual variance therefore consists of the impact of the variance in labor hours and labor rate.

Total variance	(−) $2,100
Variance due to wage rate	(+) 1,200
Variance due to labor hours	(−) $3,300

This indicates that the labor hours in excess of the budget were costing $3,300 per month and were being lessened by the lower hourly rate that was actually being paid; so the net impact on cost was an increase of $2,100.

The worth of this information cannot be completely appreciated unless we can determine if the additional cost incurred resulted in higher productivity or efficiency. As we demonstrated earlier, the productivity in terms of patients served decreased. But there are other forms of productivity, which reduce costs in other areas, even though direct-labor hours increase. Let's explore this possibility in our example, before we deduce that the $2,100 direct-labor cost increase is favorable or unfavorable.

Upon investigation we find that the nurses' hours increased for the following reasons:

1. Aides were being used for duties formerly performed by dietary, laundry, and housekeeping staffs. These duties were transferred to nursing because the aides were better able to do duties formerly done by other people. The following functions improved overall efficiency because it transferred compatible duties to the aides' job responsibilities:

Duty	Former Department
Straighten rooms	Housekeeping
Fold laundry	Laundry
Deliver trays	Dietary
Wash bed pans, water pitchers, wheel chairs	Housekeeping
Install bed rails	Housekeeping
Transfer patients	Administration

   This revision of job duties resulted in an increase in nursing salaries of $2,100 but it reduced salary costs in other departments.

2. The RN in Skilled was floating between the two sections. This eliminated 100 hours of LPN time. The LPN was assigned the duty of being the facility's ward clerk, in a move to improve the medical recordkeeping. This decision was necessitated because the records were deemed inadequate and not conducive to Medical Review. This deficiency was losing the facility reimbursement because the patients were not being evaluated properly and Medicaid reimbursement levels were too low.

If we find that costs decreased in other departments by more than $2,100 because of a lighter work load, and that reimbursement increased, then we can deduce that the $2,100 variance was really not unfavorable because management had managed labor in a cost effective manner and was in fact "beating" the budget in two areas.

SUMMARY

Budgeting and budget analysis is simply *good management!* (Unfortunately, good management is *on* the minds of many but *in* the minds of only a few.) Isn't it ironic that many business managers learn the hard way—they simply do not learn until they are in a crisis. Just like the wayward traveler said:

> I drove to Clarksville without a map. It took twice as long to get there as it should have. The problem was that I just didn't have time to plan the trip until I got lost.

Take your choice, live and learn or learn to live. Budgeting and budget analysis is learning while mapping the road to success.

BUDGET ANALYSIS CASE STUDY

Budget Analysis Report
Month of _____

	Actual	Budget	(+) Favorable (−) Unfavorable Variance
Revenue			
SNF			
Private	$30,000	$32,000	(−) $ 2,000
Medicaid	14,600	13,500	(+) 1,100
Medicare	2,700	4,100	(−) 1,400
Veterans	—	—	—
	$47,300	$49,600	(−) $(2,300)
ICF			
Private	$11,300	$14,200	(−) $ 2,900
Medicaid	12,500	9,600	(+) 2,900
Veterans	1,350	—	(+) 1,350
	$25,150	$23,800	(+) $ 1,350
Total revenue	$72,450	$73,400	(−) $ (950)
Ancillaries	$ 7,000	$ 6,000	(+) $ 1,000
Operating Expenses			
Direct Labor SNF			
RNs	$ 3,300	$ 2,700	(−) $ 600
LPNs	2,850	2,400	(−) 450
Aides	13,500	14,000	(+) 500
	$19,650	$19,100	(−) $ (550)
Direct Labor ICF			
RNs	$ 600	$ —	(−) $ 600
LPNs	550	1,000	(+) 450
Aides	4,100	2,700	(−) 1,400
	$ 5,250	$ 3,700	(−) $(1,550)
Total Direct Labor	$24,900	$22,800	(−) $(2,100)
Indirect Labor			
Dietary	$ 4,800	$ 5,800	(+) $ 1,000
Housekeeping	1,600	1,800	(+) 200
Laundry	1,000	1,000	—
Maintenance	900	900	—
Total Indirect Labor	$ 8,300	$ 9,500	(+) $ 1,200

	Actual	Budget	(+) Favorable (−) Unfavorable Variance
Other Direct Labor			
Activities	$ 1,300	$ 1,300	$ —
Rehabilitation	1,200	1,200	—
Physical Therapy	200	200	—
Total Other Direct Labor	$ 2,700	$ 2,700	$ —
Controllable Overhead			
Supplies			
Food	$ 7,500	$ 7,000	(−) $ 500
Medical	4,000	3,700	(−) 300
Cleaning	300	300	—
Laundry	100	200	(+) 100
Repairs	—	1,000	(+) 1,000
Utilities	3,900	3,000	(−) 900
Employee benefits	4,500	4,000	(−) 500
Total Controllable Overhead	$20,300	$19,200	(−) $ 1,100
Fixed Overhead			
Administrative			
Salaries	$ 5,000	$ 5,000	$ —
Supplies	150	150	—
License, etc.	50	50	—
Insurance	900	900	—
Professional fees	300	250	(−) 50
Telephone	200	200	—
Data processing	100	100	—
Working capital interest	50	50	—
Organization cost	100	100	—
Capital Cost			
Depreciation	600	600	—
Mortgage interest	—	—	—
Real estate taxes	1,500	1,500	—
Rent	11,700	11,700	—
	$20,650	$20,600	(−) $ 50
Total Operating Expense	$76,850	$74,800	(−) $ 2,050
Net Income or (Loss) from Nursing Home Operations	$ 2,600	$ 4,600	(−) $ 2,000

Problem:
1. Why did bottom line come in below budget?
2. What factors effect the variance in:
   Revenue
   Controllable expenses
   Fixed expenses
3. Why is this exercise so important?

Variance Analysis

    Variance analysis is a management tool that can help you control your costs, motivate your employees, and isolate small problems before they get bigger. The accounting procedures for variance analysis can be very complicated, but the basic principles are not.

DEFINITION OF VARIANCE ANALYSIS

Variance analysis is a method of analyzing differences between *expected* results and *actual* results. These differences are called *variances*.

THE BASIC STEPS IN VARIANCE ANALYSIS

First, you set *standards*. Assume, for example, that you are an ICF facility. If each patient day requires 2½ hours of direct labor at $5 per hour, your standard is $12.50 of direct labor cost per patient day.

Next, compare your actual results to your standard. If actual labor cost for 100 patient days is $13,050, you have an *unfavorable* variance of $550. According to your standard, the 100 patient days should have cost only $12,500 (100 units × $12.50 per day). The $550 difference is an unfavorable variance because your profits are $550 less than they would have been had you produced the service at standard labor cost.

Finally, you *analyze* the variance. In our example, there are two possible explanations for it. One is a *quantity variance,* which means you used more than 2½ hours of labor to care for each patient. The other is a *price variance,* which means your labor cost more than $5 per hour. Your unfavorable variance of $550 could have been caused by either of these or by both in combination.

CALCULATING PRICE AND QUANTITY VARIANCES

There are simple formulas for calculating each type of variance. If the actual labor time for the 100 days was 300 hours, the *quantity variance* is:

Quantity variance = (Standard hours − Actual hours) × Standard wage rate
                       = (250 hours − 300 hours) × $5.00 per hour
                       = −$250 unfavorable variance

In other words, the 100 days should have taken 250 hours to produce (100 days × 2½ hours per day) but actually took 300 hours. This inefficient use of labor in effect cut into profits by $250 per day. The unfavorable quantity variance was made even larger by an unfavorable price variance. If actual labor cost was $6.00 per hour, the *price variance* was:

Price variance = (Standard rate − Actual rate) × Actual hours
               = ($5.00 − $6.00) × 300 hours
               = −$300 unfavorable variance

Price and quantity variances together explain the total direct-labor variance:

Price variance = (Standard price − Actual price) × Actual quantity
Quantity variance = (Standard quantity − Actual quantity) × Standard price

CALCULATING VARIANCES FOR DIRECT SUPPLY (MATERIAL) COST

The procedure is the same as for direct-labor cost. Set a standard specifying the quantity and price of the direct supplies required for each patient day. Then compare the standard with the actual supply costs and analyze the variances.

128 Basic Accounting and Budgeting for Long-Term Care Facilities

The analysis again focuses on *price* and *quantity* variances. Favorable variances increase your profits above standard, and unfavorable ones cut profits. The formulas for supply variances are like those for labor variances:

Unfavorable quantity variance	−$250
Unfavorable price variance	−300
Total unfavorable direct-labor variance	−$550

Together, price and quantity variances will account for the total supply variances.

CAN OVERHEAD COSTS BE ANALYZED WITH VARIANCE ANALYSIS?

Variance analysis also works for overhead costs, but the procedure differs from that for labor and material costs. The difference occurs because there are two different kinds of overhead costs—fixed and variable. Your *fixed costs,* like rent or depreciation, do not change as your production level changes. *Variable costs,* like indirect labor, vary with production volume. Each patient day service you provide "absorbs" (or is allocated) some portion of your fixed and variable overhead costs.

THE BASIC STEPS FOR ANALYZING OVERHEAD VARIANCES

First, you set a *standard absorption rate.* This is the overhead cost that should be absorbed by each patient day when you produce at normal or standard volume.

For example, assume fixed overhead costs of $1,000, variable overhead costs of $20 per day, and standard volume of 100 patient days. You find your absorption rate simply by dividing fixed overhead by standard volume ($1,000 / 100 days — $10 per day) and adding the $10 to your variable overhead of $20. Your standard absorption rate is $30. If you produce at exactly standard volume, all your overhead—fixed and variable—will be absorbed by the 100 patient days.

Once you have your standard absorption rate, you compare actual overhead cost with standard and then explain any differences using specific variances.

THE DIFFERENCE BETWEEN STANDARD AND ACTUAL OVERHEAD COST

Two variances—*volume* variances and *spending* variances—explain the difference between standard and actual overhead cost. You get a volume variance if you do not produce at exactly standard volume because you will absorb too much or too little fixed overhead.

If, for example, you have 90 patient days instead of 100, each should absorb $11.11 of fixed overhead ($1,000/90 days). Instead, in your estimate each absorbs only $10 of fixed overhead, since your absorption rate was based on a standard volume of 100 days. You have an *unfavorable volume variance* of $100 because the 90 days have absorbed only $900 (90 units × $10) out of $1,000 of fixed overhead.

You can get the same result using the *volume variance equation:*

Volume variance = Absorbed overhead − Standard overhead

In this case, absorbed overhead is $2,700 (90 units × $30 absorption rate) while standard overhead is $2,800 [$1,000 fixed overhead + ($30 variable overhead × 90 units)]. The equation yields the unfavorable volume variance of −$100 ($2,700 − $2,800 = −$100).

The other overhead variance, the *spending variance,* occurs if actual overhead costs, either fixed or variable, differ from standard. If you have 90 patients and the actual overhead cost is $2,600, the spending variance is:

Spending variance = Standard overhead − Actual overhead
 = $2,800 − $2,600
 = + $200 favorable

The total overhead variance is then the difference between absorbed and actual overhead:

Total overhead variance = Absorbed overhead − Actual overhead
 = $2,700 − $2,600
 = + $100 favorable

RELATING VARIANCES TO EACH OTHER AND TO A NURSING HOME'S COSTS

The chart in Exhibit 4-3 shows the relationships between variances. Reading from left to right, any differences between your actual and expected costs can be explained in terms of labor, material, or overhead variances. These are explained by more detailed variances like price or spending variances.

Exhibit 4-3 illustrates a facility's variances, each of which ultimately affects your costs and your profits. Moreover, favorable and unfavorable variances often offset each other. When this happens, it can disguise a cost-control problem and keep you from doing something about it until it becomes severe.

Exhibit 4-3 Relationships Between Variances

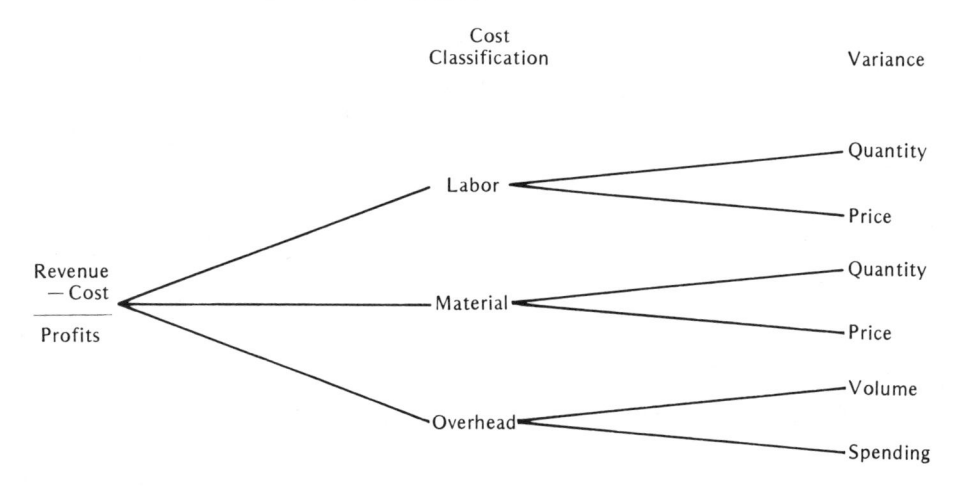

```
                        Cost
                    Classification              Variance

                                                    Quantity
                         Labor
                                                    Price

Revenue                                             Quantity
 − Cost                Material
 ─────                                              Price
 Profits
                                                    Volume
                       Overhead
                                                    Spending
```

SUMMARY

Variances can be used in other ways to manage a facility better. You can use variance analysis whenever you compare actual results with standard or budgeted results.

Variance analysis by itself is not a cure-all. It is a tool that must be combined with the judgment of experienced administrators to be useful, and it often provides just the *starting point* for further evaluation of problems.

A full-fledged system of variance analysis takes time, special recordkeeping, updating of supply and labor standards, and so forth. You should use it to evaluate only costs that are important enough to justify the added expense.

Try to *integrate* your variance analysis with other managerial controls and incentives. If an employee has control over a particular cost, make him responsible for developing standards, working to the standards, and explaining variances from the standards.

CHAPTER 5
Capital Budgeting

How do you decide in which assets your nursing home should be investing? The answer to this question will reveal a great deal about your long-term prospects for success, because sound investment decisions ultimately are the foundation for profitability. The most effective tool to help you make these decisions is *capital budgeting*.

How is Capital Budgeting Used?

Capital budgeting is based on the assumption that, as a business manager, you have investment options available, and it is used to help you evaluate the options and choose those which are best suited to your business. The following steps outline the process of capital budgeting:

1. *Establish a business plan.* Capital budgeting decisions should be made in the context of an overall long-range plan for your business. Unless you have such a plan, there is no way to determine what investments you need to make or what assets you need to acquire.
2. *Establish an investment evaluation system.* After deciding that certain types of investments are consistent with your business plan, measure the financial attractiveness of the available options. The evaluation system you choose should be suitable for analyzing all types of capital investments, regardless of their duration.
3. *Evaluate and rank investment alternatives.* Since your capital investment budget will almost always be smaller than the total cost of investments you find attractive, you should establish a ranking system to construct a priority list for the investments.

Capital Investment Options

Since your business provides services, capital investment decisions are of two major types: decisions to maintain or replace existing equipment or facilities, and decisions to add new equipment or facilities.

REPLACEMENT DECISIONS

Other than cost, factors to consider in making an asset replacement decision include:

1. *Consumer demand*—Before replacing worn-out capital assets, satisfy yourself that the services generated by the facility will continue to be sought by customers in future years.
2. *Asset flexibility*—If you anticipate a decline in consumer acceptance of your long-term care services during the expected life of the replacement asset, the asset should be adaptable to other uses to justify its acquisition.
3. *Obsolescence risks*—Replacement decisions will often require that you judge the likelihood that movable equipment will become obsolete during its expected life.

CAPACITY DECISIONS

Whenever a capital asset acquisition allows you to increase your service output beyond existing levels or allows you to move into new areas, the acquisition should be thought of as capacity expansion. Unless you are adding equipment very similar to that already in use, a new capacity decision is generally more difficult to make than a replacement decision because you may not have access to the cost and operating data that is often available for making replacement decisions. You will also have to consider the same factors of consumer demand, asset flexibility, and risk of obsolescence.

New capacity decisions can be categorized in terms of the effect such decisions will have on your overall operations:

1. *Increasing existing output*—The most straightforward capacity decision involves acquiring assets to increase the output of existing services. Acquisition of the additional assets presumes that you have already exhausted other options for expansion (such as day care or meals on wheels) or that you have decided that expansion is the only way to meet demand.
2. *Horizontal integration*—Horizontal integration means adding capacity that allows you to generate more services similar to those presently provided.
3. *Vertical integration*—Vertical integration occurs when expansion allows you to move into another form of long-term care, such as home health services.
4. *Full diversification*—If an expansion decision results in moving you into a new branch of business, you will be involved in the process of diversification. Since diversification decisions often have the greatest potential for a positive or negative impact on your business, they require the greatest study in relation to your overall business plan.

Evaluation of Capital Investment Options

The techniques used for evaluating capital investment options vary significantly in terms of their sophistication and complexity. You should understand each of the three major evaluation techniques and know how and when to use them. In some circumstances, you will use these tools to evaluate a number of investment options that can be developed simultaneously, such as expansion and diversification ideas, and at other times, you will be using them to choose among options such as replacement or reconditioning decisions.

CASH FLOW METHOD

Regardless of the capital budgeting technique you use, your analysis will require *after-tax* cash flows. This example shows how to compute after-tax cash flows:

Patient revenue	$100.00
Cost	
Supply costs	$40
Labor costs	30
Depreciation	20
	−90.00
Profit before tax	$10.00
Tax (with 46% rate)	−4.60
Profit after tax	$5.40
Depreciation	+ 20.00
After-tax cash flow	$ 25.40

Depreciation is added back to "profit after tax" because it is a noncash deduction taken for tax purposes only. Because you did not actually pay the depreciation amount, you still have it as part of your cash flow. The outflow of the dollars occurred when you purchased the assets now being depreciated.

PAYBACK METHOD

The payback method for making capital budgeting decisions is based on the amount of time needed for you to recover your initial investment out of after-tax cash flows. This time is the *payback period*.

A PAYBACK EXAMPLE

Assume that you have the opportunity to invest in an expansion project with the following after-tax cash flows for each additional bed:

Year	(Outflows)	Inflows	Net Flow
0	$(15,000)	$ -0-	$(15,000)
1	-0-	5,000	5,000
2	-0-	8,000	8,000
3	-0-	10,000	10,000

At the end of Year 2, $2,000 of the investment remains to be recaptured ($15,000 − $5,000 − $8,000 = $2,000). Since $10,000 of after-tax inflows are generated during the third year, the payback period ends during that year. The exact answer is found by assuming that the $10,000 is generated evenly throughout the year and then dividing $2,000 by $10,000 to compute the fractional part of the third year necessary for the investment recapture. This fraction is one-fifth. The payback period is two and one-fifth years.

The main disadvantage of the payback method is that it does not take into account the time value of money. This method treats dollars received in Year 3 the same as dollars spent in Year 0, even though a dollar in Year 0 is worth more than a dollar received in Year 3. A second disadvantage of this method is that it might eliminate sound investments that do not have an acceptable payback period but have substantial cash flows in later years. For this reason, there has been a steady decline in the use of the payback method without consideration of the value of money. As a result it is being replaced by discounted cash flow methods.

Even though it has several major disadvantages, the payback method is useful in conjunction with discounted cash flow methods. These methods evaluate the investment's worth, and the payback method may then be used to determine how long your investment funds will be subject to risk during the time that cash inflows have not recaptured the full investment.

NET PRESENT VALUE METHOD

The essence of the "present value" is to evaluate projects on the basis of *today's* dollars, even though the projects may involve revenues and expenses spread over a number of years. For this reason, the technique is known as a *discounted cash flow* method.

THE TIME VALUE OF MONEY

The net present value method of analysis was developed to take into account the time value of money, which exists as interest is accrued for the use of the money. If no interest were paid, the following equation would be valid: $1 (today) = $1 (in two years) = $1 (in three years). But because of interest, $1 today is worth more than $1 a year from now or two years from now.

THE DISCOUNT RATE

To compute the *present value* of an investment—its worth in today's dollars—an appropriate interest rate known as the *discount rate* is selected. For example, by using 10 percent as the discount rate, you can compute today's value of $1 to be received one and two years from now: $1 × .909 (discount factor for one year at 10 percent) = $0.909; $1 × .826 (discount factor for two years at 10 percent) = $0.826.

The discount factor is found in a present value table and is selected on the basis of the interest rate being used and the period of time being studied. You can now compare the present value of all three amounts:

$1 To Be Received	Present Value
Today	$1.00
In one year	$0.909
In two years	$0.826

You should choose to receive $1 today rather than $1 next year.

THE COST OF CAPITAL

The appropriate discount rate to use in capital budgeting analysis is the *cost of capital,* which represents the weighted-average cost of all sources of capital for your business. Unless your investments earn at least as much as your cost of capital, they will impair your facility's financial base. For example, if the cost of capital is

8 percent and you are investing money in projects paying 5 percent, you are losing 3 percent on each investment. This is the spiral nursing homes now seem to be facing.

Calculating the cost of capital is one of the most complicated tasks you will face as a business manager because traditional methods only allow you to make an educated guess. You must determine the after-tax cost of each source of capital and then compute a weighted average for these costs.

COST OF DEBT

Use the cost of debt that you would incur if funding a new project today. Suppose this cost is 9 percent. To compute the cost on an after-tax basis (interest is deductible), multiply it by $(1 - t)$, where t is your tax rate. If $t = 46\%$, your after-tax debt cost is $9\% \times (1 - .46) = 4.86\%$.

COST OF EQUITY (STOCK)

This cost represents the return required by the owners of the business. It is already in after-tax dollars because payments to owners that are returns on their investments are not tax deductible. A useful technique for estimating your cost of equity follows:

1. Find the current average return on risk-free investments, such as U.S. Treasury bills and notes.
2. Estimate the extra return required by investors to compensate them for the *business risks* facing your facility. Business risks include such factors as the strength of competition, product viability, and market conditions.
3. Estimate the extra return required by investors to compensate them for the *financial risks* facing your business. Financial risks include the extent of your debt repayment obligations. The more debt you have to repay, the riskier your financial condition becomes in a downturn.
4. Add the extra returns estimated in steps 2 and 3 to the risk-free rate. This is your cost of equity.

WEIGHTED AVERAGE

Assume that your after-tax cost of debt is 5 percent and that your cost of equity is 10 percent. If 75 percent of your capital comes from equity and 25 percent of it comes from debt sources, your weighted-average cost of capital is found like this:

After-Tax Cost			Weight		
Debt	5%	×	25%	=	1.25%
Equity	10%	×	75%	=	7.50%
Weighted-average cost of capital				=	8.75%

A NET PRESENT VALUE EXAMPLE

Suppose you wish to evaluate a bed expansion project with the following characteristics:

1. Initial cash outflow = $25,000 per bed
2. After-tax cash inflows:

Year	Per Bed Inflow
1	$2,500
2	4,000
3	6,000
4	7,000
5	8,000

Assuming a weighted-average cost of capital of 10 percent, the following table shows how to compute the net present value of this investment, which is the total present value of all inflows and outflows. Outflows are treated as negative numbers.

Year	Per Bed Inflow/(Outflow)		Discount Factor		Per Bed Present Value
0	($25,000)	×	1.000	=	($25,000)
1	2,500	×	0.909	=	2,273
2	4,000	×	0.826	=	3,304
3	6,000	×	0.751	=	4,506
4	7,000	×	0.683	=	4,781
5	8,000	×	0.621	=	4,968
	Total = Net Present Value			=	($5,168)

The result tells you that the investment has a negative net present value, and this means the return over the five years is less than your cost of capital. If your investment plans require that you make a profit in five years, you should reject the project because you will lose $5,168 per bed, in terms of today's dollars, if you go ahead with the investment.

If the investment yielded a net present value of zero, its return would be equal to your cost of capital, and investing in it would not impair your home's finances. If the investment has a net present value greater than zero, its return exceeds your cost of capital, and it merits serious consideration.

An important lesson to learn from this example is that the next present value of the investment is negative even though the undiscounted cash inflows, which total $27,500, exceed the original cost of $25,000. This result occurs because of the *timing* of the cash inflows. The further into the future each inflow is received, the less each dollar of that inflow is worth in terms of today's dollars.

THE INTERNAL RATE OF RETURN METHOD

The internal rate of return method also uses discounted cash flow techniques. The goal of this method is to find the discount rate that will produce a net present value of zero for the investment under consideration. This discount rate is known as the *internal rate of return* and represents the actual return on your investment.

GRAPHIC ANALYSIS

The internal rate of return can be seen in the graph (Exhibit 5-1):

Exhibit 5-1 Internal Rate of Return

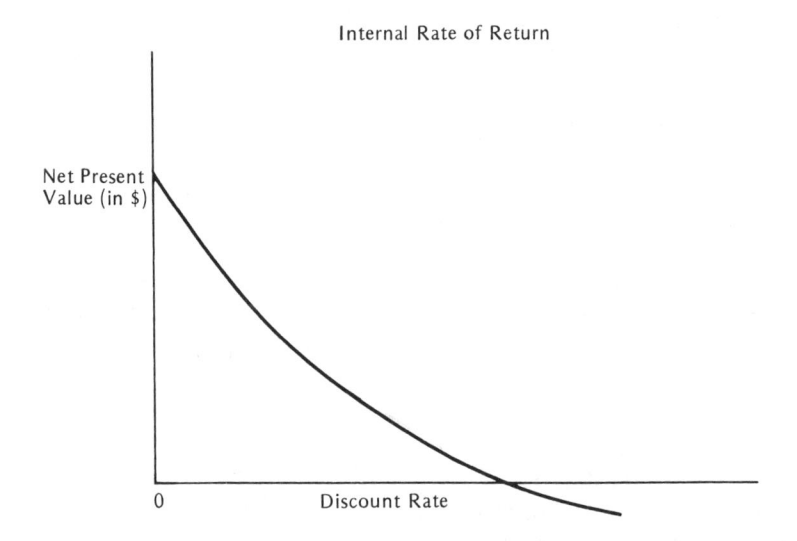

When the discount rate is zero, the net present value is simply the undiscounted difference between cash outflows and inflows. As the discount rate increases, the net present value of the investment decreases. At the point where the net present value curve crosses the discount rate line, you will find the internal rate of return because that discount rate yields a net present value of zero.

HOW TO FIND THE INTERNAL RATE OF RETURN

The only way to find the internal rate of return is through a trial-and-error process. You can use the discount factor approach, an electronic calculator with financial capability, or a computer to assist you. The following is an example of how to find the internal rate of return using discount factors:

1. Initial cash outflow = ($187.00)
2. After-tax cash inflows:

Year	Inflow
1	$100
2	107

The first step is to assume a discount rate and discount the flows to arrive at a trial value. If you start with 6 percent, your discount table would look like this:

Year	Cash Flows		Discount Factors (for 6%)		
0	($187.00)	×	1.000	=	($187.00)
1	100.00	×	0.943	=	94.30
2	107.00	×	0.890	=	95.23
	Net Present Value			=	$2.53

Six percent is not quite high enough to reduce the net present value to zero. You may wish to try 7 percent as your next discount rate, and it will produce the following table:

Year	Cash Flows		Discount Factors (for 7%)		
0	($187.00)	×	1.000	=	($187.00)
1	100.00	×	0.935	=	93.50
2	107.00	×	0.873	=	93.41
	Net Present Value			=	$(0.09)

The internal rate of return is close to 7 percent because the net present value at that discount rate is only negative by 9¢. The true value will lie just under 7 percent, but for purposes of this example, 7 percent can be considered as the internal rate of return.

Choosing an Investment

Having used one or more of the three basic techniques for evaluating your capital budget options, you now need to rank the options in order to decide which ones to choose.

1. *Nonfinancial ranking* involves measuring the investments against your overall business plan and determining if they belong to investment categories that are consistent with your needs.
2. *Financial ranking* requires you to refer back to the three basic evaluation techniques.
3. *Ranking by payback.* Under the payback method, investment options are compared according to the length of their payback periods. A project with a payback of two years is ranked higher than one with a payback of three years. Some businesses set a cutoff period and reject all investments which have paybacks beyond that period. This is dangerous since large cash inflows may occur after the cutoff.
4. *Ranking by net present value.* One way to use net present value analysis to rank projects is to establish a priority list based on the net present value of each investment, with the highest net present value receiving the top priority.

5. *Ranking by the internal rate of return.* To rank by the internal rate of return on investments, simply arrange the internal rates in descending order; the investment having the highest internal rate of return is the most attractive financially.

Another way of using net present value analysis involves computing a *profitability index* for each investment. The profitability index is defined as follows:

$$\frac{\text{Present value of after-tax inflows}}{\text{Present value of after-tax outflows}}$$

Investments are then ranked according to their profitability index, with the investment having the highest index being first. For example, suppose the total present value of inflows for a day care project is $28,918 and the total present value of outflows is $17,900. The profitability index equals:

$$\frac{\$28,918}{\$17,900} = 1.62$$

This means that day care will generate $1.62 in after-tax inflows, measured in today's dollars, for each dollar of after-tax outflows, also measured in today's dollars.

MAKING THE BEST INVESTMENT DECISIONS FOR YOUR NURSING HOME

Capital budgeting is designed to help you make the best investment decisions for your business. The most effective technique involves discounted cash flow analysis. The time you spend familiarizing yourself with this technique will greatly improve your home's potential for long-range profitability.

When facing capital budgeting decisions you should use all three methods, for they produce different priority lists. You should also focus again on the riskiness of each project to help you make a choice.

Remember, an investment with a high net present value or internal rate of return may be much riskier than one with an average projected return. Your attitude toward taking a risk should moderate the rate of return prospects.

Once you have made your investment decisions the capital budget will consist of a summary of your planned expenditures and expected financing. See example in Exhibit 5-2.

The substance of the plan is to make the needed replacements, expand the existing therapy capacity, and diversify into day care and home health services. The replacements required little analysis because the roof leaked and the equipment was obsolete and the investment had to be made to stay in business. On the other hand, the expansion of the therapy room and the diversification into other services required extensive rate of return analysis to justify the assumption of added risk. The investors and the bankers would not make their decision without a complete capital budget on the pay back period using discounted cash flow projections. The following final financing arrangements were founded on an internal rate of return of 10 percent above the cost of capital which was considered commensurate with the risk.

		%
Working capital	$25,000	3.7%
New financing	50,000	7.4
Refinancing	400,000	59.3
New invested capital	200,000	29.6
Total capital investment in diversification	$675,000	100.0%

Exhibit 5-2 Planned Expenditures and Expected Financing Summary

	Year 1	Year 2	Year 3	Year 4	Year 5
1. Planned Expenditures					
New roof	$30,000				
Therapy room		$80,000			
Day care center			$75,000		
Home health service				$100,000	
Pediatric wing					$500,000
Movable equipment replacements	10,000	10,000	–	25,000	–
Total Expenditures	$40,000	$90,000	$75,000	$125,000	$500,000
2. Expected Financing					
Working capital	$20,000	$20,000	$25,000	$25,000	$ –
Debt capital					
New financing	20,000	40,000	50,000	–	–
Re-financing	–	–	–	–	400,000
Invested capital	–	20,000	–	100,000	100,000
	$40,000	$80,000	$75,000	$125,000	$500,000

CHAPTER 6
Cash Flow Budgeting

Cash flow is like "Old Faithful" at Yellowstone Park. So long as there is a source of sustenance Old Faithful will spout its gusto regularly. However, if its resources disappear, Old Faithful will disappear. Cash flow works on the same principle. Before cash can flow it must be made available. The objective of a cash flow budget is to determine when cash will be available so the outflow can be planned. Therefore, the cash resources must be budgeted first.

The budgeting of cash resources, more commonly known as cash receipts, can be done in a number of different ways. It can be done by taking the prior year's monthly cash receipt book totals and using them as the basis for budgeting next year's monthly cash receipt figures. This is the least sophisticated way of budgeting anticipated cash resources. Another way is to take the total budgeted revenue for the year, remove the effect of beginning and ending receivables so you have a cash basis revenue figure, and divide it by 12 to get expected monthly cash receipt figures. This method is not much better than the first method. Still another method is to take the budgeted monthly revenues and presume that the collection of that budgeted revenue will be in the following month, and the cash receipts budget for a particular month will be the revenue billed for the prior month.

The best method of budgeting cash receipts is a combination of all of the preceding methods. Following are the steps to be carried out in budgeting cash receipts:

1. List the budgeted revenues by source of payment. In other words, list monthly budgeted revenues by private pay, Medicare, Medicaid, and other sources.
2. Determine when each will be collected. This should be set up in a work paper form so the numbers can be put into a particular column. See Exhibit 6–1. The private pay revenues for routine care will be collected in the month billed. The Medicare and Medicaid billings should be put into the collection period that can be historically justified. Bad accounts and the likelihood of uncollectible accounts should be eliminated from Accounts Receivable before predicting cash receipts.
3. Cash receipts from sources other than patients should be predicted as best as possible. For example, beauty shop income, income from sale of meals to employees, vending machine income, and so on, should be put into the month for which they are collected.
4. Any settlements with third parties for prior years should be predicted and put into the particular month.
5. Any anticipated patient refunds that will reduce the potential cash to be used for expenses should be removed from Receivables or included in the cash disbursements budget. Either method is acceptable.

Once these figures are itemized it is an easy matter of laying out the cash receipts budget. See Exhibit 6–2.

The cash disbursements budget is a little more complex. Cash is expended for a variety of purposes. It is paid out in the form of wages, merchandise purchases for inventory, or for instant use. It is paid out for purchase of services. It is expended

Exhibit 6-1 Medicaid Cash Receipts Budget

Line No.		Budgeted Revenue	(1) Accounts Receivable Balance	(2) January	(3) February	(4) March	(5) April	(13) December
1								
2		Beginning Receivable	$150,000	$110,000	$70,000			
3								
4	Jan	$100,000	140,000		80,000	$20,000		
5	Feb	90,000	110,000			80,000	$10,000	
6	Mar	110,000	120,000				100,000	
7	Apr	120,000	130,000					
8	May	115,000	135,000					
9	June	115,000	140,000					
10	July	120,000	150,000					
11	Aug	140,000	175,000					$10,000
12	Sept	125,000	185,000					
13	Oct	110,000	155,000					20,000
14	Nov	100,000	130,000					75,000
15	Dec	90,000	115,000					
16	Total Bills $1,335,000							
17	Total Cash $1,370,000			$110,000	$120,000	$100,000	$110,000	$105,000
18								
19		Beginning receivable	150,000					
20								
21		Budgeted revenue	1,335,000					
22								
23		Budgeted cash receipts	(1,370,000)					
24								
25		Ending receivables	$115,000					

Note:
This type of worksheet would be used for all sources of cash receipts
- Private
- Medicare and Medicaid
- Sundry income

Actual cash receipts and accounts receivable should be compared to the cash budget monthly to gauge progress.

to pay payroll taxes, insurance, real estate taxes, and utilities. It is used to pay off the mortgage and to service the debt. Almost all expenditures are paid by a specified time. If that specified time were the same for all expenditures, the cash disbursement budget would be as simple a matter as the cash receipts budget. However, when a nursing home is in a tight cash position, every bill that it receives

143 Cash Flow Budgeting

Exhibit 6-2 Cash Receipts Budget

Line	Source	Total	(1) January	(2) February	(3) March	(4) April	(13) December
1	Budget						
2	Patient Revenue						
3	Medicaid	$137000-	$11000-	$12000-	$10000-	$11000-	$10500-
4	Medicare	25000-	2000-	2500-	1000-	2000-	2000-
5	Private	100000-	9000-	8500-	9000-	9000-	7500-
6	Other	5000-	400-	400-	500-	500-	500-
7		267000-	22400-	23400-	20500-	22500-	20500-
8	Nonpatient Revenue						
9	Beauty shop	900-	80-	80-	70-	80-	80-
10	Sale of meals	800-	80-	80-	60-	80-	50-
11	Vending machines	120-	10-	10-	10-	10-	10-
12	Laundry	180-	10-	20-	10-	20-	20-
18	Total Budgeted						
19	Cash Receipts	$269000-	$22580-	$22590-	$20650-	$22690-	$20660-
21	Actual						
22	Patient Revenue						
23	Medicaid		$20000				
24	Medicare		1000				
25	Private		8500				
26	Other		400				
27			29900				
28	Nonpatient Revenue						
29	Beauty shop		100				
30	Sale of meals		90				
31	Vending machines		20				
32	Laundry		10				
36	Total Actual Cash Receipts		$30120				
38	Variance		$ 7540				
39	Mix		2040				
40	Occupancy		2500				
	Cash Flow		3000				

and every bill that it pays may be treated differently. The art of debtmanship, as it is called in the credit bureau circles, is to determine which bills must be paid first; or more simply who could hurt you the most if you did not pay their bill. So for the cash disbursements budget a specified list of expenditures must be made. These should be listed according to their payment characteristics. For example, a nursing home's cash disbursements could be arrayed as follows:

1. Salaries and wages
2. Payroll taxes

3. Purchases for inventory
4. Purchases for instant use
5. Principal and interest payment
6. Rent payment
7. Payment of real estate taxes
8. Payment of utilities
9. Payment of insurance
10. Payment for consultant services
11. Payment of dividends
12. Payment of Medicare settlement
13. Payment of income taxes, interest, and penalty costs
14. Payment of miscellaneous items not included above

The next step would be to list the budgeted expense for these items for the next year. To have an accurate cash forecast, the budget of these items must be done on a monthly basis. The budget of operating expenses represents the amount of expense incurred for the month, but not necessarily the amount of the cash to be expended to pay for those expenses.

The next step is to plot out how the budgeted expenses and purchases will be paid. Exhibits 6–3 and 6–4 show that exercise. As can be seen from the work sheets, the line items are categorized as to when they will be paid in relation to when they are incurred. In many cash budgets the preparer fails to anticipate the slowdown of payment if the total amount of revenue being put into the bank is not adequate to cover expenditures. So as a result, the cash flow budget becomes a cash deficit budget or a deficit spending budget. So, when we are putting together the cash flow projection, we will be very careful, at any point where the cash balance is not adequate to cover all expenditures, to decide whether we borrow money and put more cash in the bank, accelerate collections on receivables, or slow down the payments on accounts payable. If this sort of planning is not done, the cash budget is not going to be usable. Exhibit 6–5 is the monthly comparison of cash disbursement to cash receipts. Many companies do this exercise for the thrill of having done it and being able to say they have done it, but they really do not use it. You can see from the information provided that if you were to adhere to the cash budget as strictly as possible, the likelihood of accomplishing the operating goals is improved. Another benefit of cash budgeting is to allow the business manager to anticipate peaks and valleys in the cash flow and act accordingly. For example, if the cash budget indicates an excess cash outflow in the month of June due to real estate taxes that must be paid, but it is covered by a cash surplus accumulated prior to that date, the business manager can expect to have adequate cash in the bank to cover the real estate tax bill. If building a cash surplus has not been planned, the money must be borrowed on a short-term basis and revenues increased to start building a cash

Cash Flow Budgeting

Exhibit 6-3 Cash Disbursements Budget

Line No.	Type of Payer or Supplier	Budget Total	January	February	March	April	December	Line No.
1								1
2	Salaries							2
3	Jan 90,000		$90,000 -					3
4	Feb 90,000			$90,000 -				4
5	Mar 100,000				$100,000 -			5
6	Apr 110,000					$110,000 -		6
7	May 110,000							7
8	June 100,000							8
9	July 100,000							9
10	Aug 120,000							10
11	Sept 115,000							11
12	Oct 100,000							12
13	Nov 90,000							13
14	Dec 90,000	$1,215,000 -					$90,000 -	14
15								15
16	Payroll taxes							16
17	Purchases —							17
18	Inventory (Exhibit 6-4)	54,000 -	4,000 -	5,500 -	4,000 -	4,500 -	4,000 -	18
19	Floor	12,000 -	1,000 -	900 -	800 -	1,000 -	1,500 -	19
20	Principle and Interest	24,000 -	2,000 -	2,000 -	2,000 -	2,000 -	2,000 -	20
21	Rent	1,200 -	100 -	100 -	100 -	100 -	100 -	21
22	Utilities	17,000 -	2,000 -	2,000 -	1,500 -	1,000 -	2,000 -	22
23	Insurance	4,800 -	400 -	400 -	400 -	400 -	400 -	23
24	Consultants	1,200 -	100 -	100 -	100 -	100 -	100 -	24
25	Dividends	500 -	500 -					25
26	Medicare settlement	1,000 -				500 -		26
27	Real Estate Taxes	300 -						27
28	Income Taxes	2,400 -			400 -			28
29	Miscellaneous	2,400 -	200 -	200 -	200 -	200 -	200 -	29
30								30
31								31
32	Total Budgeted Cash Disbursements	$245,000 -	$193,000 -	$20,200 -	$19,500 -	$20,800 -	$193,000 -	32

Note: There would be a subschedule for each line item that varied in the amount paid per month. See Exhibit 6-4 for purchases.

surplus to pay off the bank loan and to start accumulating a surplus for the next time around.

The saying—it takes cash to pay bills—will always be true. The business may be doing very well from an accrual accounting standpoint, but may be in dire trouble because it is not able to create the resources to pay the bills of the business quickly enough. The cash flow budget helps the administrator bridge the gap

Exhibit 6-4 Purchases Cash Disbursements Budget Inventory

Line No		Budgeted Purchases	Accounts Payable Balance	January	February	March	April	December	Line No
1	Beginning Payables		$60,000	$40,000	$20,000				1
2									2
3	Jan	$40,000	60,000		35,000	$5,000			3
4	Feb	45,000	50,000			35,000	$10,000		4
5	Mar	50,000	60,000				35,000		5
6	Apr	45,000	60,000						6
7	May	50,000	65,000						7
8	June	55,000	65,000						8
9	July	40,000	60,000						9
10	Aug	40,000	40,000						10
11	Sept	45,000	40,000					$10,000	11
12	Oct	35,000	45,000					5,000	12
13	Nov	40,000	45,000					25,000	13
14	Dec	45,000	50,000						14
15	Total								15
16	Purchases $530,000								16
17									17
18	Total Cash								18
19	Payments $540,000			$40,000	$55,000	$40,000	$45,000	$40,000	19
20									20
21	Beginning Payables		60,000						21
22									22
23	Budgeted Purchases		530,000						23
24									24
25	Budgeted Cash Disbursements		(540,000)						25
26									26
27	Ending Payables		$50,000						27

Note:
This type of worksheet would be used for all types of payments to creditors on account.
Actual cash payments and accounts payable should be compared to the cash budget monthly to gauge progress.

between accrual accounting and cash management. The administrator who does a good job in cash management will have adequate working capital. Adequate working capital after the initial investment should come from cash flow. Unfortunately, many companies start out undercapitalized and must do a much better job in cash management than if they started with adequate capital. Generally speaking, the nursing home industry is a highly leveraged business which requires very strict management of cash.

Exhibit 6–6 is a graphic example of what happens in a nursing home in terms of cash flow. As you can see the expenditures for supplies, materials, labor, and overhead costs such as interest, depreciation, and administrative expenses are expended first. These expenses are incurred as services are provided. For that a charge is assessed to the patient. In the case of a private patient, the service charge is collected in advance. This is positive cash flow because the collection is made

Cash Flow Budgeting

Exhibit 6-5 Summary Cash Budget

Forecasted Cash Flow

Line No		Total	January	February	March	April	December	Line No
1	Beginning Cash	$100,000	$100,000	$132,800	$156,700	$168,200	$326,400	1
2								2
3								3
4	Cash Receipts Budget	2,690,000	225,800	225,900	206,500	226,900	206,600	4
5								5
6								6
7	Cash Disbursements Budget	2,450,000	193,000	202,000	195,000	208,000	193,000	7
8								8
9								9
10	Ending Cash	340,000	132,800	156,700	168,200	187,100	340,000	10
11								11
12								12
13								13
14	Actual Cash	$	$100,000	$160,000	$	$	$	14
15								15
16	Variance		(32,800)	3,300				16
17								17
18	Analysis of Variance							18
19	Accounts Receivable							19
20	Increase (Over Budget)		20,000					20
21	Decrease (Under Budget)		-	2,000				21
22	Accounts Payable							22
23	Increase (Over Budget)		-	1,300				23
24	Decrease (Under Budget)		12,800					24
25	Other —		-					25
27			$ 32,800	$ 3,300				27

before the expense is incurred. With third-party payers the services are provided, the bill is prepared and submitted to the payer and they pay; someday. This type of cash flow is negative because the cost is incurred and paid for, and collection comes later. This is the reason for working capital. It is to finance the business until the revenue is turned to cash. The discount of customary charges to a level that the Medicare and Medicaid Programs pay is also negative cash flow because the private pay patients charge results in full cash collections. Cash flow planning is the balancing of the cash cycle. As you can see from the exhibits, the quicker you

Exhibit 6-6 Cash Flow Cycle

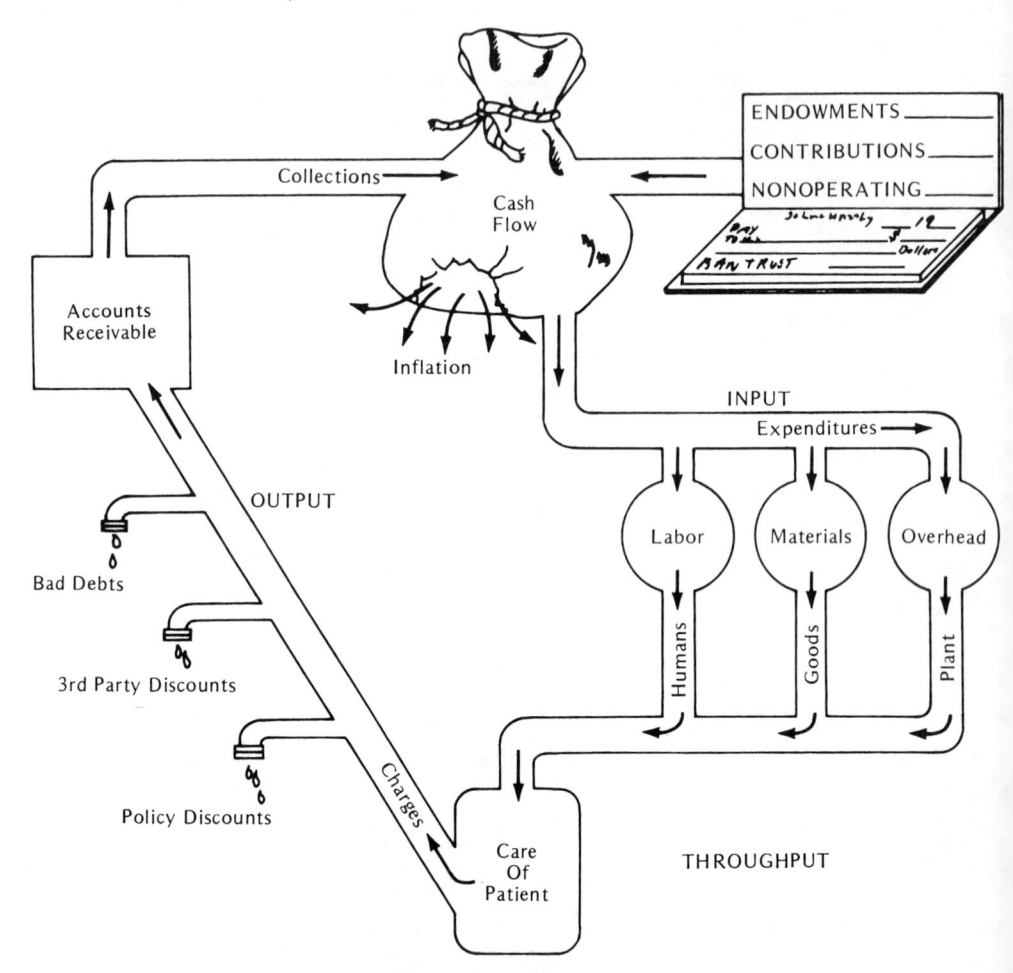

collect the revenue, the more stable the cash position will be. The longer it takes you to assess, submit, and collect the bill, the more unstable the cash position will be and the higher your working capital requirements will be. The return on investment also must be higher in this situation to provide adequate working capital.

CHAPTER 7
Financial Reports

Objectives of Management Reporting

Good management is *on* the minds of many but *in* the minds of only a few. This is a truism that happens to be true. Management needs information to be good. It needs current information to be timely. It needs accurate information to be right. The information should come in systematic and regular stages:

Stage One—Daily	*Stage Two—Monthly*	*Stage Three—Annually*
Productivity	Balance sheet	Financial statements
Revenues	P/L statement	Tax returns
Receipts	Cash flow	Cost reports
Expenses	Production reports	Prospective budget report
Expenditures	Cost analysis report	Prospective pricing structure
Cash balances		

Components of Management Reporting

These reports must be timely to be useful. The following is a rule-of-thumb calendar for timeliness:

STAGE ONE—DAILY

Report	Target Date
Productivity report	By noon of next day
Revenue report	By noon of next day
Cash report	By noon of next day
Payables report	By noon of next day
Staffing report	By 9:00 AM of next day

STAGE TWO—MONTHLY

Report	Target Date
Balance sheet	By 10th of following month
P/L statement	By 10th of following month
Cash flow statement	By 10th of following month
Production report	By end of 1st day of following month
Cost analysis report	By 10th of following month

STAGE THREE—ANNUALLY

Report	Target Date
Financial statements	By end of second month following year-end
Tax returns	By 15th of third month following year-end
Cost reports	By 15th of third month following year-end

150 Basic Accounting and Budgeting for Long-Term Care Facilities

Prospective budget report   Two months before year-end
Prospective pricing structure   One month before year-end

To be effective the reports must be put in the hands of those that can use them. The following is a rule-of-thumb line-up for use of the reports:

STAGE ONE—DAILY

Report	Primary Manager	Secondary Manager
Productivity report	Administrator	Director of nursing
Revenue report	Administrator	Chief accountant
Cash report	Administrator	Chief accountant
Payables	Administrator	Chief accountant
Staffing report	Administrator	Director of nursing

STAGE TWO—MONTHLY

Report	Primary Manager	Secondary Manager
Balance sheet	Administrator*	Chief accountant
P/L statement	Administrator*	Chief accountant
Cash flow statement	Administrator*	Chief accountant
Production report	Administrator	Director of nursing
Cost analysis report	Chief accountant	Administrator

*and the Board of Directors if they meet monthly.

STAGE THREE—ANNUALLY

Report	Primary Manager	Secondary Manager
Financial statements	Board of Directors	Shareholders
Tax returns	Chief accountant	Administrator
Cost reports	Chief accountant	Administrator
Prospective budget	Board of Directors	Administrator
Prospective pricing structure	Board of Directors	Administrator

Stage One—Daily

Productivity reporting must be done daily to be effective. The objective is to control the units going into production at a predetermined level so costs do not outrun the price. In a nursing home this consists of controlling the following:

Production Unit (Input)	Control Device
Nursing hours	Staffing plan and nursing hours report
Housekeeping hours	Staffing plan and hours worked
Maintenance hours	Staffing plan and hours worked

Dietary meals	Count of patient meals and guest meals served
Laundry pounds	Soiled laundry weighed
Production Unit (Output)	*Control Device*
Physical therapy	Report of PT hours or modalities
Medications	Count number of medications administered
Patient days of care	
By payer	Patient billing
By level of care	Patient census

The production quotas should be predetermined in doing the planning for the budget. The closer the planning gets to the actual daily activities the more accurate the estimates will be.

Granted all this takes time, but good management takes effort. However, the results are always, without fail, commensurate to the effort. The pitfall of production scheduling and reporting is that it creates paperwork and paperwork in itself is nonproductive. This can be resolved by assigning the patient production reporting to a ward clerk, who can also be assigned medical recordkeeping duties, and by assigning the employee production reporting to the department head as a part of their administrative responsibilities. (See Exhibits 7–1 through 7–10 for sample reports.)

Ultimately, as the production scheduling and reporting procedures become routine, an incentive system of rewards for the attainment of or the beating of quotas can be implemented. The true accomplishment of cost control is through a practical system of production quotas and incentives that also accomplish patient care objectives.

Stage Two—Monthly

Monthly reporting must be timely to be effective. The objective is to convert productivity reports to financial values which can be used by management to monitor its operations game plan. The reports should be prepared from the accounting records by no later than the tenth of the following month. The monthly reports consist of the following:

Description	*Purpose*
Balance Sheet	Determination of net worth and changes in the assets and liabilities as of a certain date. Demonstrates the turnover rate of assets and the rate of return on those assets.
P/L Statement	Determination of the results of the business enterprise for a particular period of time in relation to the plan for operations. Demonstrates the amount each share of ownership earned.

Cash Flow Statement	Determination of the reasons for the change in the cash balances. Demonstrates the sources of cash and uses of cash in the business cycle.
Production Report	Determination of the degree that potential capacity is being attained. Demonstrates the actual attainment of production to meet quotas that are adequate to produce budgeted revenue.
Cost Analysis Report	Determination of the cost of each unit of service produced. Demonstrates the cost of providing the business' product.
Ratio Analysis Report	Financial analysis of the relationship of the various components of the financial reports.

Financial management is a continuing process. It must be done consistently and systematically if it is to be effective. The accounting system and the management information system (reports) must be up-to-date, accurate, and grouped in such a way that management can understand and use them. See the sample monthly report in Exhibit 7–11.

Financial Ratios

Once the accounting records are of a quality that will allow for the preparation of monthly balance sheets, P/L statements, and cash flow statements, the administrator should expect to receive an analysis of the financial statements. The financial analysis should come in a summary form for concise review by the administrator. The management reports can be condensed, so only the relevant and controllable facts are presented to the administrator. The components for this ratio analysis would be the balance sheet, the rate of return, and the P/L statement. (See Exhibit 7–12 for the formulas.)

I. Balance Sheet
   A. Current ratio
   B. Acid test
   C. Proprietary ratio
   D. Accounts receivable turnover
   E. Inventory turnover
II. Rate of Return
   F. Book value per share
   G. Rate of earnings on total capital
   H. Rate of earnings on proprietary equity
III. P/L Statement
   I. Operating ratio
   J. Number of times fixed charges earned
   K. Net income ratio

Exhibit 7-1 Summary Production Report

Summary Production Report

	Budget Total	January	February	March	First Quarterly Total	Second Quarterly Total	Third Quarterly Total	Fourth Quarterly Total	Annual Total
Routine Nursing Services									
Skilled days— Private Medicare Medicaid									
Intermediate days— Private Medicaid									
Residential days— Private									
Ancillary Service									
Pharmacy prescriptions									
Lab procedures									
Physical therapy hours									
Recreation procedures									
Rehab procedures									
General Services									
Dietary meals									
Laundry pounds									
Housekeeping hours									
Maintenance hours									
Nursing Hours—Skilled									
Registered Licensed Aides									
Nursing Hours Intermediate									
RN LPN Aide									
Nursing Hours—Residential									
LPN Aide									

Exhibit 7-2 Sample Census

DATE	Census on Previous Day Male / Female	Admissions Male / Female	Discharges Male / Female	Transfer Male / Female	Census at End of Day Male / Female	Total Census
1	50 / 68				50 / 68	118
2	50 / 68	Riddle, M			50 / 68	118
3	50 / 68	Waters, L. / Waters, V	Waters, L.		50 / 70	120
4	50 / 70	Waters, L.			51 / 70	121
5	51 / 70		Blome, E.		51 / 71	122
6	51 / 71				51 / 71	122
7	51 / 71			Riddle, M.	51 / 70	121
8	51 / 70				51 / 70	121
9	51 / 70				51 / 70	121
10	51 / 70			Jenkins, M.	51 / 70	121

Average Census — Divide total by days in month
Percent Capacity — Divide average census by capacity

 green — Medicare
 red — Skilled
 circled — Expired
 blue — Intermediate
 black — VA contract

Exhibit 7-2 (cont.)

(5) Intermediate				(6) Skilled				(7) Shelter				(8) Medicare		(9) VA Contract				LINE No.
Private		Medicaid		Private		Medicaid		Private		Medicaid				Intermediate		Skilled		
Beg. Total	End. Total	Beg. Total	End. Total	Beg. Total	End. Total	Beg. Total	End. Total	Beg. Total	End. Total	Beg. Total	End. Total	Beg. Total	End. Total	Beg. Total	End. Total	Beg. Total	End. Total	
35	35	37	37	9	9	28	28	5	5	2	2	-0-	-0-	2	2	-0-	-0-	1
35	35	37	37	9	9	28	28	5	5	2	2	-0-	-0-	2	2	-0-	-0-	2
35	35	37	39	9	9	28	28	5	5	2	2	-0-	-0-	2	2	-0-	-0-	3
35	35	39	40	9	9	28	28	5	5	2	2	-0-	-0-	2	2	-0-	-0-	4
35	36	40	40	9	9	28	28	5	5	2	2	-0-	-0-	2	2	-0-	-0-	5
36	36	40	40	9	9	28	28	5	5	2	2	-0-	-0-	2	2	-0-	-0-	6
36	36	40	39	9	9	28	28	5	5	2	2	-0-	-0-	2	2	-0-	-0-	7
36	36	39	39	9	9	28	28	5	5	2	2	-0-	-0-	2	2	-0-	-0-	8
36	36	39	39	9	9	28	28	5	5	2	2	-0-	-0-	2	2	-0-	-0-	9
36	35	39	39	9	10	28	28	5	5	2	2	-0-	-0-	2	2	-0-	-0-	10

155

Exhibit 7-3 Sample Staffing Plan

STAFFING PLAN

NURSING STATION NO.

FULL-TIME EQUIVALENT STAFF – 3 PM to 11 PM

Day	1	2	3	4	5	6	7	8	9	10	11	12	13	14	15	16	17	18	19	20	21	22	23	24	25	26	27	28	29	30	31	Total Staff	Total Hours
Certified Section																																	
RNs																																	
LPNs																																	
Aides																																	
Totals																																	
Noncertified Section																																	
Skilled																																	
RNs																																	
LPNs																																	
Aides																																	
Intermediate																																	
RNs																																	
LPNs																																	
Aides																																	
Residential																																	
LPNs																																	
Aides																																	
Totals																																	

Exhibit 7-4 Sample Production Record: Nursing

Production Record
Department: Nursing—RNs
Production Unit: Hours

Month	Staffing Hours				Average Labor Rate	Estimated Nursing Costs
	Skilled	Intermediate	Residential	Total		
1						
2						
3						
4						
5						
6						
7						
8						
9						
10						
11						
12						

Note: Budgeted production statistics would be based on prior year actual from this report adjusted for any significant expected change in occupancy.

Exhibit 7-5 Sample Production Record: Housekeeping and Maintenance

Production Record
Department: Housekeeping and Maintenance
Production Unit: Hours

Month	Rooms		Administrative Areas	Physical Therapy	Pharmacy	Beauty and Barber	Total Hours
	Certified	Non Certified					
		SNF / ICF					
1							
2							
3							
4							
5							
6							
7							
8							
9							
10							
11							
12							
Actual							
Budget							

NOTE: This information can be gathered on a sample bais (say one week/quarter).

Exhibit 7-6 Sample Production Record: Dietary

	Production Record				
Department: Dietary					
Production Unit: Meals served					

	Patients		Employee	Guest	Total
Month	Certified	Non Certified			
1		SNF	ICF			
2						
3						
4						
5						
6						
7						
8						
9						
10						
11						
12						
Totals						

NOTE: Budgeted dietary production units would be based on prior year actual from this report adjusted for any significant expected change in occupancy.

Exhibit 7-7 Sample Production Record: Laundry

	Production Record						
Department: Laundry							
Production Unit: Pounds of dirty laundry							

	Certified Section				Non-Certified Section		
Month	Private	Medicare	Medicaid	Total	Private	Medicaid	Total
1							
2							
3							
4							
5							
6							
7							
8							
9							
10							
11							
12							
Totals							

NOTE: Budgeted production statistics would be based on prior year actual from this report adjusted for any significant expected change in occupancy.

Exhibit 7-8 Sample Production Record: Physical Therapy

	Production Record								
Department: Physical therapy								
Production Unit: Treatment Hours								
	Licensed Personnel				Assistants			
Month	Private	Medicare	PA	Total	Private	Medicare	PA	Total
1								
2								
3								
4								
5								
6								
7								
8								
9								
10								
11								
12								
Totals								

NOTE: Budgeted production statistics would be based on prior year actual from this report adjusted for any significant expected change in occupancy.

Exhibit 7-9 Sample Production Record: Pharmacy

	Production Record							
Department: Pharmacy							
Production Unit: Number of Prescriptions							
	Certified Section				Non-Certified Section		
Month	Private	Medicare	PA	Total	Private	Medicaid	Total
1							
2							
3							
4							
5							
6							
7							
8							
9							
10							
11							
12							
Totals							

NOTE: Budgeted production statistics would be based on prior year actual from this report adjusted for any significant expected change in occupancy.

Exhibit 7-10 Sample Patient Census Report

Patient Census Report
Nursing Station No.

*Care	Room No.	Name	1	2	3	4	5	6	7	8	9	10	11	12	13	14	15	16	17	18	19	20	21	22	23	24	25	26	27	28	29	30	31	Resident Days
		Private Pay																																
S	107	John Doe	x	x	x	x	x	x	x	x	x	x	x	x	x	x	x	x	x	x	x	x	x											31
S	108	Mary Doe																						x	x	x	x	x	x	x	x	x	x	10
S	109		x	x	x	x	x	x	x	x	x	x	x	x	x	x	x	x	x	x	x	x	x	x	x	x	x	x	x	x	x	x	x	31
S	110		x	x	x	x	x	x	x	x	x	x	x	x	x	x	x	x	x	x	x	x	x	x	x	x	x	x	x	x	x	x	x	31
I	121		x	x	x	x	x	x	x	x	x	x	x	x	x	x	x	x	x	x	x	x	x	x	x	x	x	x	x	x	x	x	x	31
I	122		x	x	x	x	x	x	x	x	x	x	x	x	x	x	x	x	x	x	x	x	x	x	x	x	x	x	x	x	x	x	x	31
I	123		x	x	x	x	x	x	x	x	x	x	x	x	x	x	x	x	x	x	x	x	x	x	x	x	x	x	x	x	x	x	x	31
I	124						x	x	x																									7
		Total Private	7	7	7	7	7	7	7	6	6	6	6	6	7	7	7	7	7	7	7	7	7	7	6	6	6	6	6	6	6	6	6	203
		PA (Medicaid)																																
S	115		x	x	x	x	x	x	x	x	x	x	x	x	x	x	x	x	x	x	x	x	x	x	x	x	x	x	x	x	x	x	x	31
S	116		x	x	x	x	x	x	x	x	x	x	x	x	x	x	x	x	x	x	x	x												20
I	117		x	x	x	x	x	x	x	x	x	x	x	x	x	x	x	x	x	x	x	x	x	x	x	x	x	x	x	x	x	x	x	31
I	118		x	x	x	x	x	x	x	x	x	x	x	x	x	x	x	x	x	x	x	x	x	x	x	x	x	x	x	x	x	x	x	31
		Total PA	4	4	4	4	4	4	4	4	4	4	4	4	4	4	4	4	4	4	4	4	3	3	3	3	3	3	3	3	3	3	3	113
		Medicare																																
S	130		x	x	x	x	x	x	x	x	x	x																						10
S	131		x	x	x	x	x	x	x	x	x	x	x	x	x	x	x	x	x	x	x	x	x	x	x	x	x	x	x	x	x	x	x	31
S	132		x	x	x	x	x	x	x	x	x	x	x	x	x	x	x	x	x	x	x	x	x	x	x	x	x	x	x	x	x	x	x	31
S	133		x	x	x	x	x	x	x	x	x	x	x	x	x	x	x	x	x	x	x	x	x	x	x	x	x	x	x	x	x	x	x	31
S	134		x	x	x	x	x	x	x	x	x	x	x	x	x	x	x	x	x	x	x	x	x	x	x	x	x	x	x	x	x	x	x	31
S	135																					x	x	x	x	x	x	x	x	x	x	x	x	20
		Total Medicare	6	6	6	6	6	6	6	6	6	6	5	5	5	5	5	5	5	5	5	5	4	4	4	4	4	4	4	4	4	4	4	154
		Totals	17	17	17	17	17	17	17	16	16	16	15	15	16	16	16	16	16	16	16	16	14	14	13	13	13	13	13	13	13	13	13	470

* Level of Care
I Intermediate
S Skilled

Exhibit 7-11 Sample Balance Sheet and Statements of Income and Cash Flow

J. L. Rhoads & Co., P.C.

Queenwood Professional Building
81 E. Queenwood Road Morton, Illinois 61550

Telephone 309/266-7686

Retirement Village, Inc.
BOARD OF DIRECTORS

    The accompanying balance sheet of Retirement Village, Inc., as of 5/31/80 and the related statements of income and cash flow for the period then ended have been compiled by us.

    A compilation is limited to presenting, in the form of financial statements, information that is the representation of management. We have not audited or reviewed the accompanying financial statements and, accordingly, do not express an opinion or any other form of assurance on them.

    Management has elected to omit substantially all of the disclosures, including a statement of fund balance and changes in financial position, required by generally accepted accounting principles. If the omitted disclosures were included in the financial statements, they might influence the user's conclusions about the company's financial position, results of operations, and changes in financial position. Accordingly, these financial statements are not designed for those who are not informed about such matters.

                                           J. L. RHOADS & CO., P.C.
                                           Certified Public Accountants

Morton, Illinois
6/23/80

RETIREMENT VILLAGE, INC.

Accounting Period: 05

Page 1

BALANCE SHEET
5/31/80

	5/31/80	4/30/80	Increase (Decrease)
ASSETS			
CURRENT ASSETS			
Cash	$227,766.36	$44,309.49	$183,456.87
Savings Accts. & C.D.s	$439,139.52	$449,475.69	($10,336.17)
Marketable Securities	$12,618.38	$12,618.38	$0.00
Unexpended Bond Proceeds	$66,105.61	$64,249.36	$1,856.25
Accts. Rec.—Private Patients	$86,739.82	$62,717.66	$24,022.16
Accts. Rec.—Medicaid	$51,125.01	$42,536.05	$8,588.96
Accts. Rec.—Medicaid Pending	$2,440.50	$7,880.84	($5,440.34)
Accts. Rec.—Other	$0.00	$0.00	$0.00
Hill-Burton Receivable	$8,194.00	$8,194.00	$0.00
Real Estate Contracts Rec.	$7,058.87	$7,107.79	($48.92)
Physician Fees - Clearing	$40,238.48	$35,275.27	$4,963.21
Accrued Interest Receivable	$927.50	$927.50	$0.00
Unexpired Insurance	$1,779.75	$1,779.75	$0.00
TOTAL CURRENT ASSETS	$944,133.80	$737,071.78	$207,062.02
CAPITAL ASSETS			
Land	$96,017.50	$96,017.50	$0.00
Land Improvements	$25,172.43	$25,172.43	$0.00
Buildings	$5,085,287.42	$5,087,287.42	($2,000.00)
Equipment	$879,261.56	$878,776.32	$485.24
Less Accumulated Depreciation	($1,503,365.29)	($1,488,457.29)	($14,908.00)
Construction in Progress	$280,161.31	$210,185.51	$69,975.80
Bond Consultation Fees	$54,143.65	$54,143.65	$0.00
TOTAL CAPITAL ASSETS	$4,916,678.58	$4,863,125.54	$53,553.04
TOTAL ASSETS	$5,860,812.38	$5,600,197.32	$260,615.06

162

RETIREMENT VILLAGE, INC.

Accounting Period: 05

BALANCE SHEET
5/31/80

	5/31/80	4/30/80	Increase (Decrease)
LIABILITIES AND CAPITAL			
LIABILITIES			
CURRENT LIABILITIES			
Notes Payable - Current	$0.00	$0.00	$0.00
Mortgages Payable - Current	$28,878.70	$33,379.82	($4,501.12)
Bonds Payable - Current	$0.00	$0.00	$0.00
Accounts Payable - Trade	$84,894.22	$43,476.35	$41,417.87
Payroll Deductions	$459.44	$321.88	$137.56
Accr. Salaries & Wages Pay.	$53,519.97	$88,851.75	($35,331.78)
Payroll Taxes	($106.68)	($126.09)	$19.41
Accrued Interest Payable	$68,228.72	$68,228.72	$0.00
Due To/From Guests Trust Funds	$16,022.91	$16,144.39	($121.48)
Burial Funds Payable	$9,000.00	$9,000.00	$0.00
Unfulfilled Entrance Fees Pay.	($964.30)	$30,000.00	($30,964.30)
Deferred Annuity Gifts	$68,801.83	$68,801.83	$0.00
TOTAL CURRENT LIABILITIES	$328,734.81	$358,078.65	($29,343.84)
LONG-TERM LIABILITIES			
Notes Payable - Term	$0.00	$0.00	$0.00
Mortgages Payable - Term	$691,229.02	$691,229.02	$0.00
Bonds Payable - Term	$1,083,324.00	$1,047,474.00	$35,850.00
Life Care Commitment	$2,061,705.94	$2,104,141.77	($42,435.83)
TOTAL LONG-TERM LIABILITIES	$3,836,258.96	$3,842,844.79	($6,585.83)
TOTAL LIABILITIES	$4,164,993.77	$4,200,923.44	($35,929.67)
CAPITAL			
Village Equity	$2,265,448.47	$2,017,809.60	$247,638.87
Reserve - Life Care Commit.	($775,175.21)	($775,175.21)	$0.00
Net Income (Loss)	$205,545.35	$156,639.49	$48,905.86
TOTAL CAPITAL	$1,695,818.61	$1,399,273.88	$296,544.73
TOTAL LIABILITIES AND CAPITAL	$5,860,812.38	$5,600,197.32	$260,615.06

Accounting Period: 05

RETIREMENT VILLAGE, INC.
INCOME STATEMENT

Page 1

	CURRENT PERIOD 5/1/80 - 5/31/80 Amount	Per Patient Day	YEAR - TO - DATE 1/1/80 - 5/31/80 Amount	Per Patient Day
PATIENT SERVICES REVENUE				
SHELTERED CARE				
Holden Center	$37,711.44	$4.11	$205,233.80	$4.58
TOTAL SHELTERED CARE	$37,711.44	$4.11	$205,233.80	$4.58
SKILLED CARE				
Wesley I	$17,425.40	$1.90	$114,946.23	$2.57
Wesley I—Medicaid Pending	$4,594.71	$0.50	$12,475.55	$0.28
Wesley II	$41,861.39	$4.57	$181,107.76	$4.04
Dycus	$14,467.87	$1.58	$87,623.60	$1.96
TOTAL SKILLED CARE	$78,349.37	$8.55	$396,153.14	$8.84
INTERMEDIATE CARE				
Wesley I	$36,857.16	$4.02	$167,980.42	$3.75
Wesley II	$901.29	$0.10	$16,366.10	$0.37
Dycus	$21,261.27	$2.32	$91,447.99	$2.04
Holden Center	$0.00	$0.00	$0.00	$0.00
TOTAL INTERMEDIATE CARE	$59,019.72	$6.44	$275,794.51	$6.16
ANCILLARY SERVICES				
Physical Therapy	$785.50	$0.09	$3,834.50	$0.09
Speech Therapy	$0.00	$0.00	$90.14	$0.00
Occupational Therapy	$0.00	$0.00	$0.00	$0.00
Medical Supplies	$91.56	$0.01	$598.79	$0.01
Drugs	$66.60	$0.01	$313.20	$0.01
Oxygen	$0.00	$0.00	$0.00	$0.00
Physicians Fees	$270.00	$0.03	$1,500.00	$0.03
Other Medical	$0.00	$0.00	$264.40	$0.01
TOTAL ANCILLARY SERVICES	$1,213.66	$0.13	$6,601.03	$0.15
LESS UNCOMPENSATED CARE				
Uncompensated Care—Cont. Fees	($18,338.91)	($2.00)	($119,530.16)	($2.67)
Cost Adj—Life Care Commitment	($15,456.00)	($1.69)	($38,640.00)	($0.86)
Recognized Rev—Life Care Com.	$57,891.83	$6.31	$144,729.59	$3.23
Medicare Discount	$0.00	$0.00	$0.00	$0.00
Patient Refunds	$0.00	$0.00	$0.00	$0.00
TOTAL UNCOMPENSATED CARE	$24,096.92	$2.63	($13,440.57)	($0.30)

164

Accounting Period: 05

RETIREMENT VILLAGE, INC.
INCOME STATEMENT

	CURRENT PERIOD 5/1/80 - 5/31/80 Amount	Per Patient Day	YEAR - TO - DATE 1/1/80 - 5/31/80 Amount	Per Patient Day
TOTAL PATIENT SERVICES REVENUE	$200,391.11	$21.86	$870,341.91	$19.43
Independent Living Revenue	$3,688.00	$0.40	$24,070.89	$0.54
Other Operating Revenue	$4,098.00	$0.45	$14,349.77	$0.32
TOTAL OPERATING REVENUE	$208,177.11	$22.70	$908,762.57	$20.28
OPERATING EXPENSE				
HEALTH CARE SERVICES				
Holden Center (Sheltered Care)	$43,611.48	$4.76	$173,776.10	$3.88
Wesley I	$38,431.26	$4.19	$133,714.17	$2.98
Wesley II	$70,163.94	$7.65	$282,051.44	$6.30
Dycus	$39,048.34	$4.26	$164,722.67	$3.68
Holden Center (Intermediate Care)	$178.13	$0.02	$413.29	$0.01
Nursing Administration	$4,156.30	$0.45	$22,238.24	$0.50
Social Rehabilitation	$4,772.83	$0.52	$21,543.39	$0.48
Physical Rehabilitation	$2,567.27	$0.28	$12,314.67	$0.27
Speech Rehabilitation	$0.00	$0.00	$400.00	$0.01
Apartments	$5,326.31	$0.58	$24,733.07	$0.55
Cottages	$3,797.46	$0.41	$16,465.86	$0.37
TOTAL HEALTH CARE SERVICES	$212,053.32	$23.13	$852,372.90	$19.02
Support Services (Unallocated)	($1,358.11)	($0.15)	$43,970.76	$0.98
TOTAL SUPPORT SERVICES (UNALLOCATED)	($1,358.11)	($0.15)	$43,970.76	$0.98
CAPITAL COSTS				
Depreciation	$8,643.00	$0.94	$43,215.00	$0.96
Interest	$4,226.88	$0.46	$45,568.70	$1.02
TOTAL CAPITAL COSTS	$12,869.88	$1.40	$88,783.70	$1.98
Other Operating Expense	$1,197.38	$0.13	$14,378.84	$0.32
TOTAL OPERATING EXPENSE	$224,762.47	$24.51	$999,506.20	$22.31
NET INCOME (LOSS) FROM OPERATIONS	($16,585.36)	($1.81)	($90,743.63)	($2.03)

Accounting Period: 05

RETIREMENT VILLAGE, INC.

INCOME STATEMENT

Page 3

	CURRENT PERIOD 5/1/80 - 5/31/80 Amount	Per Patient Day	YEAR - TO - DATE 1/1/80 - 5/31/80 Amount	Per Patient Day
NON-OPERATING INCOME / EXPENSE				
Investment Earnings	$5,322.66	$0.58	$12,244.12	$0.27
Special Gifts-Wills & Bequests	$0.00	$0.00	$0.00	$0.00
Conference Apportionment—Reg.	$5,910.25	$0.64	$24,437.78	$0.55
Conference Apport. - Special	$9,349.19	$1.02	$84,537.48	$1.89
Special Gifts—All Other	$44,208.95	$4.82	$169,744.73	$3.79
Donated Oil Royalty Income	$578.17	$0.06	$3,994.73	$0.09
Bake Sales & Bazaars	$0.00	$0.00	$618.60	$0.01
Other	$122.00	$0.01	$711.54	$0.02
TOTAL NON-OPERATING INCOME (EXPENSE)	$65,491.22	$7.14	$296,288.98	$6.61
NET INCOME (LOSS)	$48,905.86	$5.33	$205,545.35	$4.59
Patient Days	9,169		44,803	

166

RETIREMENT VILLAGE, INC.

Accounting Period: 05

STATEMENT OF CASH FLOW

Page 1

	CURRENT PERIOD 5/1/80 - 5/31/80	YEAR-TO-DATE 1/1/80 - 5/31/80
CASH—BEGINNING BALANCE:		
Cash In Bank - Operating	$24,558.10	$51,357.87
Cash In Bank - Building	$640.96	$640.96
Cash In Bank - Gift Shop	$1,856.04	$1,856.04
Cash In Bank - Trust Funds	$15,894.39	$7,900.00
Petty Cash Funds - Trust Fund	$250.00	$5,974.77
Petty Cash Funds - Operating	$1,110.00	$1,110.00
Imprest Payroll	($0.00)	$0.00
TOTAL CASH—BEGINNING BALANCE	$44,309.49	$68,839.64
NET INCOME (LOSS)	$48,905.86	$205,545.35
ADD EXPENSES REQUIRING NO OUTLAY OF CASH:		
Acc. Depr.—Land Improvements	$105.00	$525.00
Acc. Depr.—Bldgs.—Original	$2,250.00	$11,250.00
Acc. Depr.—Bldgs.—New	$2,052.00	$10,260.00
Acc. Depr.—Bldgs.—Dycus	$1,528.00	$7,640.00
Acc. Depr.—Cottages	$1,283.00	$6,415.00
Acc. Depr.—Bldgs.—Houses	$199.00	$995.00
Acc. Depr.—Bldgs.—Apartments	$660.00	$3,300.00
Acc. Depr.—Bldgs.—House Tr.	$24.00	$120.00
Acc. Depr.—Bldgs.—Wesley Ctr	$14.00	$70.00
Acc. Depr.—Bldg. Improvements	$1,261.00	$6,305.00
Acc. Depr.—Equip.,Furn & Fix.	$4,200.00	$21,000.00
Acc. Depr.—Home & Cott. Furn.	$586.00	$2,930.00
Acc. Depr.—Apartment Furn.	$150.00	$750.00
Acc. Depr.—Office Equipment	$78.00	$390.00
Acc. Depr.—Trans. Equipment	$518.00	$2,590.00
TOTAL NON-CASH EXPENSES	$14,908.00	$74,540.00
TOTAL CASH FROM OPERATIONS	$63,813.86	$280,085.35
OTHER SOURCES (USES) OF CASH		
Savings Account - Prudential	$0.00	$0.00
Savings Account - Building	$0.00	$3,200.00
Savings Account - Bonds	$10,336.17	$25,359.28
Savings Account - Chapel	$0.00	$0.00
Investment - C.D.s	$0.00	($81,300.00)
Investment - Burial C.D.s	$0.00	$2,000.00
Investment - Stocks	$0.00	$1,425.00
Investment - Bonds	$0.00	$0.00
Reserve For Bond Redemption	($1,856.25)	($58,635.62)
Accts. Rec.—Private Patients	($24,022.16)	$12,079.58
Accts. Rec.—Medicaid	($8,588.96)	($51,125.01)
Accts. Rec.—Medicaid Pending	$5,440.34	($2,440.50)
Accts. Rec.—Other	$0.00	$0.00
Hill-Burton Receivable	$0.00	$0.00

Accounting Period: 05

RETIREMENT VILLAGE, INC.
STATEMENT OF CASH FLOW

Page 2

	CURRENT PERIOD 5/1/80 - 5/31/80	YEAR-TO-DATE 1/1/80 - 5/31/80
Real Estate Contracts Rec.	$48.92	$81,647.27
Physician Fees - Clearing	($4,963.21)	($40,238.48)
Accrued Interest Receivable	$0.00	$0.00
Unexpired Insurance	$0.00	$593.25
Land	$0.00	$0.00
Land Improvements	$0.00	$0.00
Buildings - Original	$0.00	$0.00
Buildings - New	$0.00	$0.00
Buildings - Dycus	$0.00	$0.00
Buildings - Cottages	$0.00	$0.00
Buildings - Houses	$2,000.00	$2,000.00
Buildings - Apartments	$0.00	$0.00
Buildings - House Trailer	$0.00	$0.00
Buildings—Wesley Ctr.—8 Bed	$0.00	$0.00
Building Improvements	$0.00	($50.00)
Equip., Furniture & Fixtures	($178.00)	($1,794.25)
Home and Cottage Furnishings	$0.00	($2,121.30)
Apartment Furnishings	$0.00	($1,235.00)
Office Equipment	($307.24)	($4,654.41)
Transportation Equipment	$0.00	$1,055.00
Constr. In Progress—General	($45,442.19)	($124,366.22)
Constr. In Progress—Basement	($49.12)	($19,390.60)
Constr. In Progress—1st Floor	($3,191.44)	($10,597.32)
Constr. In Progress—2nd Floor	($3,433.21)	($11,039.96)
Constr. In Progress—3rd Floor	($17,589.16)	($40,172.78)
Constr. In Progress—Attic	($270.68)	($287.18)
Bond Consultation Fees	$0.00	$0.00
Notes Payable - Current	$0.00	($274,500.00)
Mortgages Payable - Current	($4,501.12)	($22,246.30)
Bonds Payable - Current	$0.00	$0.00
Accounts Payable - Trade	$41,417.87	$21,401.63
Hospitalization Ins. Payable	$0.00	$0.00
Group Life Ins. Payable	$79.56	$418.83
Wage Assignments	$0.00	$0.00
Payroll Deduction - Bonds	$0.00	$0.00
Employees Pension Fund Payable	$0.00	$0.00
Tax Sheltered Annuities Pay.	$58.00	$8.00
Accr. Salaries & Wages Pay.	($35,331.78)	$23,958.97
FICA Taxes Payable	$0.00	($41.06)
Federal Income Taxes Pay.	$0.00	($25.14)
Illinois Income Taxes Pay.	$19.41	($40.48)
State U.C. Taxes Payable	$0.00	($7,739.56)
Accrued Interest Payable	$0.00	$18,628.61
Due To/From Guests Trust Funds	($121.48)	($1,051.86)
Burial Funds Payable	$0.00	$0.00
Unfulfilled Entrance Fees Pay.	($30,964.30)	($964.30)
Deferred Annuity Gifts	$0.00	$0.00
Notes Payable - Term	$0.00	$0.00
Mortgages Payable - Term	$0.00	$0.00

RETIREMENT VILLAGE, INC.

STATEMENT OF CASH FLOW

Accounting Period: 05

	CURRENT PERIOD 5/1/80 - 5/31/80	YEAR-TO-DATE 1/1/80 - 5/31/80
Bonds Payable - Term	$35,850.00	$329,574.00
Life Care Commitment	($42,435.83)	($106,089.59)
Village Equity	$247,638.87	$247,638.87
Reserve - Life Care Commit	$0.00	($30,000.00)
TOTAL OTHER SOURCES (USES) OF CASH	$119,643.01	($121,158.63)
NET INCREASE (DECREASE) OF CASH	$183,456.87	$158,926.72
CASH—ENDING BALANCE		
Cash In Bank - Operating	$208,136.45	$208,136.45
Cash In Bank - Building	$640.96	$640.96
Cash In Bank - Gift Shop	$1,856.04	$1,856.04
Cash In Bank - Trust Funds	$15,772.91	$15,772.91
Petty Cash Funds - Trust Fund	$250.00	$250.00
Petty Cash Funds - Operating	$1,110.00	$1,110.00
Imprest Payroll	($0.00)	($0.00)
TOTAL CASH—ENDING BALANCE	$227,766.36	$227,766.36

RETIREMENT VILLAGE, INC.
INDEPENDENT LIVING

Accounting Period: 05

INCOME STATEMENT

	CURRENT PERIOD 5/1/80 – 5/31/80		YEAR – TO – DATE 1/1/80 – 5/31/80	
	Amount	Per Patient Day	Amount	Per Patient Day
INDEPENDENT LIVING REVENUE				
Apartments	$2,428.00	$1.43	$20,290.89	$2.37
Cottages	$1,260.00	$0.74	$3,780.00	$0.44
TOTAL INDEPENDENT LIVING REVENUE	$3,688.00	$2.17	$24,070.89	$2.81
OPERATING EXPENSE				
Standard Meal Cost	$812.70	$0.48	$4,564.20	$0.53
Housekeeping Salaries	$190.67	$0.11	$1,064.45	$0.12
Housekeeping Supplies	$0.00	$0.00	$0.00	$0.00
Personal Laundry Expense	$0.00	$0.00	$0.00	$0.00
Maintenance Work Order Expense	$119.47	$0.07	$1,700.12	$0.20
Utilities	$1,313.34	$0.77	$8,745.34	$1.02
Television Expense	$76.84	$0.05	$252.28	$0.03
Training & Education	$0.00	$0.00	$0.00	$0.00
Administrative Overhead	$2,003.29	$1.18	$4,356.68	$0.51
Depreciation – Apartments	$810.00	$0.48	$4,050.00	$0.47
Standard Meal Cost	$0.00	$0.00	$0.00	$0.00
Housekeeping Salaries	$0.00	$0.00	$0.00	$0.00
Housekeeping Supplies	$0.00	$0.00	$0.00	$0.00
Personal Laundry Expense	$0.00	$0.00	$0.00	$0.00
Maintenance Work Order Expense	$133.12	$0.08	$797.81	$0.09
Utilities	$1,112.45	$0.66	$7,199.58	$0.84
Television Expense	$38.48	$0.02	$242.44	$0.03
Training & Education	$0.00	$0.00	$0.00	$0.00
Administrative Overhead	$1,423.41	$0.84	$2,776.03	$0.32
Depreciation – Cottages	$1,090.00	$0.64	$5,450.00	$0.64
TOTAL OPERATING EXPENSE	$9,123.77	$5.38	$41,198.93	$4.82
NET INCOME (LOSS) FROM OPERATIONS	($5,435.77)	($3.21)	($17,128.04)	($2.00)

Patient Days—Independent Living   1,696   8,556

RETIREMENT VILLAGE, INC.
RESIDENTIAL -- SHELTERED CARE

Accounting Period: 05

INCOME STATEMENT

	CURRENT PERIOD 5/1/80 - 5/31/80 Amount	Per Patient Day	YEAR - TO - DATE 1/1/80 - 5/31/80 Amount	Per Patient Day
SHELTERED CARE REVENUE				
Holden Center - Private	$32,634.24	$13.65	$183,808.44	$15.25
Holden Center - Medicaid	$5,077.20	$2.12	$21,425.36	$1.78
TOTAL SHELTERED CARE REVENUE	$37,711.44	$15.77	$205,233.80	$17.03
OPERATING EXPENSE				
R.N. Salaries & Wages	$792.64	$0.33	$1,376.35	$0.11
LPN Salaries & Wages	$1,680.41	$0.70	$10,275.52	$0.85
Aides & Orderlies Sal. & Wages	$796.68	$0.33	$5,331.74	$0.44
Nursing Supplies	$0.00	$0.00	$0.00	$0.00
Oxygen Expense	$0.00	$0.00	$0.00	$0.00
Drugs	$0.00	$0.00	$0.00	$0.00
Medical Supplies	$0.00	$0.00	$0.00	$0.00
Administrative Overhead	$16,387.87	$6.85	$32,648.91	$2.71
Physicians' Services	$0.00	$0.00	$0.00	$0.00
Standard Meal Cost	$10,869.51	$4.55	$55,811.59	$4.63
Housekeeping Salaries	$2,074.42	$0.87	$11,218.81	$0.93
Housekeeping Supplies	$281.33	$0.12	$605.39	$0.05
Personal Laundry Expense	$143.97	$0.06	$769.19	$0.06
Maintenance Work Order Expense	$1,001.28	$0.42	$4,736.12	$0.39
Utilities	$5,218.37	$2.18	$29,029.88	$2.41
Television Expense	$0.00	$0.00	$147.60	$0.01
Training & Education	$0.00	$0.00	$0.00	$0.00
Depreciation	$4,365.00	$1.83	$21,825.00	$1.81
TOTAL OPERATING EXPENSE	$43,611.48	$18.24	$173,776.10	$14.42
NET INCOME (LOSS) FROM OPERATIONS	($5,900.04)	($2.47)	$31,457.70	$2.61

Patient Days—Residential & Sheltered Care   2,391   12,053

RETIREMENT VILLAGE, INC.
NURSING CARE
INCOME STATEMENT

Accounting Period: 05

	CURRENT PERIOD 5/1/80 - 5/31/80		YEAR - TO - DATE 1/1/80 - 5/31/80	
	Amount	Per Patient Day	Amount	Per Patient Day
PATIENT SERVICES REVENUE				
SKILLED CARE				
Wesley I - Private	$14,452.48	$2.84	$82,773.87	$3.42
Wesley I - Medicaid	$2,972.92	$0.58	$32,172.36	$1.33
Wesley II - Private	$18,283.50	$3.60	$78,948.50	$3.26
Wesley II - Medicaid	$23,577.89	$4.64	$102,159.26	$4.22
Dycus - Private	$10,744.00	$2.11	$64,320.25	$2.66
Dycus - Medicaid	$3,723.87	$0.73	$23,303.35	$0.96
TOTAL SKILLED CARE	$73,754.66	$14.51	$383,677.59	$15.86
INTERMEDIATE CARE				
Wesley I - Private	$25,411.79	$5.00	$116,721.50	$4.82
Wesley I - Medicaid	$11,445.37	$2.25	$51,258.92	$2.12
Wesley II - Private	$0.00	$0.00	$899.00	$0.04
Wesley II - Medicaid	$901.29	$0.18	$15,467.10	$0.64
Dycus - Private	$8,468.00	$1.67	$40,919.00	$1.69
Dycus - Medicaid	$12,793.27	$2.52	$50,528.99	$2.09
Holden Center - Private	$0.00	$0.00	$0.00	$0.00
Holden Center - Medicaid	$0.00	$0.00	$0.00	$0.00
TOTAL INTERMEDIATE CARE	$59,019.72	$11.61	$275,794.51	$11.40
ANCILLARY SERVICES				
Physical Therapy	$785.50	$0.15	$3,834.50	$0.16
Speech Therapy	$0.00	$0.00	$90.14	$0.00
Occupational Therapy	$0.00	$0.00	$0.00	$0.00
Medical Supplies	$91.56	$0.02	$598.79	$0.02
Drugs	$66.60	$0.01	$313.20	$0.01
Oxygen	$0.00	$0.00	$0.00	$0.00
Physicians Fees	$270.00	$0.05	$1,500.00	$0.06
Other Medical	$0.00	$0.00	$264.40	$0.01
TOTAL ANCILLARY SERVICES	$1,213.66	$0.24	$6,601.03	$0.27
TOTAL PATIENT SERVICES REVENUE	$133,988.04	$26.37	$666,073.13	$27.53
LESS UNCOMPENSATED CARE				
Uncompensated Care—Cont Fees	($18,338.91)	($3.61)	($119,530.16)	($4.94)
Cost Adj—Life Care Commitment	($15,456.00)	($3.04)	($38,640.00)	($1.60)
Recognized Rev—Life Care Com.	$57,891.83	$11.39	$144,729.59	$5.98

172

Accounting Period: 05

RETIREMENT VILLAGE, INC.
NURSING CARE
INCOME STATEMENT

Page 2

	CURRENT PERIOD 5/1/80 - 5/31/80		YEAR - TO - DATE 1/1/80 - 5/31/80	
	Amount	Per Patient Day	Amount	Per Patient Day
Medicare Discount	$0.00	$0.00	$0.00	$0.00
Patient Refunds	$0.00	$0.00	$0.00	$0.00
TOTAL UNCOMPENSATED CARE	$24,096.92	$4.74	($13,440.57)	($0.56)
NET PATIENT SERVICES REVENUE	$158,084.96	$31.11	$652,632.56	$26.97

HEALTH CARE SERVICES
WESLEY I

R.N. Salaries & Wages	$0.00	$0.00	$0.00	$0.00
L.P.N. Salaries & Wages	$0.00	$0.00	$0.00	$0.00
Aides & Orderlies Sal. & Wages	$0.00	$0.00	($39.00)	($0.00)
Nursing Supplies	$0.00	$0.00	$0.00	$0.00
Oxygen Expense	$103.60	$0.02	$1,039.02	$0.04
Drugs	$6,034.23	$1.19	$15,405.33	$0.64
Medical Supplies	$1,091.55	$0.21	$6,471.90	$0.27
Training & Education	$0.00	$0.00	$0.00	$0.00
Administrative Overhead	$14,444.83	$2.84	$28,079.59	$1.16
Physicians' Services	$0.00	$0.00	$0.00	$0.00
Utilities	$2,985.84	$0.59	$16,612.66	$0.69
Laundry Expense	$1,281.57	$0.25	$6,146.60	$0.25
Housekeeping Salaries	$2,614.37	$0.51	$11,841.32	$0.49
Television Expense	$53.16	$0.01	$325.66	$0.01
Standard Meal Cost	$8,747.26	$1.72	$42,962.23	$1.78
Personal Laundry Expense	$79.01	$0.02	$431.37	$0.02
Maintenance Work Order Expense	$598.26	$0.12	$3,673.30	$0.15
TOTAL WESLEY I	$38,033.68	$7.48	$132,949.98	$5.50

WESLEY II

R.N. Salaries & Wages	$7,011.37	$1.38	$35,398.07	$1.46
L.P.N. Salaries & Wages	$2,551.38	$0.50	$13,310.64	$0.55
Aides & Orderlies Sal. & Wages	$21,335.09	$4.20	$105,522.93	$4.36
Nursing Supplies	$0.00	$0.00	$0.00	$0.00
Oxygen Expense	$0.00	$0.00	$0.00	$0.00
Drugs	$0.00	$0.00	$0.00	$0.00
Medical Supplies	$0.00	$0.00	$0.00	$0.00
Training & Education	$0.00	$0.00	$0.00	$0.00
Administrative Overhead	$26,374.24	$5.19	$60,742.85	$2.51
Physicians' Services	$0.00	$0.00	$0.00	$0.00
Utilities	$2,057.52	$0.40	$11,437.45	$0.47
Laundry Expense	$1,823.04	$0.36	$9,769.36	$0.40

RETIREMENT VILLAGE, INC.
NURSING CARE

Accounting Period: 05

INCOME STATEMENT

	CURRENT PERIOD 5/1/80 - 5/31/80		YEAR - TO - DATE 1/1/80 - 5/31/80	
	Amount	Per Patient Day	Amount	Per Patient Day
Housekeeping Salaries	$1,544.11	$0.30	$7,589.56	$0.31
Television Expense	$38.20	$0.01	$404.37	$0.02
Standard Meal Cost	$6,391.48	$1.26	$33,257.17	$1.37
Personal Laundry Expense	$146.27	$0.03	$731.75	$0.03
Maintenance Work Order Expense	$532.82	$0.10	$3,249.26	$0.13
TOTAL WESLEY II	**$69,805.52**	**$13.74**	**$281,413.41**	**$11.63**
DYCUS				
R.N. Salaries & Wages	$2,231.30	$0.44	$12,855.08	$0.53
L.P.N. Salaries & Wages	$1,627.01	$0.32	$7,816.55	$0.32
Aides & Orderlies Sal. & Wages	$7,693.77	$1.51	$43,908.87	$1.81
Nursing Supplies	$0.00	$0.00	$0.00	$0.00
Oxygen Expense	$0.00	$0.00	$0.00	$0.00
Drugs	$0.00	$0.00	$0.00	$0.00
Medical Supplies	$0.00	$0.00	$0.00	$0.00
Training & Education	$0.00	$0.00	$0.00	$0.00
Administrative Overhead	$14,678.29	$2.89	$34,023.75	$1.41
Physicians' Services	$0.00	$0.00	$0.00	$0.00
Utilities	$2,052.95	$0.40	$11,428.32	$0.47
Laundry Expense	$1,407.47	$0.28	$6,803.41	$0.28
Housekeeping Salaries	$1,657.61	$0.33	$8,784.34	$0.36
Television Expense	$34.12	$0.01	$161.22	$0.01
Standard Meal Cost	$6,593.58	$1.30	$33,776.88	$1.40
Personal Laundry Expense	$84.61	$0.02	$347.33	$0.01
Maintenance Work Order Expense	$754.54	$0.15	$4,355.93	$0.18
TOTAL DYCUS	**$38,815.25**	**$7.64**	**$164,261.68**	**$6.79**
HOLDEN CENTER (3rd FLOOR)				
R.N. Salaries & Wages	$0.00	$0.00	$0.00	$0.00
L.P.N. Salaries & Wages	$0.00	$0.00	$0.00	$0.00
Aides & Orderlies Sal. & Wages	$0.00	$0.00	$0.00	$0.00
Nursing Supplies	$0.00	$0.00	$0.00	$0.00
Oxygen Expense	$0.00	$0.00	$0.00	$0.00
Drugs	$0.00	$0.00	$0.00	$0.00
Medical Supplies	$0.00	$0.00	$0.00	$0.00
Training & Education	$0.00	$0.00	$0.00	$0.00
Administrative Overhead	$0.00	$0.00	$0.00	$0.00
Physicians' Services	$0.00	$0.00	$0.00	$0.00
Utilities	$0.00	$0.00	$0.00	$0.00
Laundry Expense	$0.00	$0.00	$0.00	$0.00
Housekeeping Salaries	$0.00	$0.00	$0.00	$0.00
Television Expense	$167.40	$0.03	$317.68	$0.01

RETIREMENT VILLAGE, INC.
NURSING CARE
INCOME STATEMENT

Accounting Period: 05

Page 4

	CURRENT PERIOD 5/1/80 - 5/31/80 Amount	Per Patient Day	YEAR - TO - DATE 1/1/80 - 5/31/80 Amount	Per Patient Day
Standard Meal Expense	$0.00	$0.00	$0.00	$0.00
Personal Laundry Expense	$0.00	$0.00	$0.00	$0.00
Maintenance Work Order Expense	$10.73	$0.00	$95.61	$0.00
TOTAL HOLDEN CENTER (3rd FLOOR)	$178.13	$0.04	$413.29	$0.02
NURSING ADMINISTRATION				
Nursing Admin. Sal. & Wages	$3,626.43	$0.71	$18,833.90	$0.78
Medical Records Salaries	$529.87	$0.10	$2,814.33	$0.12
In-Service Training Salaries	$0.00	$0.00	$440.01	$0.02
Medical Director	$0.00	$0.00	$0.00	$0.00
Medical Records Consultant	$0.00	$0.00	$150.00	$0.01
Utilization Review Fees	$0.00	$0.00	$0.00	$0.00
Office Supplies & Expense	$0.00	$0.00	$0.00	$0.00
Training & Education	$0.00	$0.00	$0.00	$0.00
TOTAL NURSING ADMINISTRATION	$4,156.30	$0.82	$22,238.24	$0.92
REHABILITATION SERVICES				
Activities Salaries & Wages	$4,022.81	$0.79	$19,381.98	$0.80
Social Rehab. Salaries & Wages	$0.00	$0.00	$0.00	$0.00
Activity Consultants	$125.00	$0.02	$250.00	$0.01
Social Service Consultants	$0.00	$0.00	$375.00	$0.02
Supplies & Expense	$193.62	$0.04	$902.83	$0.04
Religious Supplies & Expense	($5.50)	($0.00)	$44.18	$0.00
Training & Education	$162.88	$0.03	$315.38	$0.01
Maintenance Work Order Expense	$274.02	$0.05	$274.02	$0.01
Physical Therapy Aides Sal.	$1,343.91	$0.26	$6,201.26	$0.26
Physical Therapy Assist. Sal.	$915.33	$0.18	$4,950.23	$0.20
Physical Therapy Consultants	$300.00	$0.06	$1,100.00	$0.05
Physical Rehab. Supplies	$0.00	$0.00	$0.00	$0.00
Training & Education	$0.00	$0.00	$0.00	$0.00
Maintenance Work Order Expense	$0.00	$0.00	$0.00	$0.00
Laundry Expense	$8.03	$0.00	$63.18	$0.00
Speech Therapy Salaries	$0.00	$0.00	$0.00	$0.00
Speech Therapy Consultants	$0.00	$0.00	$400.00	$0.02
Speech Therapy Supplies	$0.00	$0.00	$0.00	$0.00
Training & Education	$0.00	$0.00	$0.00	$0.00
Maintenance Work Order Expense	$0.00	$0.00	$0.00	$0.00
TOTAL REHABILITATION SERVICES	$7,340.10	$1.44	$34,258.06	$1.42
TOTAL HEALTH CARE SERVICES	$158,328.98	$31.15	$635,534.66	$26.27

RETIREMENT VILLAGE, INC.
NURSING CARE
INCOME STATEMENT

Accounting Period: 05

	CURRENT PERIOD 5/1/80 - 5/31/80 Amount	Per Patient Day	YEAR - TO - DATE 1/1/80 - 5/31/80 Amount	Per Patient Day
SUPPORT SERVICES				
DIETARY				
Kitchen Salaries & Wages	$16,749.33	$3.30	$87,791.43	$3.63
Dietary Consultant	$150.00	$0.03	$600.00	$0.02
Food Costs	$14,679.16	$2.89	$75,419.31	$3.12
Supplies	$1,866.14	$0.37	$6,818.26	$0.28
Training & Education	$0.00	$0.00	$38.00	$0.00
Maintenance Work Order Expense	$0.00	$0.00	$0.00	$0.00
Laundry Expense	$50.91	$0.01	$324.17	$0.01
LESS: Meal Cost Allocation	($33,414.53)	($6.58)	($170,372.07)	($7.04)
TOTAL DIETARY	$81.01	$0.02	$619.10	$0.03
HOUSEKEEPING				
Housekeeping Salaries & Wages	$889.94	$0.18	$4,621.96	$0.19
Housekeeping Supplies	$654.35	$0.13	$4,527.10	$0.19
Maintenance Work Order Expense	$41.12	$0.01	$41.12	$0.00
TOTAL HOUSEKEEPING	$1,585.41	$0.31	$9,190.18	$0.38
LAUNDRY				
Laundry Salaries & Wages	$3,818.14	$0.75	$19,815.12	$0.82
Laundry Supplies & Soaps	$1,269.44	$0.25	$4,180.46	$0.17
Linens	$0.00	$0.00	$873.15	$0.04
Training & Education	$0.00	$0.00	$0.00	$0.00
Maintenance Work Order Expense	$21.20	$0.00	$21.20	$0.00
Utilities	$477.85	$0.09	$3,166.94	$0.13
LESS: Personal Laundry Cost Alloc.	($5,024.88)	($0.99)	($25,386.36)	($1.05)
TOTAL LAUNDRY	$561.75	$0.11	$2,670.51	$0.11
MAINTENANCE				
Maintenance Salaries & Wages	$936.15	$0.18	$1,909.81	$0.08
Maintenance Supplies	$1,113.35	$0.22	$4,342.18	$0.18
Training & Education	$0.00	$0.00	$20.00	$0.00
Purchased Repairs & Maint.	$11,137.25	$2.19	$15,021.76	$0.62
Other Television Expense	$0.00	$0.00	$22.37	$0.00
LESS: Work Order Cost Alloc.	$0.00	$0.00	$0.00	$0.00
TOTAL MAINTENANCE	$13,186.75	$2.59	$21,316.12	$0.88
UTILITIES				
Electricity & Gas	$13,605.16	$2.68	$79,779.35	$3.30

RETIREMENT VILLAGE, INC.
NURSING CARE
INCOME STATEMENT

Accounting Period: 05

	CURRENT PERIOD 5/1/80 - 5/31/80 Amount	Per Patient Day	YEAR - TO - DATE 1/1/80 - 5/31/80 Amount	Per Patient Day
Water	$1,290.16	$0.25	$6,871.82	$0.28
Garbage Services	$173.00	$0.03	$865.00	$0.04
Pest Control	$150.00	$0.03	$600.00	$0.02
LESS: Utilities Cost Allocation	($15,218.32)	($2.99)	($87,620.17)	($3.62)
TOTAL UTILITIES	$0.00	$0.00	$496.00	$0.02
ADMINISTRATION				
Administrator's Salary	$1,373.29	$0.27	$3,411.05	$0.14
Directory of Ministry Salary	$2,043.98	$0.40	$10,615.42	$0.44
Office & Recep. Sal. & Wages	$6,063.47	$1.19	$25,584.77	$1.06
Office Supplies & Expense	$1,145.46	$0.23	$2,453.62	$0.10
Bank Charges	$0.00	$0.00	$0.00	$0.00
Office Equipment Rental	$0.00	$0.00	$0.00	$0.00
Printing & Forms	$418.32	$0.08	$1,904.87	$0.08
Data Processing Costs	$174.13	$0.03	$567.70	$0.02
Postage	$401.81	$0.08	$1,000.27	$0.04
Telephone	$695.02	$0.14	$3,379.32	$0.14
Dues & Subscriptions	$39.15	$0.01	$316.49	$0.01
Advertising & Promotion	$1,676.29	$0.33	$7,603.07	$0.31
Auto & Truck Expense	$802.13	$0.16	$5,194.98	$0.21
Travel	$44.88	$0.01	$905.23	$0.04
Dir. of Ministry Travel & Exp.	$148.83	$0.03	$1,232.73	$0.05
Training & Education	$395.00	$0.08	$395.00	$0.02
Licenses, Permits & Fees	$14.50	$0.00	$14.50	$0.00
Insurance - Fire & Casualty	$0.00	$0.00	$0.00	$0.00
Insurance - Liab. & Malpractice	$0.00	$0.00	$5,048.00	$0.21
Insurance - Other	$2,262.20	$0.45	$2,855.45	$0.12
Conference Expense	$0.00	$0.00	$47.50	$0.00
Methodist Foundation	$500.00	$0.10	$2,000.00	$0.08
Legal Fees	$10,245.31	$2.02	$12,839.68	$0.53
Auditing Fees	$0.00	$0.00	$0.00	$0.00
Management Consultants	$6,063.90	$1.19	$30,245.71	$1.25
Bond Expense	$18.78	$0.00	$424.48	$0.02
Miscellaneous Expense	$374.95	$0.07	$2,001.23	$0.08
Maintenance Work Order Expense	$0.00	$0.00	$0.00	$0.00
LESS: Administration Cost Allocation	($59,739.97)	($11.76)	($130,544.90)	($5.40)
TOTAL ADMINISTRATION	($24,838.57)	($4.89)	($10,503.83)	($0.43)
EMPLOYEE BENEFITS				
Payroll Taxes - FICA	$8,673.64	$1.71	$31,086.35	$1.28
State U.C.	$0.00	$0.00	$32.40	$0.00
Hospitalization Insurance	$0.00	$0.00	$0.00	$0.00

RETIREMENT VILLAGE, INC.
NURSING CARE

Accounting Period: 05

INCOME STATEMENT

Page 7

	CURRENT PERIOD 5/1/80 - 5/31/80		YEAR - TO - DATE 1/1/80 - 5/31/80	
	Amount	Per Patient Day	Amount	Per Patient Day
Workmen's Compensation Ins.	$5,600.00	$1.10	$5,295.15	$0.22
Employee Pension Plan	$483.40	$0.10	$3,691.36	$0.15
Moving Expenses	$0.00	$0.00	$900.00	$0.04
Director of Ministry Housing	$300.00	$0.06	$1,200.00	$0.05
Administrator's Housing	$499.92	$0.10	$1,249.79	$0.05
Employee Physicals	$15.00	$0.00	$745.00	$0.03
LESS: Employee Benefits Cost Alloc.	($15,571.96)	($3.06)	($32,082.91)	($1.33)
TOTAL EMPLOYEE BENEFITS	$0.00	$0.00	$12,117.14	$0.50
TOTAL SUPPORT SERVICES	($9,423.65)	($1.85)	$35,905.22	$1.48

CAPITAL COSTS
DEPRECIATION

Depr. - Land Improvements	$105.00	$0.02	$525.00	$0.02
Depr. - Bldgs. - Nursing Care	$5,844.00	$1.15	$29,220.00	$1.21
Depr. - Bldg. Improvements	$1,261.00	$0.25	$6,305.00	$0.26
Depr. - Equip., Furn. & Fix.	$4,200.00	$0.83	$21,000.00	$0.87
Depr. - Office Equipment	$78.00	$0.02	$390.00	$0.02
Depr. - Transportation Equip.	$518.00	$0.10	$2,590.00	$0.11
LESS: Depr. - Cost Allocation	($6,265.00)	($1.23)	($31,325.00)	($1.29)
TOTAL DEPRECIATION	$5,741.00	$1.13	$28,705.00	$1.19

INTEREST

Interest Exp. - Notes Payable	$0.00	$0.00	$2,715.00	$0.11
Interest Expense - Mortgage	$4,226.88	$0.83	$21,393.70	$0.88
Interest Expense - Bonds	$0.00	$0.00	$21,460.00	$0.89
TOTAL INTEREST	$4,226.88	$0.83	$45,568.70	$1.88
TOTAL CAPITAL COSTS	$9,967.88	$1.96	$74,273.70	$3.07
NET INCOME (LOSS) FROM OPERATIONS	($788.25)	($0.16)	($93,081.02)	($3.85)

Patient Days—Nursing Care		5,082		24,194

178

A. CURRENT RATIO
The formula for the derivation of the current or working capital ratio is:
$$\frac{\text{Current assets}}{\text{Current liabilities}}$$
This relationship is important to the short-term creditor, as it measures the borrower's ability to meet current obligations. A ratio of 200 percent or 2 to 1 was long considered satisfactory regardless of the industry. In recent years, the use of this standard as a measurement of short-term debt paying ability has been refined.

The development of standard ratios for individual industries has led to the comparison of the individual company to the industry average. Working capital requirements also vary between businesses and between periods in a particular company. At the same time, recognition has been given to the importance of defining current assets as a measure of current financial strength.

The current ratio is affected by the inclusion or exclusion of specific items. The classification of short-term prepayments is a case in point. Bankers and credit analysts tend to exclude prepayments on the premise that such items ordinarily are not converted into cash during the ordinary operations of a business. Accountants, on the other hand, include prepayments on the theory that if prepayments are not paid in advance, they will require the use of current assets during the next operating cycle. The desire to present a favorable working capital position sometimes leads to "window dressing." For example, the current ratio can be improved by holding the cash book open beyond the closing date which shows more cash for the liquidation of current liabilities.

B. ACID TEST
The formula for this ratio is:
$$\frac{\text{Cash + Marketable securities + Net receivables}}{\text{Current liabilities}}$$
The acid test ratio, also called the quick ratio or the quick current ratio, measures the *immediate solvency* or debt-paying ability of a company. A ratio of 1 to 1 is usually considered adequate, since it indicates that for every dollar of current debt there is one dollar of quick assets which can be converted into cash on short notice to meet current obligations. Only securities that can readily be converted to cash should be included in the acid test ratio.

C. EQUITY (PROPRIETARY) RATIO
The formula for this ratio is:
$$\frac{\text{Stockholders' equity}}{\text{Total liabilities + Stockholders' equity}}$$
It is frequently termed the worth-debt ratio when calculated as:
$$\frac{\text{Stockholders' equity (or } net\ worth\text{)}}{\text{Total debt (or } current\ and\ long\text{-}term\ liabilities\text{)}}$$
This ratio is one of the most important and is considered by many analysts as ranking with the current ratio in indicating credit strength. It is of great use in measuring the capital structure and the long-run solvency of a company. The

general principle to be kept in mind is that debt should be kept within limits so the business can face an adverse business depression without fear of insolvency.

The current ratio should be considered along with the proprietary ratio, particularly over an extended period. A high current ratio may not be what it seems if the company is leaning too heavily on borrowed funds to get the operating capital it needs. There is a certain point when it is relatively unimportant whether long-term capital investment is represented by borrowings or stock. The more stable the industry, the greater the amount of *debt financing* that may be done with safety. Nevertheless, the larger the proprietary ratio, the stronger the financial condition. It is significant that lending institutions have refused to sanction borrowing if it increases an already relatively high ratio of debt to total capital employed.

Subsidiary ratios computed to indicate the ratio of current assets to stockholders' equity and the ratio of plant (fixed assets) to stockholders' equity are not normally significant.

Exhibit 7-12

CONDENSED BALANCE SHEET

Assets

1. Cash
2. Temporary Investments
3. Receivables (Net)
4. Inventories
5. Prepayments
6.   Total Current Assets
7. Long-Term Investments
8. Plant and Equipment (Net)
9. Intangibles
10.   Total Assets

Liabilities and Stockholders' Equity
11. Notes Payable
12. Accounts Payable
13. Accruals
14. Deferred Income
15.   Total Current Liabilities
16. Bonds Payable
17. Mortgages Payable
18.   Total Liabilities
19. Capital Stock, Common
20. Paid-in Capital
21. Appropriated Retained Earnings
22. Unappropriated Retained Earnings
23.   Total Stockholders' Equity
24.   Total Liabilities and Stockholders' Equity

CONDENSED P/L STATEMENT

25. Net Revenues
26. Contractual Allowances
27. Operating Expenses
28. Operating Income
29. Other Income and Deductions
30. Net Income
31. Capital Costs
32. Income Taxes
33. Net Income

I. Balance Sheet Ratios	II. Rate of Return Ratios	III. P/L Statement Ratios
A. Current ratio: 6 ÷ 15	G. Rate of earnings on total capital employed: 30 ÷ 24; or (30 − 32) ÷ 24	I. Operating ratio: (26 + 27) ÷ 25
B. Acid test ratio: (1 + 2 + 3) ÷ 15		J. Number of times fixed charges earned: (30 − 32) ÷ 31
C. Proprietary ratio: 23 ÷ 24	H. Rate of earnings on proprietary equity: 33 ÷ 23	
D. Book value per share: 23 ÷ shares outstanding.		K. Net income ratio: (33 + 32) ÷ 25
E. Number of days' sales in receivables: 3 ÷ 25, times number of days cover by P/L statement		
F. Merchandise turnover 26 ÷ average inventory		

D. NUMBER OF DAYS' REVENUE IN RECEIVABLES

This relationship is calculated by dividing revenue by receivables. A more significant comparison is obtained by using the following formula:

$$\frac{\text{Accounts receivable}}{\text{Net credit revenue}} \times 365$$

The computation gives a rough estimate of the average length of time accounts are outstanding. This gives a measure for efficiency in handling the *investment in receivables*. Overinvestment in receivables may result from:

1. An overly liberal credit policy.
2. Laxity in collections.
3. Failure to write off bad accounts.

E. TURNOVER OF INVENTORY

Inventory turnover or stock-turn is derived from the formula:

$$\frac{\text{Inventory expensed}}{\text{Average inventory of supplies}}$$

or

$$\frac{\text{Revenue from supplies}}{\text{Average inventory of supplies}}$$

The figure gives the number of times the stock is replaced during a given period. It is usually stated as number of times per year. A turnover of four times per year might be stated as three months. The comparison affords a valuable indication of *inventory control*. A relatively slow turnover may mean overinvestment in merchandise, while a rapid turnover contributes favorably to working capital, because it converts physical assets to cash.

There is a normal period for each industry in which stocks should be sold and turned into cash or receivables. Carrying goods beyond this period means that extra financial burdens are incurred which must be covered out of profit.

F. BOOK VALUE PER SHARE

The owner's dollar equity in the net assets of a company is measured by the book value per share of outstanding stock. The formula for this ratio is:

$$\frac{\text{Stockholders' equity}}{\text{Number shares outstanding}}$$

Book value represents the amount payable to each share if the business is liquidated and the amount realized on the sale of assets is exactly equal to the values reported on the balance sheet. Thus, book value is essentially a *liquidation concept* based on *going-concern values*. However, as Finney and Miller point out, book value has little significance as an indicator of actual liquidating value since the balance sheet is not expressed in realizable values or as a measure of the value of the shares of a going concern. The latter is greatly affected by profits. Book value also does not mean market or par value.

When there is only one class of stock, book value is determined by dividing the total stockholders' equity by the number of shares outstanding. When more than one class of stock is outstanding, the computation becomes more involved as the rights of each class must be considered in light of the articles of incorporation and state laws.

G. RATE OF EARNINGS ON TOTAL CAPITAL EMPLOYED

One formula for this ratio is:

$$\frac{\text{Total net business income \textit{(before interest and income taxes)}}}{\text{Total liabilities} + \text{Stockholders' equity \textit{(or total assets)}}}$$

The numerator of the ratio should be restricted to operating income, and capital invested in nonoperating assets should be excluded from the denominator.

This ratio provides an indication of the economic productivity of capital. It is a measure of the earning power of the corporation as a business entity. As such it provides a *standard measure of operating efficiency,* which may be applied regardless of the type of business. An important variation of this ratio is the *rate of earnings on invested capital,* determined by dividing total net corporate income by stockholders' equity plus long-term liabilities. This ratio represents earning power from the standpoint of the suppliers of capital (both borrowed and invested) excluding income taxes.

The rate of earnings on stockholders' equity is frequently expressed in terms of *earnings per share* by dividing net income to stockholders by the number of shares of stock outstanding.

H. RATE OF EARNINGS ON STOCKHOLDERS' EQUITY

The ratio is derived as follows:

$$\frac{\text{Net income to stockholders}}{\text{Stockholders' equity \textit{(including appropriations of retained earnings)}}}$$

This comparison is also referred to as the profits-worth ratio. It is a measure of the earning power of the business from the proprietary or stockholders' point of view.

Cost of borrowed capital (interest) and the share of earnings taken by income and profits taxes have been deducted; the remainder of income is available for reinvestment or for distribution to owers.

In the single proprietorship or partnership, this computation (after deduction of appropriate amount for salaries) gives the imputed *yield on owners' investment*. The percentage remaining after deducting the prevailing interest rate for borrowed long-term capital would be the rate of excess earnings which might be attributed to managerial ability. In the case of a corporation having only one class of stock, the investor can make use of this ratio to measure the attractiveness of the stock as an investment.

I. OPERATING RATIO
This ratio is derived by:

$$\frac{\text{Total operating expenses (excluding capital costs)}}{\text{Net revenue}}$$

Total operating expenses include all costs—salaries, supplies, and operating overhead. This comparison is a significant *index of operating efficiency*. This ratio should ideally be used for each department. Together with the corresponding ratio of operating income to capital employed, it will measure the ultimate success of operations.

J. NUMBER OF TIMES FIXED CHARGES EARNED
The formula used for this ratio is:

$$\frac{\text{Total net corporate income less income taxes}}{\text{Interest and depreciation charges}}$$

Net business income after deduction of income taxes gives the amount of earnings accruing to creditor-investors and stockholders as a group. The fixed charges on borrowed and invested capital include interest and depreciation for the period. This ratio can also be calculated using earnings before income taxes.

This ratio is a measure of the financial strength of an organization, thus indicating the desirability of the company as an investment. A stable ratio is as desirable as a high one.

A variation of this ratio is termed the "margin of safety." This is computed by dividing the remainder of net income after interest by the amount of net income available for interest.

A calculation of "number of times fixed charges earned" may be made including required dividends on preferred stock. The needs of stockholders, however, are more often met by a separate calculation showing the *number of times dividends earned*. This ratio may be computed for each class of stock carrying regular dividend payments.

K. RATIO OF NET INCOME TO REVENUE
The formula for this ratio is:

$$\frac{\text{Net income to stockholders (before income taxes)}}{\text{Net revenue}}$$

This ratio measures the rate of return on net revenue. The percentage indicates the number of cents which remain of each dollar after considering all income statement items, excluding income taxes.

To many, a high rate of return on net revenue is necessary for successful operations. This view is not entirely sound. To evaluate properly the significance of the ratio, consideration should be given to such factors as the volume, the total capital employed, and the turnover of total assets. A low rate of return combined with rapid turnover and large sales volume may result in satisfactory earnings. The nursing home industry is an example of a slow turnover of assets and moderately low sales volume which requires a higher rate of return.

SUMMARY

A ratio in itself is meaningless. It becomes significant only when compared to a standard. The standard may be only a general mental conception of what is adequate or normal, or one gained by analysis from past experience. Standards are of two principal types—standards *internally* developed and those *externally* developed.
1. Ratios of the industry of which the company is a member.
2. Ratios of competing companies.
3. Past experience.
4. General relationships based on observation and past experience.

INTERNAL STANDARDS

Past performance provides the principal basis for the construction of internal standards. They are of greatest significance in regulating the operating efficiency of an enterprise. They provide:
1. Measures by which to gauge the success of past operations.
2. Guides by which to regulate present performance.
3. Goals by which to set future estimates.

Thus the development of internal standards is intimately tied to budget control.

In cost accounting and budgeting, internal standards are used as a means of control and as indicators of the quality of performance. It is also possible to set up standards to control receivables, inventories, fixed assets, capitalization, and profits of a business. Through the use of such standards, management can be told why the various relationships regarded as being important are not at the percentage levels at which they were anticipated. These serve as a measuring device to call attention to abnormalities. The two methods of analysis are very closely related. The budget is being used to control detailed operations, while the use of standard ratios attempts to make sure certain profit-making relationships are maintained. Internal standard ratios that are soundly set up from standard costs or budgets provide an accurate type of standard for comparison purposes.

EXTERNAL STANDARDS

The strength and success of an organization is based on how well it can compete in the marketplace. External standard ratios should be the indicator of how well a business is competing.

The principal weakness of external standards lies in the fact that comparisons should be made only between things which are comparable. Standard ratios are fairly comparable only when:

1. A large number of financial reports for the same fiscal period are available.
2. The organizations furnishing the reports are financially sound.
3. The organizations operate under similar geographic conditions.
4. Reports are of recent date.
5. Deviations of the individual ratios from the average ratio are not too great.
6. Accounting methods throughout the industry are substantially uniform.
7. Business policies which influence ratios are substantially uniform.
8. Services handled or produced and sold are substantially similar.

The most serious difficulty in the development of dependable standard ratios lies in the degree of *incomparability of the original data.*

Financial Analysis

BALANCE SHEET

A company's balance sheet (Exhibit 7–13) tells you the results of the business endeavor from inception to the present time. It represents the equity position of the business for all transactions to date. Therefore, it is the indicator of the long-run stability of the business, taking into consideration the short-run results that are shown on the P/L statement. The primary stability indicators on the balance sheet generally are:

- Working capital (current assets less current liabilities)
- Investment in capital assets (plant and equipment)
- Equity capital (equity investment plus or minus the profit or loss from the business)
- Debt capital (long- and short-term financing)

WORKING CAPITAL

The time it takes to convert the product or services produced to cash requires capital. Generally the production comes before the sale and the cash paid out comes before the cash is collected; to finance this period of time a business needs working capital. Working capital is the excess of current assets (cash, accounts receivable, and inventory) over current liabilities (accounts payable and short-term debt). In other words, a business needs to pay its payroll and its bills currently, prior to the collection for the sale of its product. If it is not capable of paying its bills on a timely basis, the success potential of the business is impaired.

Exhibit 7-13 Sample Balance Sheet

Statement 1
Nursing Center, Inc.
Balance Sheet
November 30, 1976

Assets

Current Assets			
Cash on hand		$ 500 (2)	
Patient's Accounts Receivable	$ 82,551		
Less—Estimated doubtful accounts	1,000	81,551 (2)	(9)
Supply inventories, at cost		9,883(10)	
Prepaid expenses		4,472	$ 96,406 (1)
Long Term Investment, at Cost			2,250
Property and Equipment, at Cost			
Land		$ 27,790	
Land improvements	$ 15,527		
Buildings	859,197		
Equipment	202,347		
Total Historical Cost	$1,077,071		
Accumulated depreciation	491,295	585,976	613,766 (4)
Total Assets			$712,422 (5)
Restricted Cash Held in Escrow for Patients			$ 5,976

Liabilities and Equity Capital

Current Liabilities			
Bank overdraft		$ 1,539	
Accounts Payable		9,538	
Current portion of long term debt		5,844	
Accrued salaries		3,546	
Accrued property taxes		24,209	
Accrued interest		773	
Accrued insurance		74	
Income taxes		7,000	$ 52,523 (1)
			(2)
Long Term Liabilities			
Notes payable		$ 76,644	
Mortgage note payable less			
current portion shown above		185,974	262,618 (3)
Equity Capital			
Capital stock	$200,000		
Paid-in capital	12,150		
Treasury stock	(75,000)	$137,150	

Retained earnings
　Beginning of period　　　　　　　　　　$230,016
　Net income for the period　　　　　　　　30,115　　　　260,131　　　397,281 (3)
　　Total Liabilities and Equity Capital　　　　　　　　　　　　　　　$712,422

Patient's Funds Held in Escrow　　　　　　　　　　　　　　　　　　$ 5,976

Highlights
(1) *Current ratio* ($96,406 ÷ $52,533) = 1.84
(2) *Acid test* ($81,551 + 500 ÷ $52,533) = 1.56
(3) *Debt to equity ratio* ($262,618 ÷ $397,281) = 66%
(4) *Net fixed investment turnover rate* ($904,500 ÷ $613,766) = 1.47; *Gross fixed investment turnover rate* ($904,500 ÷ $1,007,071 = .87)
(5) *Total asset turnover rate* ($904,500 ÷ $712,422) = 1.27; before depreciation ($904,500 ÷ [$712,422 + $491,295]) = .75
(6) *Return on total investment* (debt and equity) ($30,115 ÷ $376,875 × 1.47) = 11.75%; ($30,115 ÷ $376,875 × 1.27) = 10.16%; ($30,115 ÷ $376,875 × .75) = 5.99%
(7) *Return on equity investment* ($30,115 = $7,000 + $8,158 ÷ $376,875 × 1.47) = 17.76%; ($45,273 ÷ $376,875 × 1.27) = 15.24%
(8) *Debt service coverage* ($30,115 + $18,572 + $3,158 = $56,845 × 12/5 = $136,428 ÷ $47,953) = 2.85
(9) *Days revenue in accounts receivable* ($376,185 ÷ 153 days = $2,458 revenue per day $81,551 ÷ $2,458 = 33 days revenue in accounts receivable)
(10) *Inventory turnover rate* ($93,500 supply purchases ÷ $9,883 = 9.46)

The amount of working capital (cash, inventory, accounts receivable minus accounts payable) required varies from business to business. Bankers feel comfortable with twice as much in current assets as in current liabilities. This rule of thumb is not rigid but has validity for the nursing home business which is high in labor costs and low in capital costs.

The amount of working capital needed also is related to the business objectives and philosophy. For example, if the objective was to show a rapid growth in earnings, the decision might be to sell more services by expanding the services offered. This would increase the amount of accounts receivable and, most likely, the capital investment. To finance this growth long-term borrowing must be negotiated. In doing this the working capital and borrowings have increased to expand revenue and earnings. This type of strategy is only successful if the accounts receivable are collected so the borrowings can be repaid. The manner in which the amount of working capital is determined and the ratio of current assets to current liabilities follows:

　Current assets (those expected to be used in one year)
　　Cash　　　　　　　　　　　　　　　　　　　　　　$20,000
　　Accounts receivable　　　　　　　　　　　　　　　　80,000
　　Inventory　　　　　　　　　　　　　　　　　　　　100,000
　　　　　　　　　　　　　　　　　　　　　　　　　　$200,000

Current liabilities (those expected to be paid in one year)
Accounts payable   (20,000)
Short-term debt   (80,000)
Working capital $100,000

Current ratio $\dfrac{\$200,000}{\$100,000} = 2 \text{ to } 1$

INVESTMENT IN CAPITAL ASSETS

The amount that has been invested in a business can be determined from its balance sheet. That investment will normally consist of:

- Property
- Plant
- Equipment
- Working capital

The manner in which the business investment is financed is very important to the success of the business. In other words, the more stable the financing, the more stable the potential of success. The investment is normally financed as follows:

- Equity capital (owners' capital in the form of cash or inventory)
- Borrowed capital (debt capital in the form of bank loans or owners' loans)
- Short-term credit (in the form of vendors' accounts payable)

The more the investment amounts to, the higher the amount of profit margin required to return to the business adequate cash to reward investors. The reward is commonly called dividends or *return on investment*. The degree of the reward to investors is a function of the profit margin and its relationship to the amount of the investment. For example, a business with a very low capital investment can pay a higher *rate* of return to investors than can the business with a high capital investment, if the profit margins as a percent of sales are the same.

		Company A	Company B
Revenue		$1,000,000	$2,000,000
Cost		900,000	1,800,000
Profit Margin		$100,000	$200,000
	% of sales	10%	10%
Value of investment		$1,000,000	$4,000,000
Return on investment		10%	5%

In this example, Company B, with the higher investment in relation to sales, must generate a higher percentage profit margin, if it is expected to compete with Company A in the investment market.

The investment in capital assets is normally subject to deterioration and eventually the capital investment must be replaced. In other words, a plant gets old and will need to be rebuilt. This loss of useful value is called depreciation. Depreciation expense represents the amount of capital that is needed to come out of revenues to replace capital assets. This is sometimes referred to by economists as return *of* investment. In an accounting sense, depreciation represents the amount that would be required to replace the same asset at its original cost. This is called accounting depreciation or historical depreciation.

Economists and financial analysts adjust the historical depreciation for the inflation factor. In other words, they adjust the accounting depreciation expense for the change in the value of the dollar and any significant change in technology since the date of purchase. This is done to determine profitability after economic depreciation. For example:

	Historical Cost	Replacement Cost
Plant	$1,000,000	$2,000,000
Equipment	500,000	1,000,000
	$1,500,000	$3,000,000
Historical depreciation		
Plant (50-year life)	$20,000	
Equipment (10-year life)	50,000	
	$70,000	
Economic depreciation		
Plant (50-year life)		$40,000
Equipment (10-year life)		140,000

The difference of $110,000 represents the economic depreciation expense that *must* come out of business revenues, either now or later, if the business is to continue.

In theory the economic depreciation is as much a cost of doing business as payroll and purchases and must be recognized as such. In practice businesses many times ignore this factor and assume that it will be covered out of retained earnings or covered by additional financing at a later date. In sound business circles, economic depreciation is taken into consideration in establishing product prices and restraint in paying dividends, so retained earnings can be accumulated to cover the economic costs.

If the business is mainly labor intensive with little capital investment, inflation is a factor that is absorbed each period and economic depreciation is not as relevent.

EQUITY CAPITAL

The amount that the owners (investors) put into the business in the form of cash, goods or services, represents the equity capital in the business. The results of the business' activity from inception to the date of the balance sheet are the retained earnings. The equity and retained earnings less all dividends paid to date represent the total capital still in the business. For example:

Equity capital		$100,000
Retained earnings	$500,000	
Less dividends	(200,000)	300,000
Total capital of business		$400,000

DEBT CAPITAL

The amount that the owners borrow to help finance the business is called debt capital. The borrowings can be short-term or long-term. Generally, the short-term (to be repaid within one year) financing will be unsecured or secured by uncollected accounts receivable and/or inventory on hand. The debt incurred to finance working capital is the most common short-term financing. The long-term (to be repaid over a period in excess of a year) financing will almost always be secured by mortgages on the property, plant, or equipment being financed. Long-term financing, therefore, is almost always used to acquire capital assets.

The interest expense paid on the borrowings is called the debt service and the principal payment is called debt reduction.

SUMMARY

The analysis of the balance sheet should answer the following questions:
- Is there adequate working capital?
- What is the value of the investment and what is the return on that investment?
- How much equity capital is in the business and how much total capital is still in the business?
- What is the return on equity investment?
- What is the amount of debt capital in relation to the equity capital?
- Can the debt service and debt reduction be paid out of the company's accumulated capital after dividends?

If these questions can be answered, the long-run financial stability of the business can pretty well be predicted. See the sample balance sheet in Exhibit 7–14.

CASH FLOW STATEMENT

The cash flow statement (Exhibit 7–15) is the summation of the business transactions resulting in an increase or decrease in the cash balance of the company. For example, let's review a cash flow statement of a company that is making a profit but is in a cash bind.

Profit for the year	$100,000
Adjustment for items not requiring cash	
Depreciation	100,000
Amortization	50,000
	$250,000
Increase in accounts receivable	(50,000)
Decrease in inventory	100,000
	$300,000
Decrease in accounts payable	200,000
Cash provided by operations	$100,000

Debt principal payment	(200,000)
Purchase of equipment	(300,000)
Bank loans	100,000
Additional equity investment	200,000
Decrease in cash for the year	$(100,000)
Cash at beginning of year	50,000
Cash at end of year	$(50,000)

This example demonstrates why cash flow analysis is the best method for analyzing a business' liquidity. In other words, can the business effectively convert the fruits of its labor into cash in a timely manner? Since it takes cash to pay the bills and run the business, this type of analysis is probably the most important indicator of business success.

In this case the business is in jeopardy if it cannot arrange for short-term financing. An in-depth analysis would probably show that not enough capital was put into the business to finance the capital investment and profits are not sufficient to cover the debt service, debt reduction, and purchase of equipment.

P/L STATEMENT

A nursing home's P/L statement tells you what has happened in the business during the accounting period it covers. In theory, it tells you the amount of revenue made by the facility, the expenses it incurred, and the profit which resulted. It shows the results of the equity investment for one year. It is often called the transition of the equity investment, transition meaning the continuation of a going business concern from one operating period to the next.

Income statements are supposed to be prepared in accordance with generally accepted accounting principles (GAAP). However, certain accounting methods can distort the performance of the business. The astute administrator knows what the P/L statement reveals and what it obscures about the operations of his business and knows how to use the P/L statement to assess his facility's profitability. Also, the astute analyst can evaluate the results of a business operation through financial analysis. The following is an explanation of the financial analysis of the P/L statement.

FINANCIAL ACCOUNTING STRATEGY

A well-run nursing home has a definite strategy. It also has a *financial accounting strategy,* which is usually designed to *make it appear* that management is achieving its business objectives. Suppose, for instance, that a company has rapid growth in earnings as its principal objective. By choosing to recognize revenue as soon as possible and to defer accrual of expenses as long as possible, management can increase reported profits, even though the cash flow of the firm is unchanged. Thus, the business can be made to appear to be growing faster than it really is, at least temporarily.

Financial accounting strategy is often also designed to make a company appear to behave as investors would prefer it to behave. For example, investors as a group will pay a higher relative price for the shares of a company which has a stable

Exhibit 7-14 Sample Balance Sheet

Assets	1977	1976	Increase (Decrease)
Current Assets:			
Cash	$(50,000)	$ 50,000	$(100,000)
Accounts receivable less allowance for bad debts	150,000	100,000	50,000
Inventory	100,000	200,000	(100,000)
Marketable securities	25,000	25,000	—
Prepaid expenses	10,000	10,000	—
Total current assets	$ 235,000	$ 385,000	$(150,000)
Capital Assets:			
Land	$ 100,000	$ 100,000	$ —
Plant	1,500,000	1,500,000	—
Equipment	600,000	300,000	300,000
Total capital assets	$2,200,000	$1,900,000	$ 300,000
Less accumulated depreciation	450,000	350,000	100,000
Net capital assets	$1,750,000	$1,550,000	$ 200,000
Organization costs, less Amortization	$ 150,000	$ 200,000	$ (50,000)
Total assets	$2,135,000	$2,135,000	$ —

Ratios

Current ratio	÷ $235,000	$385,000
	$290,000	$390,000
	= .81 to 1	.99 to 1
Acid test	÷ $125,000	$175,000
	$290,000	$390,000
	= .43 to 1	.45 to 1
Debt to equity ratio	÷ $1,300,000	$1,500,000
	$1,700,000	$1,700,000
Debt	= 76%	88%
Equity	= 24%	22%
Return on equity	÷ $100,000	$100,000
	$400,000	$200,000
	= 25%	50%
Return on shareholders investment	÷ $100,000	$100,000
	$545,000	$245,000
	= 18%	41%

Asset turnover rate	÷ $2,000,000 $2,135,000 = .94	$1,900,000 $2,135,000 .89	

			Increase
Liabilities and Capital	*1977*	*1976*	*(Decrease)*
Current Liabilities:			
Accounts payable	$ 100,000	$ 300,000	$(200,000)
Notes payable to banks	100,000	—	100,000
Accrued expenses	50,000	50,000	—
Income taxes	40,000	40,000	—
Total current liabilities	$ 290,000	$ 390,000	$(100,000)
Long Term Debt			
Mortgage note payable	$1,300,000	$1,500,000	$(200,000)
Capital:			
Equity investment	$ 400,000	$ 200,000	$ 200,000
Retained earnings—			
Beginning of year	$ 45,000	$ (55,000)	$ 100,000
Profit for the year	100,000	100,000	—
Total retained earnings	$ 145,000	$ 45,000	$ 100,000
Total capital	$ 545,000	$ 245,000	$ 300,000
Total liabilities and capital	$2,135,000	$2,135,000	$ —
Return on assets	(1) ÷ $ 94,000 $2,135,000 = 4.4%	(1) $ 89,000 $2,135,000 4.2%	
Return on investment in capital assets	(1) ÷ $ 94,000 $2,200,000 = 4.3%	(1) $ 89,000 $1,900,000 4.7%	
Inventory turnover rate			
Cost of goods sold	÷ $1,500,000	$1,550,000	
Average inventory	$ 150,000 = 10.0	$ 200,000 7.8	
Receivable turnover rate			
Sales	÷ $2,000,000	$1,900,000	
Average accounts receivable	$ 125,000 = 16.0	$ 100,000 19.0	
Days revenue in receivables	23 days	19 days	

(1) Net income times asset turnover rate

Exhibit 7-15 Sample Summary Cash Flow Statement

Statement 3
Nursing Center, Inc.
Summary Cash Flow Statement

	November	Year to Date
Funds Provided		
Net income	$ 5,922	$30,115
Add: Depreciation	3,714	18,572
	$ 9,636	$48,687
Bank loan	—	30,000
Decrease in accounts receivable	5,000	10,000
Total funds provided	$14,636	$88,687
Funds Used		
Purchase of equipment	$ 6,000	$15,000
Repair roof	—	30,000
Pay mortgage payments	3,500	17,500
Decrease in current liabilities	5,000	20,000
Total funds used	$14,500	$82,500
Cash flow	$ 136	$ 6,187
Beginning cash balance	(1,675)	(7,726)
Ending cash balance (overdraft)	$(1,539)	$(1,539)

earnings pattern than they would for the shares of a company with the same average earnings, but an erratic pattern. Exhibit 7-16 illustrates this point.

Average earnings for Firm A and for Firm B are the same, but since Firm A has a stable pattern of earnings, its shares will command a higher price in the market. If Firm B has uncollectible accounts receivable which must be written off, its managers would be smart to postpone taking the loss until a period when earnings are high. This practice will not change long-term average earnings, but it will make earnings appear less volatile than they actually are.

You should determine your financial strategy and attempt to meet your business objectives by structuring your income reporting as best fits your needs. This is all according to GAAP, of course.

REVENUE RECOGNITION

The first step in analyzing a P/L statement (Exhibit 7-17) is to determine whether the method for recognizing revenue accurately reflects the nature of the business. Consider the ordinary nursing home operation. When should the revenue from the services be recognized? Is income earned when the patient is admitted? When the service is provided? When the service is collected?

Exhibit 7-16 Graph of Average Earnings Per Share

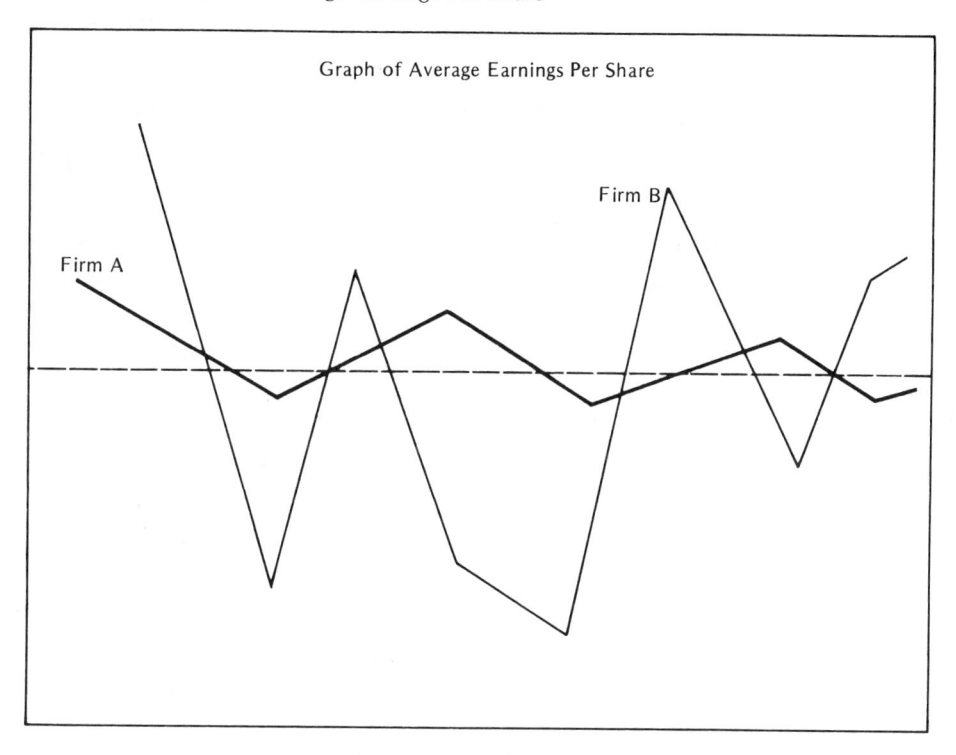

Graph of Average Earnings Per Share

Firm A

Firm B

The company should recognize revenue *when it is earned,* that is, when the service is provided to the patient. Keep in mind that the period in which revenue is earned is not necessarily the same as the period in which payment is received.

Here are the most commonly used *revenue recognition methods:*
- Recognition at the time of billing for the delivery of service—accrual basis.
- Recognition when billing is collected—cash basis.

The footnotes to the P/L statement should tell you which method is used.

Determine also what allowances are made for contractual discounts and bad debts. Obviously, the importance of these allowances varies with the type of third-party contracts that the home has. Ordinarily, such allowances are based on historical experience. But changes in policy can make historical experience inapplicable. A change in credit policy may lead to increased revenue but also aggravate collection problems.

Revenue recognition may pose a problem in the nursing home industry, for it raises some major accounting issues in the treatment of contractual discounts and cost settlements. When you analyze a P/L statement, make a judgment about how reliable the revenue figure is by assuring yourself that a fair recognition method is used and that adequate allowances for contractual discounts and uncollectible accounts have been made.

CONTRACTUAL ALLOWANCES

The Medicare and the Medicaid programs do not pay customary charges. This means that they pay a different price than the private pay patient pays for the same service. The reasons for this have been explained elsewhere in the book, but generally speaking their reasoning is that they should receive a volume discount, and that the health care providers should not make a windfall profit from government patients. If the nursing home cannot collect customary charges for a Medicare or a Medicaid patient, a discount must be recognized. Since this discount arises from a contract the provider signs with the Medicare and/or the Medicaid programs, it is referred to as the contractual allowance or the contractual discount. According to generally accepted accounting principles, the value of the services being provided should be valued in the accounting records at a customary price. The thinking here is to record the amount of potential revenue based on the customary pricing structure output of the nursing home. Since the gross amount of the price for Medicare and Medicaid patients will not be collected, an accounting entry must be made to remove the uncollectible amount from accounts receivable and discount the customary charge to the amount the program will pay.

Under a retrospective formula the periodic payments made by the programs do not represent the final price. The final price is determined from a cost report that the provider files at the end of its fiscal year, comparing the costs for providing the care to the amount of the interim periodic payments. The difference between the revenue that would have been realized had the patients been private paying patients and the amount the program pays represents the final discount. The accounting for this can be studied in Chapter 3.

Under a prospective reimbursement system the accounting treatment can be slightly different. Many prospective reimbursement formulas establish a group rate, group rate meaning a set price for a certain type of facility. The group rate effectively represents a contract price. In most instances, if the provider's costs are less than the contract price, they keep all or some of the difference. If their actual costs exceed the contract price, they absorb the loss. This approach is not quite as scientific as the retrospective formula. It presumes that it should cost X dollars to provide the care and establishes a ceiling, somewhat in excess of that average, to allow the cost conscious provider to compete against a contract price and earn maximum profit. This approach, if properly administered, becomes a reasonable price. In this framework the provider accepts a discounted price but knows the price in advance.

Many accountants have assumed that this situation should be accounted for in the same manner as retrospective reimbursement. The conflict arises when the facility derives 60–80 percent of its total volume from the Medicare and Medicaid programs. At that point, if they are on a prospective rate (contract price), the customary price would seem to be the price established for the programs. So, to record revenue at the price that is customarily charged to the private paying patient would create a revenue figure that is meaningless. With 60–80 percent of the volume being provided by one buyer at a set contracted price, it is not likely that the business has the potential to earn any more revenue than it already has.

The theory should state that the customary price is the price paid by the predominant buyers in the marketplace. If that predominant buyer is the private paying market and the facility is only taking Medicare or Medicaid patients to contribute to their bottom line, the customary charge expected to be recovered would be the private pay rate. Under these circumstances a complete contractual discount approach would be in order. However, where the primary buyers of the services are the Medicaid and/or Medicare programs, the contract price established by the programs is the customary price. Under this theory there would be no contractual discount. The private pay market, which would have a price in excess of the program price, would be recorded as revenue at its actual value, as would the government programs.

Many accountants have speculated that the difference between the contract price for the programs and the customary price for private paying patients should always be recorded as a discount. They term this either a volume discount or a contractual discount. This thinking fails to acknowledge the fact that the programs contribute a great deal of the volume to the marketplace. Many of the beds have been built to serve that market. To deduce that the facility could earn potential revenue on the basis of its current private pay rate is untrue. It can create the appearance of being inflationary if taken out of context. The truth of the matter is that the federal programs have enabled many homes to expand their bed capacity and their services, and they never planned to recover a higher customary private rate. As a matter of fact, their customary private rate is normally established to subsidize as much as possible the tighter margin that is required by the federal programs. So, to create revenue at a fictitious price and record a discount that really does not exist is a distortion of the gross revenue, and the contractual discount.

This theory dictates that value of the contractual discount or contractual allowance is dependent on the facility's patient mix. The facility that has a predominant private pay market should recognize the contractual discount on federal program patients. Those that predominantly serve federal program patients should not recognize a contractual discount.

PRESENTATION OF COSTS AND EXPENSES

P/L statements ordinarily divide nursing home expenses into three categories:

1. Operating expense
2. Administrative expense
3. Capital cost

Operating expenses are those expenses directly related to the cost of producing the services. They include supplies, labor, and overhead, and an allocated portion of the cost of fixed assets (depreciation of plant and equipment) and cost of capital (interest expense).

Administrative expenses are those which are associated with the accounting period in which they are incurred, rather than with specific services. These *period* expenses include the salaries of administration and business office staff, advertising, education, professional fees, and so on.

Patient revenue less operating and administrative expense appears on the P/L statement as operating income. Operating income less capital costs is usually called profit.

Financial analysts often call profit from nursing home earnings before depreciation, interest, and taxes to identify those revenues and expenses associated with the ordinary operations of the firm exclusive of the cost of capital. When capital costs are subtracted and extraordinary items are added in, we have profit before taxes.

Perhaps the most crucial accounting issue in assessing the reliability of an income statement is the valuation of the inventory and fixed assets in determining the cost of services provided. Some assets, such as labor and supplies, are completely consumed in the production of services. Other assets, such as plant and equipment, are not used up completely. Most such assets *do* have to be replaced eventually. They wear out or become obsolete. Therefore, a charge, called *depreciation,* is included in the costs to cover the expense of owning and replacing productive capacity.

For example, a plant costing $1 million and having a useful life of ten years can be depreciated at the rate of $100,000 a year (assuming no salvage value). During the first year of operation, $100,000 is charged to capital costs, and at the end of the year, the plant is listed on the balance sheet at $900,000.

Generally accepted accounting principles require that inventory, plant, and equipment be valued at acquisition cost. But in a period of inflation, the original purchase price of an asset may be far below its *replacement cost.*

If you consider the following illustration, you will see how a P/L statement can distort the profitability of a firm.

Effect of Inflation

Suppose XYZ Nursing Home has plant and equipment which cost $1,000,000 and which have a useful life of thirty years. Suppose they have to be replaced next year. Unfortunately, due to inflation, the replacement cost will be $2,000,000 for the same productive capacity. Thus, the depreciation charge will rise from $33,333 to $66,666. Here are before and after P/L statements which show how a nice profit can become marginal!

	Before Replacement	After Replacement
Revenue	$600,000	$600,000
Less:		
Operating Expense:		
Labor	200,000	200,000
Materials	100,000	100,000
Depreciation	33,333	66,666
Administrative expenses	200,000	200,000
Total Cost	533,333	566,666
Profit before taxes	$66,667	$33,333

The P/L statements of nursing homes like XYZ, which have high plant and equipment expenses, generally overstate profits. To get an idea of actual profitability, you should have your accountant estimate the average useful life of your plant and equipment and divide by two to get the average age of equipment in service. Then adjust depreciation expense upward to correct for the inflation that has occurred during the average-age period. Even though this is not a generally accepted accounting practice and should not normally be reflected in your accounting records, it will provide the owner with valuable insight into how to establish prices and manage cash flow and give the analyst a means to weigh the success of operations.

Inflation has an effect on inventory which may make the operating expenses misleading. Depending upon the valuation method used, the impact of inflation on the P/L statement may be hidden in the inventory figure on the balance sheet or in the cost of supplies figure in the P/L statement. The only way to alleviate the distortion is to properly value the goods on hand at their acquired cost. If this is not feasible, and it usually is not, a method that closely parallels your buying and production practices will come as close as possible. Your accountant will be able to assist you in selecting the proper method.

Extraordinary gains and losses result from events that are not a part of the firm's ordinary operations and include expenses (such as a major fire) or gains (such as those resulting from the sale of a piece of equipment). These items require special treatment in the P/L statement in order not to distort current period earnings. The certified public accountants have specific guidelines for reporting such transactions. See the pronouncements of the Financial Accounting Standards Board (FASB).

SUMMARY

The financial analysis of the P/L statement in the nursing home business is more important than the balance sheet, especially if the business does not have adequate equity capital. In such circumstances, the debt payment may require more earnings than what is being produced by the business. This usually means that the funds provided by earnings to cover physical deterioration of the capital assets (depreciation) are spent on debt payments and not put aside for replacement and payment of the cost of capital. If this is occurring, immediate steps are required to correct the deficient capital structure of the business. Also, the P/L statement is indicative of the short-run results of the investment and the indicator of the impact of short-run decisions on the return on investment. The long-run performance of the business can best be seen on the balance sheet which represents the equity position of the business for all the P/L transactions to date.

The administrator that takes the future seriously needs to apply certain scientific techniques to business management. No matter what the size of the business, its location, or patient mix, it needs a good approach to decision making. These analysis guides can provide administrators with insight for their decisions and financial analysts with a basis for judging the success of the business for a specific period. This is important for all because, "the difference between being a domino or being an entreprenuer is in what you do and when you do it."

THE ANALYSIS OF THE P/L STATEMENT ON A PER-PATIENT-DAY BASIS

As pointed out in previous chapters the primary production unit for nursing homes is the patient day. The patient day encompasses a 24-hour period in which the patient is provided space, meals, and health care services. The value of what the patient is receiving must be stated in terms that will convert the service to a price. The patient is occupying and utilizing the nursing home on a daily basis, providing aids to daily living to each of the patients. The logical production unit, therefore, would be the amount of cost incurred for each patient for each day the services are rendered.

Since all of the costs cannot be determined on a direct basis, because of common overhead costs, a cost per day must be estimated on the basis of daily averages. This average cost per patient day, even though not totally accurate, at least gives administrators an idea of what they should be charging for the services. The better job that the nursing home can do of costing their services, the better job the administrator can do of pricing the services. The more detailed the cost accounting system, the more accurate the price and the more predictable the profit margin.

With the patient day as the production unit and actual monthly revenue and expenses figures available from accounting records, it is an easy matter to convert the values to values per patient day. This approach will relate the revenue and the cost to the services being produced. This also will allow for a more astute analysis of the P/L statement. Let's look at an illustrated P/L statement (refer back to Exhibit 7–17) to get a grasp of what we are talking about. You can see that the gross revenue by level of care and by responsible party is individually reported according to patient-day values. The patient days used to determine the per diems are the actual patient days by the same categories. In our example you can also see, reported alongside the actual per day revenues, the budgeted per day revenues. This is the first step in instituting financial analysis of the P/L statement and an evaluation of performance in relation to the plan. At this point we will discuss the relevance of the information and in later chapters we will formulate an approach for analyzing the variances between actual and budget performance. In our example, the average overall revenue per day is $18.88. The actual operating expenses per patient day are $13.93 for nursing care and $1.34 for ancillary care, and the fixed capital expense per patient day is $1.75. After the information is compiled the question, "Is the average revenue per day adequate to cover operating expenses and capital expense and leave a reasonable profit?" should be answerable. Since higher or lower occupancy directly affects the bottom line, the review of the per diem figures will give administrators a feel for where they stand in providing the average day of care for all patients. If they are not satisfied with the performance, further analysis of specific types of patients is required.

If the facility is on a flat rate, then the patient days multiplied by that flat rate should be the same as the total revenue. If the facility is on a variable rate the average price will not be totally indicative of performance. The mix of patients will cause a distortion of the evaluation of performance. To get more specific, revenue and expenses must be related, by type of service. By converting values to a like base unit of production, the administrator can weigh specifics and not just overall averages. The per diem revenue for a certain skill level and type of patient can be indicative of actual profit potential. In business terminology this is called "product line" or "profit center" reporting.

The system that provides a quick and concise review of the average revenues per patient day, being generated by the different levels of care and different payers, gives the analyst answers and solutions to revenue shortages. The comparison of figures from month to month or from year to year or between actual and budget will provide direction as to the effect of changes in volume and the patient mix.

The per diem costs that you see by functional cost center (dietary, laundry, etc.) represent the components of the patient care costs. The usefulness of this information depends on the sophistication of the accounting and management information system. If it is providing adequate information then it is possible to evaluate the performance of each department. This can be done by reviewing productivity reports and by comparing actual per day expenses to the budget. It is then possible to find out why a department has a higher or lower level of performance than expected.

The nursing home's largest expense is salary. Salaries, converted to per patient day values for each department, allow administrators to control and manage salary expenses. A nursing home that receives this information and has a detailed job position staffing plan with a budget based on the same information will be able to track down reasons for poor performance. The home that does not get this information will never be able to determine the true cause for poor performance and may not even be aware of the problem.

Good management of costs must be in the areas that vary with changes in occupancy, changes in patient mix, or changes in the economy. These are called variable expenses or, for financial control purposes, controllable expenses. Those costs that are sunk and not influenced by the policies and procedures carried out by management, are called fixed expenses. In a nursing home these expenses usually consist of depreciation, interest, real estate taxes, insurance, and to a certain degree, utilities. These types of expenses do not vary significantly, if at all, with changes in occupancy or mix. However, an analysis of the per day fixed costs will tell you how the actual capacity is affecting the absorption of fixed costs. The presumption is that to reach a breakeven point that will produce an adequate bottom line, the facility must spread its fixed costs over an optimum number of production units. The only way to accomplish this is to determine the point where the fixed and variable costs for a certain capacity are covered by the same number of units of revenue. This is called the break-even point.

In summary, the nursing home that can analyze and control its expenses and forecast and determine its revenue is well on its way to a predictable profit. Those that ignore the principles of business eventually find themselves out of business.

Exhibit 7-17 Sample Income Statement

Statement 2
Nursing Center, Inc.
Income Statement
For The Five Months Ended November 30, 1976

	Actual Year to Date					Year to Date Budget			
	Per Patient Day	Percent of Gross Revenue	Per Patient Day ICF	Per Patient Day Shelter	Total	Total	Per Patient Day Total	Per Patient Day ICF	Per Patient Day Shelter
Routine Service Revenue	$ 18.48	93.72%	$ 19.25	$ 15.30	$370,000	$ 18.50	$ 19.30	$ 15.30
Contractual Discounts	(.84)	(4.24)	(1.04)	—	(15,000)	(.75)	(.94)	—
Net routine service revenue	$ 17.64	89.48%	$ 18.21	$ 15.30	$355,000	$ 17.75	$ 18.36	$ 15.30
Drugs and medical supplies	.82	4.15	1.02	—	15,000	.75	.94	—
Physical therapy	.39	1.96	.48	—	10,000	.50	.62	—
Other	.03	.17	.04	—	—	—	—	—
Total patient service revenue	$ 18.88	95.76%	$ 19.75	$ 15.30	$380,000	$ 19.00	$ 19.92	$ 15.30
Expense								
Operating expense								
General services	$ 5.00	25.37%	$ 5.00	$ 5.00	$ 95,000	$ 4.75	$ 4.75	$ 4.75
Health care								
Intermediate care	5.67	27.38	6.73	—	105,000	5.48	6.56	—
Shelter care		1.33	—	1.35	4,500			1.13
General administration	3.26	16.56	3.26	3.26	60,000	3.00	3.00	3.00
Total operating expenses	$ 13.93	70.64%	$ 14.99	$ 9.61	$264,500	$ 13.23	$ 14.31	$ 8.88

202

Capital Expense								
Depreciation	$ .94	4.72%	$ .94	$ .94	$ 18,600	$ .93	$ .93	$ .93
Interest	.41	2.07	.41	.41	8,200	.41	.41	.41
Real Estate taxes	.40	2.03	.40	.40	8,000	.40	.40	.40
	$ 1.75	8.82%	$ 1.75	$ 1.75	$ 34,800	$ 1.74	$ 1.74	$ 1.74
Ancillary service expense	$ 1.34	6.86%	$ 1.69	—	$ 25,000	$ 1.25	1.56	—
Total expense	$ 17.02	86.32%	$ 18.43	$ 11.36	$324,300	$ 16.22	$ 17.61	$ 10.62
Net Income Before Income Taxes	$ 1.86	9.44%	$ 1.32	$ 3.94	$ 55,700	$ 2.78	$ 2.31	$ 4.68
Provision for Income Taxes	.35	1.79	.25	.61	19,000	.95	.81	1.50
Net income for the period	$ 1.51	7.65%	$ 1.07	$ 3.33	$ 36,700	$ 1.83	$ 1.50	$ 3.18
Salaries	$ 9.67	49.04%	$ 9.95	$ 5.11	$185,000	$ 9.25	$ 9.33	$ 4.78
Patient Days								
	16,080		16,080			16,000	16,000	
Intermediate care	3,881			3,881		4,000		4,000
Shelter care	19,961					20,000		
Percent Occupancy	96%		99%	91%		97%	99%	92%

Some facilities use percentages in their analysis of the P/L statement, by relating expenses as a percentage of revenue. This is somewhat indicative of the variability of expenses, but it is not as informative as the per patient day analysis. Percentages are usually more meaningful for comparing a facility to external standards.

Since profit is the business survival kit, adequate skills and tools must be developed to assist administrators in controlling the bottom line. This can only be done by upgrading accounting and reporting systems and developing the skills to use them. This reminds me of a story I heard recently about the nursing home administrator who had taken over a losing proposition. The home was on the verge of bankruptcy. It was borrowing from time to time to meet payroll and payroll taxes. The quality of care was eroding, the patient load declining. It seemed hopeless. But the following actions were taken and the home turned around.

DIAGNOSIS: BUSINESS NEEDS HEALING

The records were put on the accrual basis of accounting. Previously the billings, the purchases, the accounts receivable, and the accounts payable were not recorded in the general ledger. The accounting records were put on a strict accrual basis. The management reports were devised to give the administrator a bird's-eye view of the nursing home's per diem costs and production levels. (The reports and records used are presented in previous chapters.) The administrator was taught how to use the information that would be available.

After about six months of posting and entering figures, the nursing home's bookkeeper had a good working knowledge of the system. The administrator also understood the records better, due to being involved in installing the system and training the bookkeeper. During this transition period, the accounting reports and the management reports were slowly pieced together. The administrator began to use these newfound skills to assist in decision making. The exercise had its side benefits in that problems were dealt with much sooner. The administrator's awareness of costs and revenue stimulated better job performance. The facility was more inclined to raise its private pay price and pursue higher reimbursement the more confident it became in the information.

The situation had been dire, but with diligent effort to upgrade the records and summarize the information into management reports the situation of negative cash flow was completely turned around. In the process, an operating budget was done and the figures were used in the management reports every month to determine how well the facility was doing towards accomplishing its profit plan.

EPILOGUE: THE BUSINESS IS HEALED

Ironically a good plan cannot be done until good accounting records are available along with a knowledge of how to use them. Many of these techniques can be self-taught. It is just a matter of purchasing reference material, such as this book, to give the administrator a resource to use in implementing a good management information system.

Stage Three—Annually

The year-end reports are more for communication purposes than for management purposes. They are mainly used to keep the shareholders and creditors informed on an annual basis. If prepared by independent accountants they may serve the purpose of reporting audited data.

The reports are more condensed and do not purport to report management data. The American Institute of Certified Public Accountants (AICPA) is the authoritative source for the annual reporting guidelines. A complete selection of authoritative material on health care can be obtained from the AICPA in New York.

The key information that annual reports communicate are:

- Net income per share
- Return on investment
- Asset turnover rate
- Working capital ratio
- Working capital change
- Debt to equity ratio
- Receivable turnover rate
- Cash flow and change in financial position

SUMMARY

The term *capital* means "the wealth, whether in money or property, accumulated by or owned or employed in business by an individual or firm." Other terms are used interchangeably, such as net worth, net equity, stockholders' investment, or interest, but none is quite as descriptive as capital. The free enterprise system, known as capitalism, is founded on the concept of business vitality through the accumulation of capital. Therefore, I have chosen to revitalize the term and use it not only in discussing the shareholders' investment but also in categorizing costs and depreciable assets.

In the analysis of a balance sheet the most critical test for a business to pass is the adequacy of the equity capital investment in relation to the debt incurred to finance working capital and capital assets. It is, therefore, necessary for all parties involved in accounting for and reporting the financial condition of nursing homes to comprehend the purpose of the numbers. This is difficult to put in perspective because there are multiple purposes due to the needs of investors, bankers, regulators, tax collectors, ad infinitum.

But when you put the purposes to the test of logic you will find that the relevance of the statements to different parties goes like this:

Report	Interested Party	Primary Interest
Balance Sheet	Investor	Return on equity treatment
	Banker	Return on debt investment

Report	Interested Party	Primary Interest
	Regulators	Value of equity
	Tax Collectors	Retained earnings
Income Statement	Investor	Earnings per share
	Banker	Earnings available to service debt
	Regulator	Mark-up to their beneficiaries
	Tax Collectors	Value of taxable income
Cash Flow Statement	Investor	Cash available for dividends
	Banker	Cash available for debt payments
	Regulator	Cash available for operations
	Tax Collectors	Cash available for tax payments

As you can see, to the investor and the banker the analysis will be directed towards the Capital section of the balance sheet, while the regulator and tax collector are bypassing the Capital section for the sake of valuing the profitability as it relates to their specific purpose. Thus, the structuring of the balance sheet through the accounting records should be geared to the needs of the investor and banker.

What do the investors and bankers want to see in the Capital section for nursing homes? They want disclosure of the following:

- Types of stock owned by investors, the class of stock, par value, number of shares, and dividend rights of each class.
- The amount of paid-in capital (excess over par value).
- The amount of stock redeemed for the treasury for later sale.
- The amount of earnings that are being reinvested in the business and the amount of earnings paid out in the form of dividends.

The values for these items must come from the accounting records based on the prior or prospective cash transactions that effect capital investment and retained earnings.

On the other hand, the regulator and tax collector can be pacified through the submission of their special forms.

CHAPTER 8
Cost Accounting

Definition of Cost Accounting

With the growth in the nursing home industry and with greater public and governmental interest in regulating nursing home conduct, it has become increasingly necessary to pay close attention to whether management has achieved maximum efficiency in every stage of the production process. The accountant has now been entrusted with the responsibility of reporting the operating costs of departments, production units, and other activities of the business. The accountant is compelled to accomplish this task with accuracy and regularity so that management can base its decisions on the information reported.

In addition to tracing the flow of costs by service unit, many other matters require the attention of the cost accountant. Among these are studies of the extent to which costs are controllable, the preparation of cost reports to aid in determining third-party reimbursement and in reducing costs and expenses, an analysis of the effect or costs of changes in the volume of production, the construction of break-even charts, estimates of future costs and future profits, limits applicable to price fixing, incentive plans, and studies of the desirability of replacing or expanding plant and equipment.

Cost accounting may be described as being that part of accounting which determines the cost of a particular department and service unit of the company. Cost accounting is not an end in itself but is the means of controlling and reducing the costs of production, marketing, and administration. From this concept it becomes apparent that cost accounting represents that tool of management which aids in the guidance of business activities and in the attainment of the objective of producing a maximum of services at a cost that will produce optimal profit to the business.

WHAT IS COST?

In connection with the preceding definition of cost accounting, it must be pointed out that the term cost is elusive. In the P/L statement the term cost describes the cost of the service that is marketed during the fiscal period. However, terms like salaries, telephone expenses, supplies, advertising, and others are not labeled costs, but expenses. The distinction in terminology is merely accounting convention, but it does explain the fundamental data in its broadest sense. More specifically, costs represent that portion of the price of services that has either not yet been utilized or has not yet expired in connection with the realization of revenue. Inventories, buildings and machinery, and prepaid expenses fall into this category of deferred expenses. Expenses, on the other hand, are the costs applied against revenue. Depreciation constitutes the best example of such expired cost. While a distinction between cost and expense is obviously needed as the basis for recording transactions, it has limitations in guiding management to intelligent decisions and profitable operations. This is true because efficient and profitable operations cannot be measured without regard to value, and cost is only one of the value concepts.

In cost accounting it is recognized that different cost concepts are acceptable in different situations. But usually too much emphasis is put on the determination of unit cost for financial accounting purposes while neglecting the use of cost concepts for managerial purposes. It should be possible to predetermine unit costs to enable management to control expenditures at the source and to channel and confine these expenditures within a tolerance set in advance by management.

HOW MUCH COST ACCOUNTING IS NEEDED?

One business may need a more extensive and elaborate accounting system than another. Some of the factors that determine accounting needs are size, nature of the business, and type of ownership and control. The nursing home industry needs are being compounded by tight profit margins and government regulations. Therefore, their cost accounting needs are becoming more extensive and elaborate.

Cost accounting adds no additional steps to the familiar accounting cycle. It elaborates, extends, and more precisely classifies the information. In order to record and present complete and adequate details of business operations, more columns are likely to be provided in the purchases journal; more departmental control accounts are needed, especially for the expense accounts; and more supporting statements are prepared. Furthermore, monthly or even weekly or daily reports are expected in addition to the annual statements that are characteristic of financial accounting. Underlying records and procedures are required such as perpetual inventories and schedules of fixed overhead, which make it possible to prepare reports promptly and without excessive expenditures of time and cost.

Cost accounting uses the principles and procedures established in financial accounting by setting up a separate analysis utilizing the general accounts. As the term implies, cost accounting consists of a system concerned with the more adequate, detailed, and precise recording and measurement of cost elements as they originate and flow through the productive process. Costing is extended to a point where the cost of materials, labor, and all other expenses is known for each unit of service.

Objectives of Cost Accounting

If cost accounting is to determine, report, and analyze the cost of a particular department and service unit, a cost scheme must be devised that will:

1. Ascertain costs by departments and units.
2. Control the expenditures connected with the production, marketing, and administration of the service.
3. Provide a basis for estimating the costs of a unit of service and for the setting of a profitable price.
4. Permit management to base operating decisions on the cost accounting information.

COST FINDING

Cost finding or cost determination in nursing homes consists of recording, classifying, and allocating the total costs of a business and absorbing these costs in departments and services. This cost finding process is based on the same information and procedures as are customarily used for general accounting. In cost finding, however, expenses and costs are further broken down into the specific activities and functions of the business.

COST CONTROL

The control of expenditures is the primary purpose of cost accounting. Accurate and prompt information given to management enables an administrator to control the costs per unit for each department. Control increases the probability of efficient use of labor, supplies, and beds. Even though the reimbursement system regulates prices to a large degree, the profit-making capacity of a business is determined by the efficiency with which costs are controlled.

The control of costs is improved through the use of standard costing and a budget. This combination of standard costs and budget, called budgetary control, requires the complete integration of cost finding and financial records. When this is achieved, cost control and cost reduction are likely.

PRICING

The use of production costs per unit can help the administrator decide on a policy for pricing services. Prices are primarily governed by the cost of production, along with the economic law of supply and demand, governmental policies, trade association practices and competition, and estimates used by management of the cost of overhead departments. The estimates may include costs based on current or future market prices of supplies and labor, and historical costs may have little price-determining influence.

MANAGERIAL DECISIONS

Cost accounting can provide management with information on:
1. Whether to provide a service or to buy it on the outside, (e.g., foodservice).
2. Whether to add a new service or to drop one that is being made now (e.g., day care to supplement a heavy Medicaid patient load).
3. Whether to expand the available floor space or to try to continue under present conditions (add beds or limit expansion).
4. Whether to accept a price below the total cost in order to absorb certain costs (the decision to be made in accepting government patients).

Cost information is of particular value to management because hasty and ill-considered decisions cause additional expenses to the business without assurance that there will be adequate revenue.

Cost Accounting Data

Much of the data for cost accounting originates outside of the accounting department. In addition to the invoices and documents supporting transactions of supplies purchased, consumed, or transferred between departments, the accountant requires reports of wage allocations, records of the worker's actual time, requisition of supplies, and staff planning schedules. Market studies and statistics regarding nursing hours per patient day by level of care constitute additional source data.

The accountant's task is to evaluate and use such data in a manner that will bring out the essential facts for management. Cost data depends on proper, correct, and timely information from all levels of the organization, so cost accounting becomes a cooperative venture involving all departments of the facility. In doing so the accountant must teach all employees to be cost conscious. This means not only to observe cost procedures and to aid in execution, but also to use them to promote greater cost control and cost reduction.

Cost Department

The cost department in a nursing home is the accounting department, which is also primarily responsible for keeping the production records for supply requisitions, labor distributions, and patients' statistics. To attain the greatest usefulness, the accounting department not only must record but must also analyze costs of production, marketing, and administration, as well as prepare reports to management and governmental agencies.

These functions can be greatly facilitated through proper delegation of functions generally assigned to the accounting department. Supplies can be recorded, supervised, and reported through a perpetual inventory system supervised by the administrator or assistant administrator. The labor distribution consists of timekeeping and payroll preparation. A payroll department should be established to compute the earnings of the employees and oversee the distribution of salary costs to the appropriate department and compare actual productivity to the staffing plans.

Other functions connected with cost accounting are budgets and cost reports. In the well-run nursing home all of these responsibilities come under the direct supervision of the controller, resulting in lines of authority and responsibility illustrated by the organization chart shown in Exhibit 8–1.

Cost Accounting and Other Functions

The patient care departments, under the direction of the administrator, plan and control the patient services. In pricing the patient services, cost estimates need to be provided for each level of care and each ancillary service before an intelligent decision can be reached in accepting or rejecting a proposed budget. Likewise the efficiency of scheduling and quality of care produced by the nursing department are measured in terms of the cost incurred.

The personnel function, which interviews, screens, and selects employees for the various job classifications and records workers' behavior and performance, is also interested in keeping efficient and satisfied workers. The wage rates and the methods of remuneration agreed on with management form the basis for determining payroll costs by department.

The cash management function, which is responsible for financial administration, relies on accounting reports in scheduling cash requirements and expectations. Accurate production and distribution costs are essential to smooth financing and planning.

Exhibit 8-1 Organization Chart for Cost Accounting Responsibilities

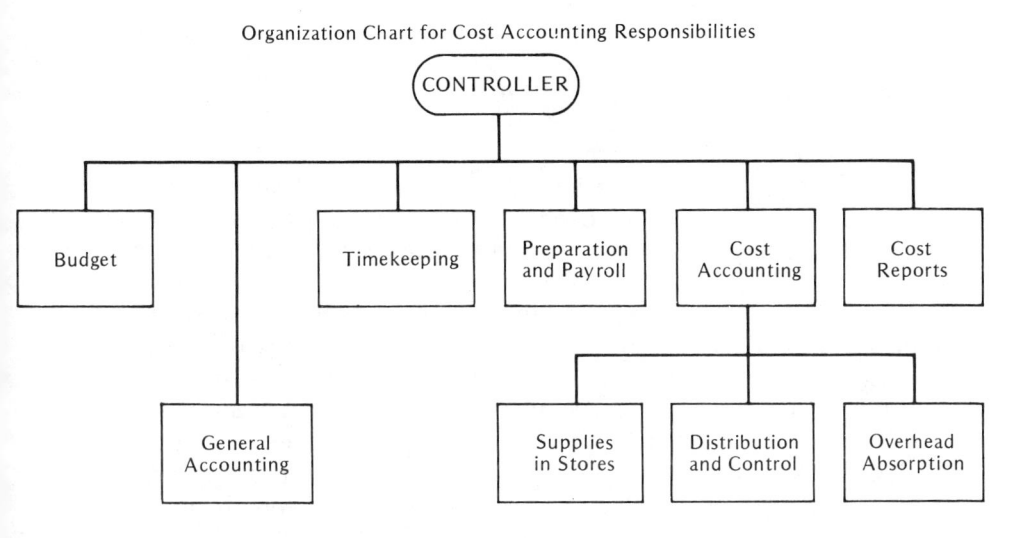

Organization Chart for Cost Accounting Responsibilities

```
                          CONTROLLER
    ┌──────────┬──────────┬──────────────┬────────────┬──────────┐
  Budget   Timekeeping  Preparation      Cost          Cost
                        and Payroll    Accounting     Reports
              ┌──────────┐         ┌──────────┬──────────────┬──────────┐
              General                Supplies   Distribution    Overhead
              Accounting             in Stores  and Control    Absorption
```

The marketing function depends on a good product at a competitive price in its dealings with prospective patients. While prices can be set by adding a chosen percentage to cost, the costs must not be ignored. Accurate production costs provide information that will show which services are most profitable and assist greatly in determining pricing decisions.

The public relations function has to maintain good relations between the facility and the public in general, patients, and patients' families. Points of contention are most likely to be prices, wages, and profits. The accounting department is often called on to provide basic information for public releases concerning these policies and practices.

The legal function needs cost accounting in keeping many affairs of the company in conformity with the law. The Wage and Hour Law, terms of union contracts, and taxes are some of the areas where the legal and cost functions need to cooperate.

Cost Accounting and Government Agencies

Cost accounting is an integral part of the Medicare and Medicaid programs. As will be seen later in this chapter, cost finding is necessary to determine:

1. The direct costs, consisting of expenditures for supplies, direct labor, and direct expenses, incurred by the home in performing the third-party contract.
2. The proper proration of any indirect costs (including a reasonable amount of management expenses) necessary for the performance of the third-party contract.

Such cost is made up of the following elements:

1. Production cost.
2. Other direct expenses.

3. Support expenses, usually termed overhead, and expenses of marketing and administration.

All program payments by Medicare and Medicaid must be cost related and are subject to audit and redetermination.

Cost and Financial Accounting

With increased emphasis on cost accounting as a means for cost control, and because the traditional methods of financial accounting do not serve this purpose, the tendency is to develop cost records independent of the financial accounting records.

Many times it was assumed that the cost department could produce costs of products, costs of manufacturing operations, or costs of services on the basis of information from production records; a tie-in with the general or financial records was considered superfluous or only partly necessary. Such an assumption is not only poorly conceived, but is also dangerous. There is a risk of substantial and frequent errors arising from the use of data from two different sources without any cross-check between them. Reports based thereon might seriously mislead management.

To avoid inaccuracies and conflict there should be a complete integration of cost and financial records, not only for the purpose of cost determination, but also for the purpose of cost control. The financial and cost accounts of a facility should be regarded as two pieces of a whole. Both utilize the same basic information, with cost accounting as the managerial refinement of financial accounting.

Financial accounting traces the flow of funds by attaching the dollars expended to the service received in exchange. When the capital is consumed and flows into the production stream, cost accounting traces these steps until all dollars expended for services find their way into the service or are considered sunk, unless recovered through the pricing mechanism. To achieve this absolute integration between cost and financial accounting, it is necessary that an accounting and cost system be structured which records, reports, and analyzes data for both financial and costing purposes.

THE ELEMENTS OF COST

The classification of costs depends largely on management objectives towards expenditures and on the character of a company's operations. For instance, the automobile used for transportation purposes by a nursing home is considered a fixed asset, while the automobiles owned by a used-car dealer are current assets. The treatment of these cost elements have important effects on balance sheet valuations, control of expense groups, cost reports, and cost analyses. The initial classification of costs will also determine the ease and accuracy with which costs are allocated to departments and services.

Total cost is defined as deductions from revenue before income taxes. In a nursing home, total cost is divided into two groups: service cost and support costs. Operating cost is often called production cost. The support costs fall again into two large divisions: indirect overhead expenses and administrative expenses. The total of operating cost and support cost is the cost to provide patient care service. The elements of cost are illustrated in Exhibit 8–2.

Production cost is the sum of the cost of direct supplies, direct labor, and direct overhead expenses. It is the figure at which the service is delivered to the patient. Indirect overhead expenses support the production costs in maintaining the patients' daily living needs. Administrative expenses include the expenses incurred in the direction, control, and administration of the company. Exhibit 8–3 illustrates the major factors that enter into total cost.

Analysis of Service Costs

The elements of service costs are listed as direct supplies, direct labor, and direct overhead expenses. Direct supplies and direct labor are combined into a classification called prime cost. Direct labor and direct overhead expenses can be combined into a classification called production cost.

FIXED, VARIABLE, AND SEMIVARIABLE EXPENSES

Some expenses vary directly in relation to changes in the volume of output (production), while others, as they are incurred, remain more or less fixed in amount. Unless the cost system defines this distinction, the costs assigned to services will not be accurate.

Variable expenses vary in direct proportion to volume. They can be assigned to operating periods with reasonable accuracy. The responsibility for variable costs lies directly with the department head. Variable costs assigned to an operating period are fully absorbed in the production cost of that period.

Exhibit 8-2 The Elements of Cost

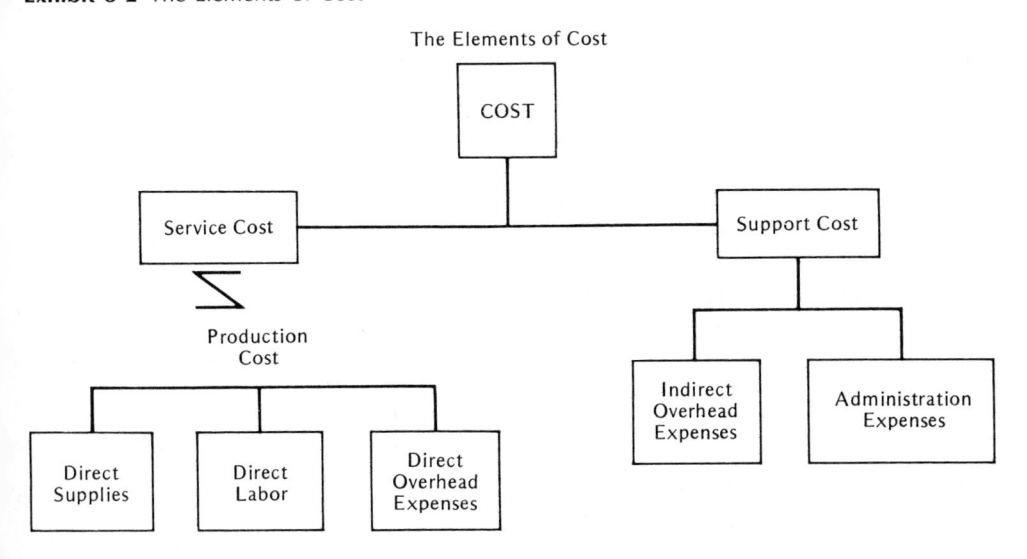

Exhibit 8-3 Analysis of Total Cost

Direct Supplies (Medical) + Direct Labor		= Prime Cost

Indirect Supplies + Indirect Labor +	Other Indirect Expenses	Direct = Overhead Expenses
↓ ↓	↓	
Includes: Includes:	Includes:	
Food Housekeeping	Rent	
Laundry supplies Dietary	Insurance—Fire	
Housekeeping Laundry	and Liability	
Supplies Maintenance	Taxes	=
	Depreciation	
	Maintenance and	
	Repairs	
	Power	
	Light	
	Heat	Production Cost

Indirect Overhead Expenses + Administrative Expenses	=	Support Cost
↓ ↓		
Includes: Includes:		
Advertising Administrative and		
Entertainment Office Salaries		
Travel Expenses Auditing Expenses		
Telephone and Telegraph Legal Expenses		
Stationary and Printing Doubtful Accounts		=
Postage Telephone and Telegraph		
Cost of Capital Stationary and		
Printing		
Postage		
Miscellaneous		
Administrative		
Expenses		Total Cost

Opportunity Cost (residual of price and cost)		+
(Ultimately the profit margin is a cost of doing business.)		Profit

		=
Cost to Consumer		Selling Price

Fixed costs do not vary in direct proportion to volume. They must be assigned to the operating periods by more or less arbitrary methods. The responsibility for fixed costs rests largely with management. Fixed costs may or may not be absorbed entirely during the operating period. The problem of assigning or not assigning fixed costs to services will be discussed later in this chapter.

Direct supplies and direct labor are usually variable in nature. The definition applies to them, but generally they are not considered in the discussion of variable and fixed costs. Direct overhead and support expenses are the items that must be most carefully examined with regard to their variable and fixed nature because they may be both semifixed or semivariable. It is impossible to budget and control these expenses successfully without understanding their tendency to be fixed or variable; this division is a necessary prerequisite to budgeting. The following departmental classification is illustrative of items that usually fall within the two categories:

Variable Overhead and Support Expenses

Dietary

Laundry

Fixed Direct Overhead and Indirect Overhead Expenses

Housekeeping

Maintenance

Administrative

USING UNIT COSTS

The determination of the cost to provide a unit of service is a basic objective of cost accounting. With the cost unit (patient day in the nursing home) selected, the question of how to accumulate these costs arises, that is, whether to compile and allocate actual costs to the units of production or whether to assign costs on a standard basis, creating variance accounts to set off the difference between the actual costs accumulated and the standard costs.

The actual or historical cost system is a procedure that collects the costs as they occur, and presents them after all services have been performed and services rendered. While the department is charged with the actual quantities and costs of supplies used and labor expended, the overhead can be allocated on the basis of some fixed rate. The use of a predetermined overhead rate shows that even the so-called "actual" cost system does not entirely live up to its name.

Because a predetermined overhead rate is used and because the system does not provide a measuring stick against which actual results can be compared, the actual cost system has been supplemented by the standard cost system. Under a standard cost system all costs are predetermined in advance of production. Services are costed on a standard basis for both quantities and dollar values. Accounts are designed to collect actual costs of the direct-cost elements. The differences en actual costs and standard costs, termed variances, are collected in separate accounts. The variances are analyzed, and management is able to move quickly to check unfavorable trends and departures from predetermined standards and from the overall profit goal.

THE COST SYSTEM AND THE BUDGET

The value of cost accounting, particularly the cost system, is greatly enhanced when it is integrated with a budget system. A budget system presents a coordinated plan of operation for the immediate future. A budget based partly on estimates and partly on past experiences depends to a great measure on the existence of accurate and reliable accounting and cost records. The cost system reveals the actual results in relation to the budget. When the cost system and budget system are coordinated they permit:

1. A comparison of the budgeted P/L statement with actual results.
2. A pro forma balance sheet compared with actual conditions.
3. A periodic comparison of actual and budgeted costs per unit of production.
4. A comparison of total operational costs with budgetary goals.

When the budget figures are based on standard costs, and when all employees are able to plan and conduct their work according to the standards, the greatest benefits of cost accounting will be derived.

PREMISE

Residents or patients receive substantially the same degree of capital and overhead costs. The patient care services vary with patient need and outcome. Thus, a system that develops fixed costs per patient day and variable costs for the labor unit will allow the payment to follow service.

Cost Distribution/Cost Centers/Cost Finding

Cost finding in nursing homes is becoming more crucial every day. The entire pricing structure is dependent on some form of cost accounting. The method selected must accomplish full absorption cost accounting, since all major services are billed to the patients as earned and no inventory is accumulated. In other words, substantially all costs incurred represent the current cost of services, since inventory of merchandise is not a very large factor. See Exhibit 8–4 for the relationship of costs to the production of revenue.

Full absorption accounting requires that costs be grouped by functional cost centers so they can be assigned to departments producing billable services to the patient. This is done by using a functional chart of accounts, which means that direct expenses for payroll, supplies, utilities, property taxes, and so on are recorded in the accounting records according to the type of service rendered to the patient. A copy of a functional chart of accounts is illustrated in Appendix 1. The costs grouped by function, are also subclassified according to responsibility and natural expense classifications. For example:

Primary Functional Classification	Secondary Responsibility Designation	Basic Natural Category
Nursing Services		
Routine service	Director of Nursing	Salaries, Supplies
Activities	Activity Director	Salaries, Supplies
Support Services		
Administration	Administrator	Salaries, Supplies, Telephone, Licenses, Professional Fees
Utilization and PSRO Review	Medical Director	Salaries, Consulting
Housekeeping	Head Housekeeper	Salaries, Supplies
Laundry	Department Head	Salaries, Linens
Dietary	Dietician	Salaries, Food, Supplies
Maintenance	Department Head	Salaries, Supplies
Ancillary Services		
Physical Therapy	Physical Therapist	Salaries, Supplies
Pharmacy	Pharmacist	Salaries, Supplies

The reporting of nursing services costs according to functional classification and subclassification looks like this:

```
Nursing Services
  Routine Services
    Director of Nursing          $15,000
    Salaries—RNs                 100,000
           —LPNs                 150,000
           —Aides                300,000
    Supplies                      10,000
      Total Routine Services   $575,000
  Activities
    Activity Director             $9,000
    Salaries                      10,000
    Supplies                       2,000
      Total Activities          $21,000
      Total Nursing Services   $596,000
```

Stratifying costs in this manner gives management the capability to assign goals and responsibilities for purposes of controlling costs. It also relates the cost to the service provided so the cost of the unit produced can be evaluated. The determination of cost of the unit produced is called cost finding. Exhibit 8–5 is an example of how the functional classification provides the information for cost finding.

Exhibit 8-4 Patient Service Cost Model

Patient Service Cost Model

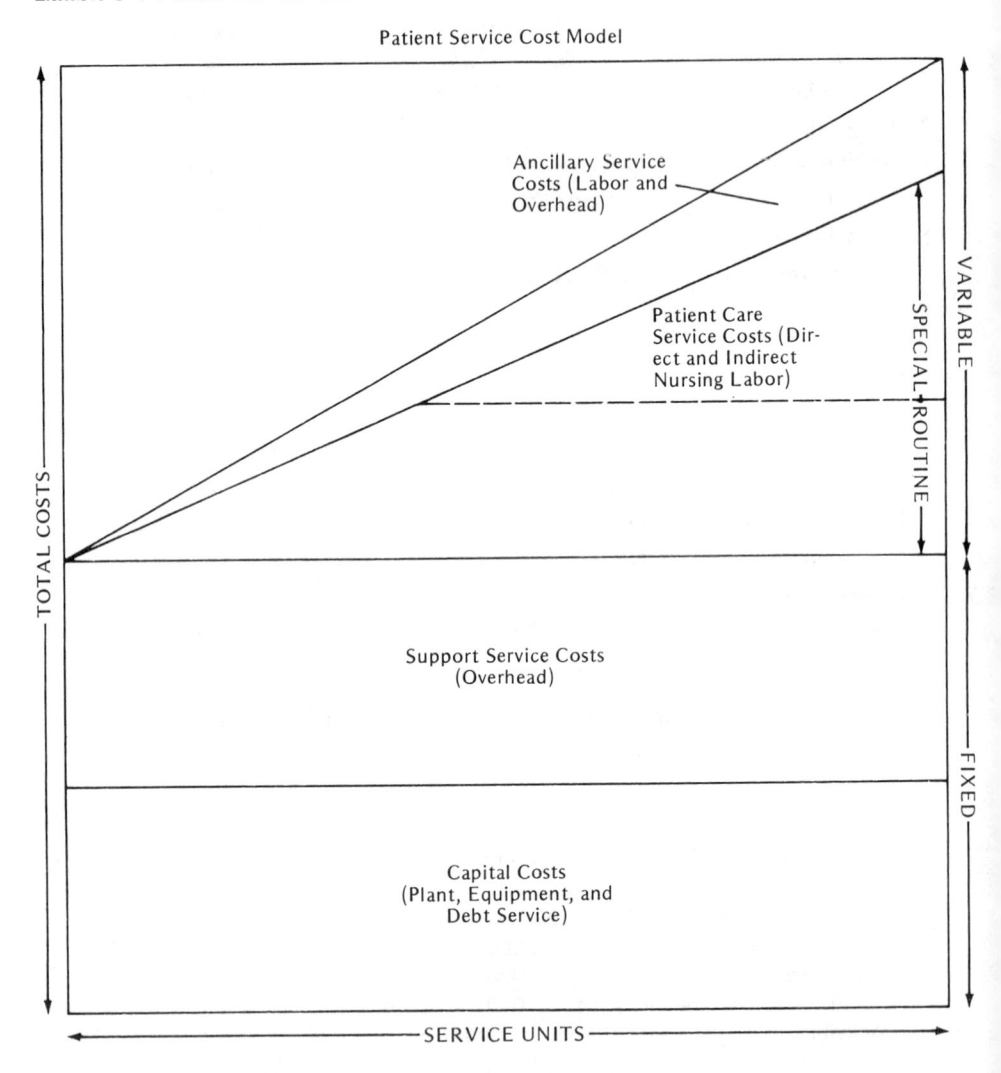

[Graph showing Total Costs vs Service Units with layers: Ancillary Service Costs (Labor and Overhead), Patient Care Service Costs (Direct and Indirect Nursing Labor), Support Service Costs (Overhead), and Capital Costs (Plant, Equipment, and Debt Service). Right side labels: VARIABLE (Special/Routine), FIXED.]

Exhibit 8-5 Sample Functional Classification Data for Cost Finding

	Total	Nursing Routine	Activities	Ancillaries Physical Therapy	Pharmacy
Salaries	$329,000	$285,000	$19,000	$15,000	$10,000
Supplies	55,000	10,000	2,000	3,000	40,000
Total Direct Cost	$384,000	$295,000	$21,000	$18,000	$50,000

Support Services (Overhead)

1. Administration	$130,000	98,800	7,800	6,500	16,900
2. Housekeeping	50,000	45,000	1,000	2,000	2,000
3. Laundry	16,000	15,200	160	480	160
4. Dietary	150,000	142,500	3,000	3,000	1,500
5. Maintenance Plant	15,000	14,400	150	300	150
6. Operation	45,000	43,200	450	900	450
7. Capital cost	100,000	96,000	1,000	2,000	1,000
	$890,000	$750,100	$34,560	$33,180	$72,160

Allocation Basis:

1. Administration is allocated on accumulated cost-direct costs percentages.

		Percent	Allocation
Routine	$295,000	76%	$ 98,800
Activities	21,000	6	7,800
PT	18,000	5	6,500
Pharmacy	50,000	13	16,900
	$384,000	100%	$130,000

2. Housekeeping is allocated on square footage or hours worked.

	Sq. Footage	Percent	Allocation
Routine	30,000	96%	$ 43,200
Activities	400	1	450
PT	500	2	900
Pharmacy	300	1	450
	31,200	100%	$ 45,000

3. Laundry is allocated on pounds of laundry.

	Pounds	Percent	Allocation
Routine	40,000	95%	$15,200
Activities	500	1	160
PT	1,000	3	480
Pharmacy	500	1	160
	42,000	100%	$16,000

Exhibit 8-5 (cont.)

4. Dietary is allocated on number of meals.

	Meals	Percent	Allocation
Routine	95,000	95%	$142,500
Activities	2,000	2	3,000
PT	2,000	2	3,000
Pharmacy	1,000	1	1,500
	100,000	100%	$150,000

5. Maintenance, operations, and capital costs allocated on square footage (also see 6 and 7).

	Square Footage	Maintenance	Operations	Capital Costs
Routine	96%	$14,400	$43,200	$ 96,000
Activities	1	150	450	1,000
PT	2	300	900	2,000
Pharmacy	1	150	450	1,000
	100%	$15,000	$45,000	$100,000

With the costs stratified by the services provided the cost per unit produced can be determined.

		Production Unit		
	Cost	Description	Quantity	Cost Per Unit
Routine	$750,000	Patient days	35,000	$21.42
Activities	34,560	Activity hours	2,500	13.82
Physical Therapy	33,180	Therapy modalities	2,000	16.59
Pharmacy	72,160	Prescriptions	7,000	10.31
	$890,000			

The cost per unit is then the basis for cost control, pricing, budgeting, long-range planning, and reimbursement.

CHAPTER 9
Cost Reimbursement

Medicare and Medicaid Reimbursement

And Then There Came Medicare and Medicaid

In nineteen sixty-six
Congress put us in a fix
They passed a law for the land
To give the needy a helping hand

The thoughts they had were good
Set by principles for which they stood
Unfortunately without regard
They misconceived, made it hard

Their thought was cost
To be paid not lost
However as the bills began to mount
Intent got lost mid the count

The numbers game was the name
With a program for costs to tame
Contain or refrain or accept the blame
Debts took on to help the lame

Freeze or moratorium imposed
Fraud and abuse said exposed
Use any means to get the votes
Feed the lions and milk the goats

Then when it gets all out of hand
Stand back and kick the sand—at
Medicare and Medicaid the law of the land.

As the poem says, "Congress put us in a fix." They passed a law that sounded very good, based on good idealistic principles. The problems arose though when the costs, which to a degree that had not been contemplated, began to escalate. The formula devised to determine how the providers of the service were paid was not based on sound business principles. The formula, retroactive cost reimbursement, was expected to pay costs incurred on a dollar-for-dollar basis. The approach was felt to be economically sound because most of the providers were not-for-profit, tax-exempt hospitals. It was felt that if the profit motive were not involved, payment of costs incurred would be sufficient. But when it became evident that the programs would also be dealing with proprietary businesses, they tacked on a factor which was called "return on providers' net equity" to compensate proprietary businesses for the profit motive.

Initially the formula worked well and paid full program costs. Certain costs were deemed unallowable, but they were not substantial. It took pressure off the institutions and the proprietary businesses because the programs were a source of new volume. It stimulated building and expansion to handle the demand. Judgments about improvements, capital acquisitions, and cost increases were easier with the federal government ready and willing to pay its full share. The mentality became that of, "If in doubt, incur the expense or spend the capital because the federal programs will pay the tab." Any remaining tab was easily passed on to the insurance companies or to the patient's family. The formula was a windfall. It provided an industry with new capital to expand its facilities and its services. It took the pressure off fund raising programs and tight budgets.

On the other hand, there was no advance funding of certain health services. Most of the services offered by the nursing homes did not qualify for insurance coverage. As a result the nursing home services had not been marketable because there was no available source of payment, other than the patient's personal funds. When the Medicare and Medicaid programs offered a source of revenue for long-term care, the demand increased sharply. And as the demand increased the capital investment and the profit motive were not far behind. Those who could not afford health services were given an opportunity receive services at a reduced price. This new volume enabled the providers to expand their facilities and services and increase their capacity. This expansion spread the fixed overhead costs over a broader base, thereby increasing profit margins and cash flow.

The profit factor based on a return on net equity, though not adequate from an economic standpoint, was a guaranteed mark-up. It did not require efficiency in operating a business. It paid the mark-up to proprietors who had invested capital and left it there. So it represented a reward for taking risk with capital, but the risk was not serious because the return was guaranteed. The problem was that a guaranteed return failed to inspire the facilities to be cost effective because there was no reward for good management.

As the federal programs expanded the available capital, it caused costs to escalate because there was no longer a reason to control costs. But ultimately the cost escalation had to stop. The tax base and the revenues could not meet the unlimited demand for services. As the reserves dwindled and the costs rose, the reimbursement methods began to take on new features which curtailed the amount the providers could be reimbursed. Some of the concepts were good but they were applied retroactively, after the provider had incurred the expense or had made the capital expenditure. This left the provider no alternatives for making meaningful management decisions, since the reimbursement decision was made after the fact and reimbursement was lost. The providers' capital began to erode, resulting in depleted capital reserves and an increased cost of administration at the government level. The overall impact of the cost cutting techniques was to level off the indiscriminate spending at the provider level. But the spending for the regulatory bureaucracy mushroomed. The regulations became more complicated; the forms and paper work required to regulate the costs and services increased tenfold.

After a decade of retroactive cost reimbursement we are now experimenting with the more businesslike method called prospective reimbursement. Prospective rate setting is the establishment of a price in advance of selling the service. This approach is used in the free enterprise system, but is balanced by the natural laws of supply and consumer demand.

In the regulated health care industry, the laws of supply and consumer demand are subverted to a multitude of regulations. There is little consumer involvement, and the public demands cost efficiency and quality. As a result, regulations are enacted without due regard for the affect on supply and demand. Unfortunately, costs have escalated until the resources have become limited. And now cost control is a priority and a negative factor in the determination of the price on a retrospective basis.

Ultimately, economics dictates that a regulated system, such as health care, needs unlimited capital; or a means of controlling the distribution of limited capital. The retrospective distribution of capital is effective only in a market with unlimited capital which will pay full costs. Then, if costs outrun the availability of capital resources, growth and expansion are stopped and eventually there would be no industry. The growth and expansion are being curtailed in the health care industry; costs are outrunning the resources.

Prospective distribution of capital appears to be the only feasible way to dole out limited capital resources. It requires that the distribution be made based on capital needs. Then if the distribution is not acceptable, negotiation can take place between the buyer and seller. In any case, the capital needs must be specified by each provider before the distribution of capital. If this takes place, limited capital is distributed to the seller based on an agreed on definition of need. The seller can determine if this is sufficient to cover costs, including inflation and profit, and the buyer can determine if this is the best way to use their limited capital. If either party finds the demands unreasonable, they can negotiate a more acceptable distribution of capital by changing:

- Demand (more units produced; reduces the fixed costs per unit)
- Supply (fewer units needed by the consumer; reduces marginal costs per unit)
- Quality (changes in production; revises the costs per unit)
- Ingredients (different mix of input or output changes costs per unit)
- Production methods (entry into the system at the most cost effective level)

The strengths of prospective rate setting are planning and definition. Essentially the buyer defines what is needed and the seller costs and prices the product. Bargaining can then take place, before the service is provided and before the cost is incurred. In this manner an agreeable price can be established. The ingredients of this negotiating process are as follows:

- A specified bill of materials (service ingredients)
- Labor content
- Overhead content
- Cost accounting and budgeting, based on historical experience
- Valuation of demand and productivity, based on historical experience.

The primary disadvantage to the prospective system is that it commits both the buyer and seller to a course of action. As the course changes, components also must change. This leads to renegotiation and, in some cases, business failures and abuses because of poor planning. However, the risk for both parties is not as high as it is with the retrospective method of capital distribution. Regardless, advanced planning is necessary and requires considerable discipline, flexibility, and education before it is effective.

To better understand the concepts of retroactive versus prospective reimbursement, let's study the following comparison:

	Retroactive	Prospective
Prior year cost	$1,000,000	$1,000,000
Unallowable cost	(100,000)	(100,000)
Next year's base cost	$ 900,000	$ 900,000
Inflation	–	100,000
Reimbursable cost	$ 900,000	$1,000,000
Payment per unit	$ 900	$ 1,000
Final reimbursement current actual cost	$ 850,000	$ 850,000
Payback	$ 50,000	$ –
Bottom line	$ –	$ 150,000

As you can see from this example the costs may be exactly the same, but the real advantage of prospective reimbursement is that the service provided is defined in advance of incurring cost, and the amount that will be paid for the services is understood. The prospective payment can include an incentive factor for the provider accomplishing efficiencies and controls that contain their actual cost.

The logic, the benefits, and the results can all be pretty well documented—prospective rate setting is much more flexible and controllable than retroactive cost reimbursement. The apprehension from the government perspective is that they lose the hold they have over the providers of service. In defining what is going to be provided and how much is to be paid before the fact, the parties are put into a position of having to negotiate, while with retroactive methods, the provider has little alternative except to accept what they can get and attempt to change the rules in the future. So from the government's perspective, even though there is not as much control over the escalation of costs, there is a concern that the providers will be in a position to balance the marketplace. It appears that the government officials relish this position; they are in control of everything, except incurred costs, under retroactive cost reimbursement.

The reimbursement methods now being used for purposes of paying the Medicare and Medicaid bills derive their cost information in accordance with Medicare Principles of Reimbursement. This requires that accounting information be reported on an accrual basis in accordance with generally accepted accounting principles. The cost figures are required to be reported in some uniform manner, on the federal or state forms. The purpose is to gather reimbursement data and provide audit trail for subsequent audits of the provider's accounting records. The cost reports use the cost center approach to reporting operating costs. The costs are reported by the department in which they are incurred. Most of the formulas use some form of cost finding to determine the cost per patient day for the service being provided. The following are some examples:

Medicare

Book costs		$1,000,000
Unallowable cost (1)		(100,000)
Allowable costs		$ 900,000
Patient care departments		$ 450,000
Service departments		450,000
Housekeeping		
Dietary		
Laundry		
Maintenance		
Administration		
		$ 900,000
Patient care—certified		$ 600,000
Patient care—noncertified		300,000
		$ 900,000

Patient care—certified	Patient Days	Percent	Amount
Medicare	10,000	33	$200,000
Nonmedicare	20,000	66	400,000
	30,000	100	$600,000

Medicare retroactive settlement	
Cost reimbursement	$ 200,000
Interim payments	
(so much per patient day)	190,000
(including payment by	
patients for coinsurance)	
Retroactive payment to provider	$ 10,000

(1) Non-patient-related and excessive costs as defined by Medicare regulations

Medicaid
Retroactive
  Basically the same as Medicare.
Prospective

Historical cost		$1,000,000
Unallowable cost		100,000
		$ 900,000
Inflation factor for operating costs		90,000
		$ 990,000
Total patient days		30,000
Adjusted patient days to get		
to a minimum occupancy (say 85%)		33,000
Cost per patient day		$30
Ceiling		$27
Reimbursement		
Medicaid patient days		15,000
Daily billing		$27
Final amount		$405,000

The methods have as their primary purpose a formal approach to establishing a controllable price for the service that the Medicare and Medicaid programs are buying. There is probably more emphasis on control than there is on providing adequate payment to allow for quality. This enigma is a result of the drastic increase in the cost of care over the last ten years; the normal price to be paid for government intervention and growth.

The cost finding techniques supporting the methods are normally similar in principle. Each attempts to attribute cost to the room and board, nursing care, and ancillary care.

Like any other business, the complexity of the methods is dependent on the degree of accuracy desired. The cost finding formulas presently have a high degree of dependence on averages. There is generally a requirement that all costs be absorbed in the period incurred for the number of patients served. (There are a few methods that strive to attribute value directly to the labor and capital cost components.) Under most methods, the average cost ultimately becomes the price for the service and any variation from that average results in more profit or loss. The government buyers are now striving to control their cost by imposing maximums on what they will pay. As the pressure to be more cost conscious builds, the concern for quality declines.

The government cost finding methods are mainly concerned with incurred costs. They are not giving adequate consideration to the declining purchasing power of the dollar. They give recognition to inflation in determining future operating expenses, but disregard inflation as it affects the capital investment. It is the policy of the government programs to limit the amount of capital expenditures as much as possible, by paying historical depreciation; and as inflation erodes the purchasing power of the dollar, the value of the investment also is depleted because capital costs are not being adequately reimbursed. When capital costs (fixed) are not fully reimbursed, there is no capital available for future repairs and expansion. The following is an example of that phenomenon.

```
Historical Cost of Capital
    Purchased value of investment    $1,000,000
    Useful life                            40 years
    Historical depreciation          $    25,000
    Debt service (25 years)          $    30,000
Economic Cost of Capital
    Purchased value                  $1,000,000
    Inflation (6 years) (36%)           360,000
        Current value                $1,360,000
        Useful life                        40 years
        Economic depreciation        $    34,000
    Investment cost
        Current value                $1,360,000
        Cost of capital percentage            9 %
                                     $   127,000
        Book interest                     30,000
        Cost of capital              $    97,000
```

Historical Cost of Capital
Depreciation	$	25,000
Interest		30,000
	$	55,000

Economic Cost of Capital
Depreciation	$	34,000
Interest		97,000
	$	131,000

In this example, if the economic cost of capital is not considered in establishing reimbursement levels, $76,000 is being lost every year to inflation. The effect of this phenomenon is astounding.

The cost reimbursement formulas must be studied in light of the health care marketplace. As pointed out before, long-term care facilities are dealing primarily with one major buyer. The federal and state programs continue to demand quality services on limited budgets. But the providers cannot investigate new technology and expand services if reimbursement methods are not more flexible. This flexibility must come from a predetermination of an acceptable amount of capital that is available to purchase health care services. Then the funds must be allocated to the different segments of the health care delivery system and distributed to the various areas of the country. The individual providers of service then can compete for the health care dollar. The distribution of capital must be based on sound specifications and cost projections pertaining to society's needs. There must also be a constant reevaluation of the regulatory process, the legislative process, and the cost of new regulations to prevent costs that cannot be absorbed.

A new approach will require an expenditure of time, effort, and dollars. But to properly structure the system, once the initial expenditure has been made and the framework established, costs can be controlled. Until this is done the problems and inefficiencies of retroactive reimbursement will continue. Costs will escalate, services will decline, capital will erode, and eventually the proper system will have to be established. The irony is that the present system does not work, but a crisis must develop before a new system is politically expedient.

APPENDIX 1
Chart of Accounts

Uniform Expense Classification Guide*

OBJECTIVE

The Expense Classification Guide serves as a reference for the uniform recording of all supplies and services expenses which are not directly billable to patients. Supplies and services billable to patients should be recorded in the ancillary cost center accounts.

HOW TO USE THE GUIDE

Each page of the guide lists various types of supplies and services according to the cost center and natural classification to which they should be charged. Some expense items may not lend themselves to being classified to a specific cost center, but to the "using" cost center. These types of expenses may have to be charged directly to the center using the expenses.

---

*Adapted from *California Long-Term Care Manual.*

EXPENSE CLASSIFICATION

Item	Cost Center Title	Code	Natural Classification Title
Abrasive floor surfacing	Plant Operation and Maintenance	5300.0	Supplies
Accounting and audit fees	Administration	5100.0	Accounting and Auditing
Ace bandages	Nursing Services	5900.0	Medical Care Materials and Supplies
Acetylene, dissolved	Plant Operation and Maintenance	5300.0	Supplies
Acids, laundry	Laundry and Linen	5500.0	Supplies
Actuarial fees	Administration	5100.0	Consulting and Management Fees
Adhesive pads	Nursing Services	5900.0	Medical Care Materials and Supplies
Adhesive remover	Nursing Services	5900.0	Medical Care Materials and Supplies
Adhesive tape	Nursing Services	5900.0	Medical Care Materials and Supplies
Admission forms	Administration	5100.0	Office and Administrative Supplies
Advertising	Administration	5100.0	Purchased Services
Air cushions, invalid	Nursing Services	5900.0	Medical Care Materials and Supplies
Airways	Nursing Services	5900.0	Medical Care Materials and Supplies
Alcohol, rubbing	Nursing Services	5900.0	Medical Care Materials and Supplies
Alcohol packets	Nursing Services	5900.0	Medical Care Materials and Supplies
Alkalies, laundry	Laundry and Linen	5500.0	Supplies
Ammonia	Housekeeping	5600.0	Cleaning Supplies
Analgesics	Nursing Services	5900.0	Pharmaceuticals
Aspirin	Nursing Services	5900.0	Pharmaceuticals
Assessments	Administration	5100.0	License and Dues Expense
Association dues	Administration	5100.0	Dues and Subscriptions
Atomizers	Nursing Services	5900.0	Medical Care Materials and Supplies
Attorney's fees	Administration	5100.0	Legal
Audit fees	Administration	5100.0	Accounting and Auditing
Autoclave tape	Nursing Services	5900.0	Nonmedical Supplies
Automatic telephone rentals	Administration	5100.0	Telephone and Telegraph
Automobile insurance premium	Administration	5100.0	Insurance Expenses

Item	Cost Center Title	Code	Natural Classification Title
Automobile license	Administration	5100.0	Automobile Expenses
Automobile rentals	Administration	5100.0	Automobile Expenses
Automobile repairs	Plant Operation and Maintenance	5300.0	Repairs and Maintenance
Badges, identification, employees	Administration	5100.0	Office and Administrative Supplies
Bags, laundry	Laundry and Linen	5500.0	Nonmedical Supplies
Bandages, elastic	Nursing Services	5900.0	Medical Care Materials and Supplies
Bandages, sterile	Nursing Services	5900.0	Medical Care Materials and Supplies
Bands, identification	Administration	5100.0	Other Nonmedical Supplies
Bank charges	Administration	5100.0	Miscellaneous Expenses
Basins, bath, emesis, face	Nursing Services	5900.0	Minor Equipment
Baskets, waste	Housekeeping	5600.0	Minor Equipment
Baskets, specimen collection, (sputum, urine, and feces)	Nursing Services	5900.0	Minor Equipment
Bath caps	Laundry and Linen	5500.0	Supplies
Bath mats	Laundry and Linen	5500.0	Supplies
Bath robes	Laundry and Linen	5500.0	Supplies
Batteries, flashlight	Maintenance	5300.0	Supplies
Bed pans	Nursing Services	5900.0	Minor Equipment
Benzalkonium chloride sol.	Nursing Services	5900.0	Medical Care Materials and Supplies
Blankets	Laundry and Linen	5500.0	Linen and Bedding
Board member expenses	Administrative Services	5100.0	Appropriate Natural Classification
Bond discount amortization	Capital Expense	7000.0	Interest Expense
Bond interest expense	Capital Expense	7000.0	Interest Expense
Bonding insurance premiums, employees	Administration	5100.0	Bonding Expenses
Bookkeeping forms	Administration	5100.0	Office and Administrative Supplies
Books, medical	Nursing Services	5900.0	Supplies
Borax	Laundry and Linen	5500.0	Supplies
Brooms	Housekeeping	5600.0	Supplies
Brushes	Housekeeping	5600.0	Supplies

Item	Category	Account	Amount
Buckets, scrub	Housekeeping	Supplies	5600.0
Building repairs by outside concerns	Plant Operation and Maintenance	Repairs and Maintenance	5300.0
Bulbs, electric light	Plant Operation and Maintenance	Supplies	5300.0
Business interruption insurance	Administration	Insurance Expense	5100.0
Business machine rentals	Administration	Rental Expense	5100.0
Business office forms	Administration	Supplies	5100.0
Buttons	Laundry and Linen	Supplies	5500.0
Canes	Physical Therapy	Medical Care Materials and Supplies	6600.0
Caps, ice (bags)	Nursing Services	Medical Care Materials and Supplies	5900.0
Carpenter tools	Plant Operation and Maintenance	Minor Equipment	5300.0
Carpeting and rugs, cleaning	Housekeeping	Purchased Services	5600.0
Carpeting and rugs, (depreciation)	Capital Expense	Depreciation and Amortization	7000.0
Cases, pillow	Laundry and Linen	Linen and Bedding	5500.0
Cash shortages, overages	Administration	Miscellaneous Expenses	5100.0
Casters	Plant Operation and Maintenance	Minor Equipment	5300.0
Catheter boxes, trays	Nursing Services	Medical Care Materials and Supplies	5900.0
Catheters, metal, rubber, etc.	Nursing Services	Medical Care Materials and Supplies	5900.0
Chart envelopes	Medical Records	Supplies	5800.0
Chart, patient	Medical Records	Supplies	5800.0
Checkbooks and vouchers checks	Administration	Office and Administrative Supplies	5100.0
Chinaware (replacement)	Dietary	Minor Equipment	5400.0
Cleaning compounds	Housekeeping	Cleaning Supplies	5600.0
Cleavers, chopping	Dietary	Minor Equipment	5400.0
Clocks, household	Nursing Services	Minor Equipment	5900.0
Clocks, interval timer	Nursing Services	Minor Equipment	5900.0
Clothes racks	Nursing Services	Minor Equipment	5900.0
Clothing, inpatients	Laundry and Linen	Supplies	5500.0
Clothing, staff	Laundry and Linen	Employee Uniforms	5500.0
Cloths, face	Laundry and Linen	Linen and Bedding	5500.0
Cloths, table	Dietary	Supplies	5400.0
Coal and coke	Plant Operation and Maintenance	Utilities—Other	5300.0
Collection fees	Administration	Collection Agencies	5100.0

Item	Cost Center Title	Code	Natural Classification Title
Compound tincture benzoin	Nursing Services	5900.0	Medical Care Materials and Supplies
Consultant fees	Dietary	5400.0	Consulting Fees
Consultant fees	Pharmacy	6000.0	Consulting Fees
Consultant fees	Physical Therapy	6600.0	Consulting Fees
Consultant fees	Medical Records	5800.0	Consulting Fees
Consultant fees	Utilization Review	5200.0	Consulting Fees
Consultant fees	Nursing Services	5900.0	Consulting Fees
Containers, false teeth	Nursing Services	5900.0	Supplies
Cotton, absorbent	Nursing Services	5900.0	Medical Care Materials and Supplies
Cotton balls	Nursing Services	5900.0	Medical Care Materials and Supplies
Cottonseed oil	Nursing Services	5900.0	Medical Care Materials and Supplies
Covers, tray or table (patients)	Dietary	5400.0	Supplies
Crutches	Physical Therapy	6600.0	Medical Care Materials and Supplies
Cuffs, blood pressure	Nursing Services	5900.0	Minor Equipment
Cups, china	Dietary	5400.0	Minor Equipment
Cups, paper, beverage	Dietary	5400.0	Supplies
Cups, paper, sputum	Nursing Services	5900.0	Medical Care Materials and Supplies
Curtains and draperies, window, cleaning	Housekeeping	5600.0	Purchased Services
Curtain and draperies, cubicle (re-placement)	Housekeeping	5600.0	Minor Equipment
Cushions, air, invalid	Nursing Services	5900.0	Medical Care Materials and Supplies
Cutters, paper	Administration	5100.0	Minor Equipment
Data processing fees	Administration	5100.0	Purchased Services
Depreciation, fixed equipment	Capital Expense	7000.0	Depreciation and Amortization
Depreciation, major movable equipment	Capital Expense	7000.0	Depreciation and Amortization
Depreciation, minor equipment	Capital Expense	700010	Depreciation and Amortization
Depressors, tongue	Nursing Services	5900.0	Medical Care Materials and Supplies
Detergents	Laundry and Linen	5500.0	Cleaning Supplies

Dextrose	Nursing Services	5900.0	Intravenous Solution
Diapers	Nursing Services	5900.0	Supplies
Dinnerware (replacement)	Dietary	5400.0	Minor Equipment
Dishes, table (replacement)	Dietary	5400.0	Minor Equipment
Dishpans (replacement)	Dietary	5400.0	Minor Equipment
Disinfectants	Housekeeping	5600.0	Supplies
Doilies, tray, paper	Dietary	5400.0	Supplies
Douche pans	Nursing Services	5900.0	Minor Equipment
Dressing tray	Nursing Services	5900.0	Minor Equipment
Dressings	Nursing Services	5900.0	Medical Care Materials and Supplies
Droppers, medicine	Nursing Services	5900.0	Medical Care Materials and Supplies
Dues, association	Administration	5100.0	Dues and Subscriptions
Dues, professional organizations	Administration	5100.0	Dues and Subscriptions
Dyes, laundry	Laundry and Linen	5500.0	Nonmedical Supplies
Earthquake insurance	Administration	5100.0	Unassigned Expenses
Education supplies, inservice	Administration	5100.0	Supplies
Electric light bulbs	Plant Operation and Maintenance	5300.0	Supplies
Electricity	Plant Operation and Maintenance	5300.0	Utilities—Electricity
Elevator inspection fees	Plant Operation and Maintenance	5300.0	Purchased Services
Elevator liability insurance	Plant Operation and Maintenance	5300.0	Insurance Expense
Elevator repairs	Plant Operation and Maintenance	5300.0	Repairs and Maintenance
Employee benefits, F.I.C.A.	Administration	5100.0	FICA
Employee benefits, unemployment insurance	Administration	5100.0	SUI and FUI
Employee benefits, parking	Administration	5100.0	Employee Benefits
Employee benefits, meals	Administration	5100.0	Employee Benefits
Employee benefits, health insurance	Administration	5100.0	Group Health Insurance
Employee benefits, life insurance	Administration	5100.0	Group Life Insurance
Employee benefits, licenses	Administration	5100.0	Employee Benefits
Employee benefits, pension	Administration	5100.0	Pension and Retirement
Employee uniforms, hospital owned	Laundry and Linen	5500.0	Uniform Expense
Enema, disposable	Nursing Services	5900.0	Medical Care Materials and Supplies

233

Item	Cost Center Title	Code	Natural Classification Title
Envelopes, paper, other	Administration	5100.0	Office and Administrative Supplies
Epsom salts	Nursing Services	5900.0	Medical Care Materials and Supplies
Equipment repair by outside concerns	Plant Operation and Maintenance	5300.0	Repairs and Maintenance
Exterminator (pest control service)	Housekeeping	5600.0	Purchased Services
Extractors, fruit juice	Dietary	5400.0	Minor Equipment
Face cloths	Laundry and Linen	5500.0	Linen and Bedding
Face masks	Nursing Services	5900.0	Medical Care Materials and Supplies
Fees, medical—Physicians	Nursing Services	5900.0	Physician Services
Fees, medical—Therapists	Physical Therapy	6600.0	Therapist Services
Fidelity bond premiums	Administration	5100.0	Insurance Expense
Fire insurance premiums	Plant Operation and Maintenance	5300.0	Insurance Expense
Flashlights and batteries	Plant Operation and Maintenance	5300.0	Supplies
Flowers, decorative	Housekeeping	5600.0	Miscellaneous Expenses
Flower pots and planters			
(1) Inside hospital	Housekeeping	5600.0	Supplies
(2) Outside hospital	Plant Operation and Maintenance	5300.0	Supplies
Food, Meat, Fish, and Poultry	Dietary	5400.0	Food
Food, Other	Dietary	5400.0	Food
Forks, kitchen	Dietary	5400.0	Minor Equipment
Forms, medical record, medical history, etc.	Administration	5100.0	Office and Administrative Supplies
Freight charges	Administration	5100.0	Freight Expense
Fuel, gas	Plant Operation and Maintenance	5300.0	Utilities—Gas
Fund raising expenses	Administration	5100.0	Fund Raising
Funnels	Plant Operation and Maintenance	5300.0	Supplies
Gas, mouth	Nursing Services	5900.0	Supplies
Garbage cans	Housekeeping	5600.0	Minor Equipment
Gas (fuel)	Plant Operation and Maintenance	5300.0	Utilities—Gas
Gasoline	Plant Operation and Maintenance	5300.0	Supplies
Gauze	Nursing Services	5900.0	Medical Care Materials and Supplies

Germicides, cleaning	Housekeeping	5600.0	Cleaning Supplies
Glass, window	Plant Operation and Maintenance	5300.0	Supplies
Glassware, kitchen, dining room	Dietary	5400.0	Supplies
Gloves, disposable	Nursing Services	5900.0	Supplies
Gloves, reusable, nonsterile	Nursing Services	5900.0	Supplies
Glue, furniture, etc.	Plant Operation and Maintenance	5300.0	Supplies
Gowns, employee	Laundry and Linen	5500.0	Employee Wearing Apparel
Gowns, patients'	Laundry and Linen	5500.0	Supplies
Grass seed	Plant Operation and Maintenance	5300.0	Supplies
Graters, food	Dietary	5400.0	Minor Equipment
Greases, lubricating	Plant Operation and Maintenance	5300.0	Supplies
Guard service fees	Plant Operation and Maintenance		Purchased Services
Hangers, coat	Housekeeping	5600.0	Supplies
Heaters	Plant Operation and Maintenance	5300.0	Minor Equipment
Holders, napkin	Dietary	5400.0	Supplies
Holders, sputum cup	Nursing Services	5900.0	Supplies
Hot packs, apparatus	Nursing Services	5900.0	Instruments and Minor Medical Equipment
Hot water bottles	Nursing Services	5900.0	Instruments and Minor Medical Equipment
Hydrogen peroxide	Nursing Services	5900.0	Medical Care Materials and Supplies
Hypodermic needles	Nursing Services	5900.0	Medical Care Materials and Supplies
I.V. set	Nursing Services	5900.0	Medical Care Materials and Supplies
I.V. supplies	Nursing Services	5900.0	Medical Care Materials and Supplies
Ice (purchased)	Dietary	5400.0	Supplies
Ice bags	Nursing Services	5900.0	Supplies
Ident-a-bands	Administration	5100.0	Supplies
Industrial engineering fees	Administration	5100.0	Consulting Fees
Ink, marking	Laundry and Linen	5500.0	Supplies
Ink, printing	Administration	5100.0	Supplies
Insect extermination expense	Housekeeping	5600.0	Purchased Services
Insecticides	Housekeeping	5600.0	Supplies

	Cost Center		Natural Classification
Item	*Title*	*Code*	*Title*
Inservice education supplies	Administration	5100.0	Educational Materials
Instruments, tray—reusable	Nursing Services	5900.0	Minor Equipment
Instruments, tray—disposable	Nursing Services	5900.0	Medical Care Materials and Supplies
Insurance:			
Boiler liability	Plant Operation	5300.0	Insurance Expenses
Bonding liability	Administration	5100.0	Insurance Expenses
Elevator liability	Plant Operation	5300.0	Insurance Expenses
Fire	Plant Operation	5300.0	Insurance Expenses
Malpractice liability	Administration	5100.0	Insurance Expenses
Unemployment	Administration	5100.0	SUI and FUI
Worker's compensation (ind. injury)	Administration	5100.0	Worker's Compensation Insurance
Intercommunication system expense	Administration	5100.0	Communication Expense
Interest expense, current working capital	Administration	5100.0	Interest Expense
Interest expense, long-term	Capital Expense	7000.0	Interest—Mortages
Jackets, orderlies	Laundry and Linen	5500.0	Uniform Expense
Jars, specimen	Nursing Services	5900.0	Supplies
Kettles, steam (kitchen)	Dietary	5400.0	Minor Equipment
Kettles, steam (patients' use)	Nursing Services	5900.0	Minor Equipment
Keys	Plant Operation and Maintenance	5300.0	Supplies
Kitchen utensils	Dietary	5400.0	Minor Equipment
Knives, bread, butcher, etc.	Dietary	5400.0	Minor Equipment
Labels, other			Supplies
Ladders	Plant Operation and Maintenance	5300.0	Minor Equipment
Lamps, electric	Plant Operation and Maintenance	5300.0	Minor Equipment
Lanterns (battery or gas type)	Plant Operation and Maintenance	5300.0	Minor Equipment
Laundering (outside concerns)	Laundry and Linen	5500.0	Purchased Services
Laxatives, simple	Nursing Services	5900.0	Pharmaceuticals
Lease costs	Capital Expense	7000.0	Rent Expense
Legal fees	Administration	5100.0	Legal

236

Licenses, car, truck (other than ambulance)	Administration	5100.0	License Expense
Lime, chlorinated	Housekeeping	5600.0	Cleaning Supplies
Linen, bed	Laundry and Linen	5500.0	Linen and Bedding
Linen, sterile	Laundry and Linen	5500.0	Linen and Bedding
Long distance telephone charges, general	Administration	5100.0	Telephone and Telegraph
Lubricating fluids	Nursing Services	5900.0	Medical Care Materials and Supplies
Lubricating jelly	Nursing Services	5900.0	Medical Care Materials and Supplies
Lumber	Plant Operation and Maintenance	5300.0	Supplies
Lye	Laundry and Linen	5500.0	Cleaning Supplies
Maalox	Nursing Services	5900.0	Pharmaceutical
Magazines	Administration	5100.0	Dues and Subscriptions
Maintenance contracts	Plant Operation and Maintenance	5300.0	Repairs and Maintenance
Mangle aprons	Laundry and Linen	5500.0	Supplies
Marking ink and labels	Laundry and Linen	5500.0	Supplies
Masks, face	Nursing Services	5900.0	Medical Care Materials and Supplies
Mats, bath	Laundry and Linen	5500.0	Other Nonmedical Supplies
Mattress covers and pads	Laundry and Linen	5500.0	Linen and Bedding
Membership dues	Administration	5100.0	Dues and Subscriptions
Mortgage, interest expense	Capital Expense	7000.0	Interest—Mortgages
Motor vehicle insurance	Administration	5100.0	Insurance
Motor vehicle license (see Licenses)			
Mouthwash, nonprescription	Nursing Services	5900.0	Medical Care Materials and Supplies
Needles, aneurysm, aspirating	Nursing Services	5900.0	Instruments and Minor Medical Equipment
Needles, spinal, hypodermic	Nursing Services	5900.0	Instruments and Minor Medical Equipment
Needles, sewing	Laundry and Linen	5500.0	Supplies
Nets, laundry	Laundry and Linen	5500.0	Supplies
Newspapers	Administration	5100.0	Dues and Subscriptions

Item	Cost Center Title	Code	Natural Classification Title
Nurses' uniforms (when hospital furnished), except students'	Laundry and Linen	5500.0	Employee Wearing Apparel
Nurses' uniforms, students'	Nursing Services	5900.0	Uniform Expense
Office supplies (printing and stationery)	Administration	5100.0	Office and Administrative Supplies
Oil, fuel	Plant Operation and Maintenance	5300.0	Utilities—Other
Oils and greases	Plant Operation and Maintenance	5300.0	Supplies
Orangewood sticks	Nursing Services	5900.0	Medical Care Materials and Supplies
Oxygen	Nursing Services	5900.0	Oxygen and Other Medical Gases
Packets—alcohol, lemon/glycerine	Nursing Services	5900.0	Medical Care Materials and Supplies
Packs, steam	Nursing Services	5900.0	Minor Equipment
Pads, bed, table, etc. (cloth)	Laundry and Linen	5500.0	Linen and Bedding
Pads, cleaning	Housekeeping	5600.0	Cleaning Supplies
Pads, laundry, mangle, press	Laundry and Linen	5500.0	Supplies
Pails, scrub	Housekeeping	5600.0	Cleaning Supplies
Paint brushes	Plant Operation and Maintenance	5300.0	Supplies
Painting, contracted	Plant Operation and Maintenance	5300.0	Repairs and Maintenance
Painters' drop clothes	Plant Operation and Maintenance	5300.0	Supplies
Paints, shellacs, varnishes	Plant Operation and Maintenance	5300.0	Supplies
Pans, baking	Dietary	5400.0	Minor Equipment
Pans, dust	Housekeeping	5600.0	Cleaning Supplies
Paper, data processing printout	Administration	5100.0	Office and Administrative Supplies
Paper, duplication machine	Administration	5100.0	Office and Administrative Supplies
Paper, shelf, toilet	Housekeeping	5600.0	Supplies
Paper, wax	Dietary	5400.0	Supplies
Paper cups	Dietary	5400.0	Supplies
Paper plates	Dietary	5400.0	Supplies
Pencils—lead, crayon, marking	Administration	5100.0	Office and Administrative Supplies
Pens	Administration	5100.0	Office and Administrative Supplies
Pension plan premiums	Administration	5100.0	Pension and Retirement

Percussion hammers	Nursing Services	5900.0	Instruments and Minor Medical Equipment
Periodicals	Administration	5100.0	Dues and Subscriptions
Pillows	Laundry and Linen	5500.0	Linen and Bedding
Pins, laundry	Laundry and Linen	5500.0	Supplies
Pins, safety, straight	Nursing Services	5900.0	Supplies
Pipettes	Nursing Services	5900.0	Supplies
Pitcher, water	Dietary	5400.0	Supplies
Plaster, building	Plant Operation and Maintenance	5300.0	Supplies
Plates, china, dinner, salad, etc.	Dietary	5400.0	Minor Equipment
Plumbing supplies	Plant Operation and Maintenance	5300.0	Supplies
Polishes	Housekeeping	5600.0	Cleaning Supplies
Postage, for general use	Administration	5100.0	Postage Expense
Postage, for specific departments	Administration	5100.0	Postage Expense
Powders, insect	Housekeeping	5600.0	Supplies
Powders, scouring	Housekeeping	5600.0	Cleaning Supplies
Power, purchased	Plant Operation and Maintenance	5300.0	Utilities
Rags, cleaning	Housekeeping	5600.0	Cleaning Supplies
Razor blades	Nursing Services	5900.0	Supplies
Razors	Nursing Services	5900.0	Supplies
Receptacles, waste	Housekeeping	5600.0	Minor Equipment
Record forms, medical	Administration	5100.0	Office and Administrative Supplies
Rental charges, duplicating machine	Administration	5100.0	Leases and Rentals
Rental charges, equipment	Capital Expense	7000.0	Leases and Rentals
Repairs to buildings and equipment (by an outside concern)	Plant Operation and Maintenance	5300.0	Repairs and Maintenance
Ribbons, typewriter	Administration	5100.0	Office and Administrative Supplies
Rubber bands	Administration	5100.0	Office and Administrative Supplies
Saucers, plant	Housekeeping	5600.0	Supplies
Scalpels	Nursing Services	5900.0	Minor Medical Equipment and Instruments
Scoops, flour, sugar, etc.	Dietary	5400.0	Minor Equipment

	Cost Center		Natural Classification
Item	*Title*	*Code*	*Title*
Service charges on equipment repairs	Plant Operation and Maintenance	5300.0	Repairs and Maintenance
Sharpeners, pencil	Administration	5100.0	Supplies
Sheep skins	Nursing Services	5900.0	Supplies
Sheet wadding	Nursing Services	5900.0	Supplies
Sheets, linen	Laundry and Linen	5500.0	Linen and Bedding
Sheets, rubber, on patients' beds	Laundry and Linen	5500.0	Supplies
Signals, communication (beepers)	Administration	5100.0	Minor Equipment
Slippers, paper	Nursing Services	5900.0	Supplies
Slips, laundry	Laundry and Linen	5500.0	Office and Administrative Supplies
Soaps, dishwashing	Dietary	5400.0	Cleaning Supplies
Soaps, floor, toilet	Housekeeping	5600.0	Cleaning Supplies
Soaps, laundry	Laundry and Linen	5500.0	Cleaning Supplies
Steam cleaner rental	Housekeeping	5600.0	Expenses
Steam, purchased	Plant Operation and Maintenance	5300.0	Utilities—Other
Sterile water	Nursing Services	5900.0	Supplies
Suction tips, disposable	Nursing Services	5900.0	Medical Care Materials and Supplies
Suppositories	Nursing Services	5900.0	Medical Care Materials and Supplies
Sutures	Nursing Services	5900.0	Instruments and Minor Medical Equipment
Swabs	Nursing Services	5900.0	Medical Care Materials and Supplies
Syringes, bulb	Nursing Services	5900.0	Medical Care Materials and Supplies
Syringes, hypo.	Nursing Services	5900.0	Medical Care Materials and Supplies
Syringes, irrigating	Nursing Services	5900.0	Medical Care Materials and Supplies
Tablets, paper	Administration	5100.0	Office and Administrative Supplies
Tape remover	Nursing Services	5900.0	Medical Care Materials and Supplies
Tape, twilled	Laundry and Linen	5500.0	Supplies
Taxes, business	Administration	5100.0	Tax Expense
Taxes, personal property	Administration	5100.0	Property Taxes
Taxes, real estate	Capital Expense	7000.0	Property Taxes
Telegraph expense	Administration	5100.0	Telephone and Telegraph

Item	Department	Account #	Account
Telephone expense	Administration	5100.0	Telephone and Telegraph
Text books, student nurses'	Administration	5100.0	Education Supplies
Thermometers, mouth, bath, rectal	Nursing Services	5900.0	Medical Care Materials and Supplies
Thermostat, wall	Plant Operation and Maintenance	5300.0	Supplies
Thread, sewing	Laundry and Linen	5500.0	Nonmedical Supplies
Throat bags	Nursing Services	5900.0	Medical Care Materials and Supplies
Time cards (payroll)	Administration	5100.0	Office and Administrative Supplies
Tips, irrigating, suction, uterine, etc.	Nursing Services	5900.0	Medical Care Materials and Supplies
Tires, car, truck	Plant Operation and Maintenance	5300.0	Supplies
Tissue, facial	Housekeeping	5600.0	Supplies
Toilet paper	Housekeeping	5600.0	Supplies
Towels, bath, face	Laundry and Linen	5500.0	Linen and Bedding
Towels, paper	Housekeeping	5600.0	Supplies
Traction rope	Nursing Services	5900.0	Medical Care Materials and Supplies
Travel expense:			
Educational	Administration	5100.0	Travel Expense
"Community" service	Administration	5100.0	Travel Expense
Board	Administration	5100.0	Travel Expense
Administration	Administration	5100.0	Travel Expense
Tray covers, paper (patients' meals)	Dietary	5400.0	Supplies
Trays, dressing	Nursing Services	5900.0	Minor Equipment
Trays, serving, patients'	Dietary	5400.0	Minor Equipment
Tubes, colon, connecting, duodenal, infusion, intravenous, etc.	Nursing Services	5900.0	Medical Care Materials and Supplies
Tubing, rubber	Nursing Services	5900.0	Supplies
Tuition, employee education	Administration	5100.0	Employee Benefits
Underpads, occasional use	Laundry and Linen	5500.0	Linen and Bedding
Uniforms, employees	Nursing Services	5900.0	Uniform Expense
Urinals, patient	Dietary	5400.0	Uniform Expense
Utensils, kitchen	Nursing Services	5900.0	Minor Equipment
Utensils, stainless steel, kitchen	Dietary	5400.0	Minor Equipment
	Dietary	5400.0	Minor Equipment

	Cost Center		Natural Classification
Item	Title	Code	Title
Vaporizers, medicinal (steam kettles)	Nursing Services	5900.0	Minor Equipment
Vases, decorative	Housekeeping	5600.0	Supplies
Vegetable oil	Dietary	5400.0	Food
Venetian blind cleaning	Housekeeping	5600.0	Purchased Services
Wash cloths	Laundry and Linen	5500.0	Supplies
Waste, cotton, wool	Plant Operation and Maintenance	5300.0	Supplies
Waste receptacles	Housekeeping	5600.0	Minor Equipment
Water	Plant Operation and Maintenance	5300.0	Utilities—Water
Water treatment compounds	Plant Operation and Maintenance	5300.0	Supplies
Wax, floor	Housekeeping	5600.0	Cleaning Supplies
Window glass	Plant Operation and Maintenance	5300.0	Supplies
Window washing expense (outside concerns)	Housekeeping	5600.0	Purchased Services
Wood, fire	Plant Operation and Maintenance	5300.0	Supplies
Wringers, mop	Housekeeping	5600.0	Minor Equipment

Retirement Village, Inc.
GENERAL LEDGER CHART OF ACCOUNTS
6/25/80

ASSETS

CURRENT ASSETS

1101-0	Cash In Bank—Operating	1417-0	Buildings—House Trailer
1102-0	Cash In Bank—Building	1418-0	Buildings—Wesley Ctr.—8 Bed
1103-0	Cash In Bank—Gift Shop	1421-0	Building Improvements
1105-0	Cash In Bank—Trust Funds	1431-0	Equip., Furniture & Fixtures
1108-0	Petty Cash Funds—Trust Fund	1432-0	Home and Cottage Furnishings
1109-0	Petty Cash Funds—Operating	1433-0	Apartment Furnishings
1110-0	Imprest Payroll	1434-0	Office Equipment
1111-0	Savings Account—Prudential	1441-0	Transportation Equipment
1112-0	Savings Account—Building	1506-0	Acc. Depr.—Land Improvements
1113-0	Savings Account—Bonds	1511-0	Acc. Depr.—Bldgs.—Original
1114-0	Savings Account—Chapel	1512-0	Acc. Depr.—Bldgs.—New
1115-0	Investment—C.D.s	1513-0	Acc. Depr.—Bldgs.—Dycus
1116-0	Investment—Burial C.D.s	1514-0	Acc. Depr.—Cottages
1117-0	Investment—Stocks	1515-0	Acc. Depr.—Bldgs.—Houses
1118-0	Investment—Bonds	1516-0	Acc. Depr.—Bldgs.—Apartments
1119-0	Reserve For Bond Redemption	1517-0	Acc. Depr.—Bldgs.—House Tr.
1121-0	Accts. Rec.—Private Patients	1518-0	Acc. Depr.—Bldgs.—Wesley Ctr
1122-0	Accts. Rec.—Medicaid	1521-0	Acc. Depr.—Bldg. Improvements
1123-0	Accts. Rec.—Medicaid Pending	1531-0	Acc. Depr.—Equip., Furn. & Fix.
1127-0	Accts. Rec.—Other	1532-0	Acc. Depr.—Home & Cott. Furn.
1128-0	Hill-Burton Receivable	1533-0	Acc. Depr.—Apartment Furn.
1140-0	Real Estate Contracts Rec.	1534-0	Acc. Depr.—Office Equipment
1141-0	Physician Fees—Clearing	1541-0	Acc. Depr.—Trans. Equipment
1146-0	Accrued Interest Receivable	1601-0	Constr. In Progress—General
1163-0	Unexpired Insurance	1602-0	Constr. In Progress—Basement

CAPITAL ASSETS

1405-0	Land	1603-0	Constr. In Progress—1st Floor
1406-0	Land Improvements	1604-0	Constr. In Progress—2nd Floor
1411-0	Buildings—Original		
1412-0	Buildings—New		
1413-0	Buildings—Dycus		
1414-0	Buildings—Cottages		
1415-0	Buildings—Houses		
1416-0	Buildings—Apartments		

1605-0	Constr. In Progress—3rd Floor		**PATIENT SERVICES REVENUE**
1606-0	Constr. In Progress—Attic		
1712-0	Bond Consultation Fees		SHELTERED CARE
		3051-0	Living Center—Private
	LIABILITIES AND CAPITAL	3052-0	Living Center—Medicaid
	LIABILITIES		SKILLED CARE
	Current Liabilities	3063-0	Wesley I—Private
2111-0	Notes Payable—Current	3064-0	Wesley I—Medicaid
2112-0	Mortgages Payable—Current	3065-0	Wesley I—Medicaid Pending
2113-0	Bonds Payable—Current	3073-0	Wesley II—Medicare—Certified Section
2121-0	Accounts Payable—Trade		
2131-0	Hospitalization Ins. Payable	3074-0	Wesley II—Medicaid—Certified Section
2132-0	Group Life Ins. Payable		
2133-0	Wage Assignments	3083-0	Dycus—Private
2134-0	Payroll Deduction—Bonds	3084-0	Dycus—Medicaid
2135-0	Employees Pension Fund Payable		
			INTERMEDIATE CARE
2136-0	Tax Sheltered Annuities Pay.	3103-0	Wesley I—Private
		3104-0	Wesley I—Medicaid
2141-0	Accr. Salaries & Wages Pay.	3143-0	Wesley II—Private
		3144-0	Wesley II—Medicaid
	Accr. Vacation Pay	3183-0	Dycus—Private
	Acc. Sick Pay	3184-0	Dycus—Medicaid
2151-0	FICA Taxes Payable	3223-0	Holden Center—Private
2152-0	Federal Income Taxes Pay.	3224-0	Holden Center—Medicaid
2153-0	State Income Taxes Pay.		
2154-0	State U.C. Taxes Payable		ANCILLARY SERVICES
2181-0	Accrued Interest Payable	3311-0	Physical Therapy
2201-0	Due To/From Guests Trust Funds	3321-0	Speech Therapy
		3331-0	Occupational Therapy
2202-0	Burial Funds Payable	3341-0	Medical Supplies
2203-0	Unfulfilled Entrance Fees Pay.	3351-0	Drugs
		3361-0	Oxygen
2251-0	Deferred Annuity Gifts	3371-0	Physicians Fees
	Long-term Liabilities	3381-0	Other Medical
2311-0	Notes Payable—Term		
2312-0	Mortgages Payable—Term		LESS UNCOMPENSATED CARE
2313-0	Bonds Payable—Term		
2401-0	Life Care Commitment	3511-0	Uncompensated Care—Cont. Fees
	CAPITAL	3512-0	Cost Adj—Life Care Commitment
2951-0	Village Equity		
2961-0	Reserve—Life Care Commit.	3513-0	Recognized Rev—Life Care Com.
2999-0	Net Income (Loss)		

3521-0	Medicare Discount	4072-0	Utilities
3551-0	Patient Refunds	4073-0	Television Expense
		4083-0	Training & Education
	INDEPENDENT LIVING REVENUE	4096-0	Depreciation

Wesley I

3648-0	Apartments	4101-0	R.N. Salaries & Wages
3649-0	Cottages	4102-0	L.P.N. Salaries & Wages
		4103-0	Aides & Orderlies Sal. & Wages
	OTHER OPERATING REVENUE	4121-0	Nursing Supplies
3911-0	Barber & Beauty Shop Income	4122-0	Oxygen Expense
		4123-0	Drugs
3912-0	Village Store Income	4124-0	Medical Supplies
3913-0	Room Rentals—Guests	4125-0	Training & Education
3921-0	Telephone Charges	4129-0	Administrative Overhead
3931-0	Burial Expense Reimbursement	4131-0	Physicians' Services
		4132-0	Housekeeping Supplies
3941-0	Exp. Reimb.—Medical Insurance	4133-0	Utilities
		4134-0	Laundry Expense
		4135-0	Housekeeping Salaries
3951-0	Cable TV Charges	4136-0	Television Expense
3961-0	Dietary—Meal Charges	4137-0	Standard Meal Cost
3971-0	Ambulance Fees	4138-0	Personal Laundry Expense
3981-0	Expense Reimbursement—Other	4139-0	Maintenance Work Order Expense
3991-0	CETA Reimbursement		

OPERATING EXPENSE

Wesley II—Certified Section

	HEALTH CARE SERVICES	4141-0	R.N. Salaries & Wages
		4142-0	L.P.N. Salaries & Wages
	Sheltered Care—Living Center	4143-0	Aides & Orderlies Sal. & Wages
		4161-0	Nursing Supplies
4001-0	R.N. Salaries & Wages	4162-0	Oxygen Expense
4002-0	LPN Salaries & Wages	4163-0	Drugs
4003-0	Aides & Orderlies Sal. & Wages	4164-0	Medical Supplies
4021-0	Nursing Supplies	4165-0	Training & Education
4022-0	Oxygen Expense	4169-0	Administrative Overhead
4023-0	Drugs	4171-0	Physicians' Services
4024-0	Medical Supplies	4172-0	Housekeeping Supplies
4029-0	Administrative Overhead	4173-0	Utilities
4031-0	Physicians' Services	4174-0	Laundry Expense
4041-0	Standard Meal Cost	4175-0	Housekeeping Salaries
4051-0	Housekeeping Salaries	4176-0	Television Expense
4052-0	Housekeeping Supplies	4177-0	Standard Meal Cost
4061-0	Personal Laundry Expense	4178-0	Personal Laundry Expense
4071-0	Maintenance Work Order Expense	4179-0	Maintenance Work Order Expense

Dycus

4181-0	R.N. Salaries & Wages
4182-0	L.P.N. Salaries & Wages
4183-0	Aides & Orderlies Sal. & Wages
4201-0	Nursing Supplies
4202-0	Oxygen Expense
4203-0	Drugs
4204-0	Medical Supplies
4205-0	Training & Education
4209-0	Administrative Overhead
4211-0	Physicians' Services
4212-0	Housekeeping Supplies
4213-0	Utilities
4214-0	Laundry Expense
4215-0	Housekeeping Salaries
4216-0	Television Expense
4217-0	Standard Meal Cost
4218-0	Personal Laundry Expense
4219-0	Maintenance Work Order Expense

ICF—Holden Center

4221-0	R.N. Salaries & Wages
4222-0	L.P.N. Salaries & Wages
4223-0	Aides & Orderlies Sal. & Wages
4241-0	Nursing Supplies
4242-0	Oxygen Expense
4243-0	Drugs
4244-0	Medical Supplies
4245-0	Training & Education
4249-0	Administrative Overhead
4251-0	Physicians' Services
4253-0	Utilities
4254-0	Laundry Expense
4255-0	Housekeeping Salaries
4256-0	Television Expense
4257-0	Standard Meal Expense
4258-0	Personal Laundry Expense
4259-0	Maintenance Work Order Expense

Nursing Administration

4261-0	Nursing Admin. Sal. & Wages
4262-0	Medical Records Salaries
4263-0	In-Service Training Salaries
4271-0	Medical Director
4272-0	Medical Records Consultant
4273-0	Utilization Review Fees
4281-0	Office Supplies & Expense
4283-0	Training & Education
4301-0	Activities Salaries & Wages
4302-0	Social Rehab. Salaries & Wages
4311-0	Activity Consultants
4312-0	Social Service Consultants
4321-0	Supplies & Expense
4322-0	Religious Supplies & Expense
4323-0	Training & Education
4371-0	Maintenance Work Order Expense

Physical Rehabilitation

4401-0	Physical Therapy Aides Sal.
4402-0	Physical Therapy Assist. Sal.
4411-0	Physical Therapy Consultants
4421-0	Physical Rehab. Supplies
4423-0	Training & Education
4471-0	Maintenance Work Order Expense
4478-0	Laundry Expense

Speech Rehabilitation

4501-0	Speech Therapy Salaries
4511-0	Speech Therapy Consultants
4521-0	Speech Therapy Supplies
4523-0	Training & Education
4571-0	Maintenance Work Order Expense

Apartments

4841-0	Standard Meal Cost
4851-0	Housekeeping Salaries
4852-0	Housekeeping Supplies
4861-0	Personal Laundry Expense
4871-0	Maintenance Work Order Expense
4872-0	Utilities
4873-0	Television Expense
4883-0	Training & Education
4889-0	Administrative Overhead
4896-0	Depreciation—Apartments

Cottages

4941-0	Standard Meal Cost
4951-0	Housekeeping Salaries

4952-0	Housekeeping Supplies	5533-0	Garbage Services
4961-0	Personal Laundry Expense	5534-0	Pest Control
4971-0	Maintenance Work Order Expense	5595-0	Utilities Cost Allocation

Administration

4972-0	Utilities
4973-0	Television Expense
4983-0	Training & Education
4989-0	Administrative Overhead
4996-0	Depreciation—Cottages

Dietary

5101-0	Kitchen Salaries & Wages
5111-0	Dietary Consultant
5121-0	Food Costs
5122-0	Supplies
5123-0	Training & Education
5171-0	Maintenance Work Order Expense
5178-0	Laundry Expense
5195-0	Meal Cost Allocation

Housekeeping

5201-0	Housekeeping Salaries & Wages
5221-0	Housekeeping Supplies
5271-0	Maintenance Work Order Expense

Laundry

5301-0	Laundry Salaries & Wages
5321-0	Laundry Supplies & Soaps
5322-0	Linens
5323-0	Training & Education
5371-0	Maintenance Work Order Expense
5373-0	Utilities
5395-0	Personal Laundry Cost Alloc.

Maintenance

5401-0	Maintenance Salaries & Wages
5421-0	Maintenance Supplies
5423-0	Training & Education
5431-0	Purchased Repairs & Maint.
5432-0	Other Television Expense
5495-0	Work Order Cost Alloc.

Utilities

5531-0	Electricity & Gas
5532-0	Water

Administration

6101-0	Administrator's Salary
6102-0	Directory of Ministry Salary
6103-0	Office & Recep. Sal. & Wages
6121-0	Office Supplies & Expense
6122-0	Bank Charges
6123-0	Office Equipment Rental
6124-0	Printing & Forms
6125-0	Data Processing Costs
6126-0	Postage
6127-0	Telephone
6128-0	Dues & Subscriptions
6129-0	Advertising & Promotion
6130-0	Auto & Truck Expense
6131-0	Travel
6132-0	Dir. of Ministry Travel & Exp.
6133-0	Training & Education
6141-0	Licenses, Permits & Fees
6151-0	Insurance—Fire & Casualty
6152-0	Insurance—Liab. & Malpractice
6153-0	Insurance—Other
6154-0	Conference Expense
6171-0	Methodist Foundation
6181-0	Legal Fees
6182-0	Auditing Fees
6183-0	Management Consultants
6184-0	Bond Expense
6185-0	Write offs
6191-0	Miscellaneous Expense
6195-0	Maintenance Work Order Expense
6196-0	Administration Cost Allocation

Employee Benefits

6271-0	Payroll Taxes—FICA
6272-0	State U.C.
6281-0	Hospitalization Insurance
6282-0	Workmen's Compensation Ins.
6283-0	Employee Pension Plan
6284-0	Moving Expenses
6291-0	Director of Ministry Housing

6292-0	Adminstrator's Housing	7911-0	Barber & Beauty Expense
6295-0	Employee Physicals	7912-0	Village Store Expense
6296-0	Employee Benefits Cost Alloc.	7913-0	Burial Exp. & Ins. Premiums
		7914-0	Resident Medical Insurance
		7915-0	Ambulance Expense

Capital Costs

NON-OPERATING INCOME/EXPENSE

7006-0	Depr.—Land Improvements		
7011-0	Depr.—Bldgs.—Nursing Care	7951-0	Savings Account Interest
7014-0	Depr.—Bldgs.—Cottages	7952-0	Cert. of Deposit Interest
7015-0	Depr.—Bldgs.—Houses	7953-0	Interest Income—Other
7016-0	Depr.—Bldgs.—Apartments	7955-0	Dividends
7017-0	Depr.—Bldgs.—House Trailer	7956-0	Vendors Commissions
7021-0	Depr.—Bldg. Improvements	7960-0	Special Gifts-Wills & Bequests
7031-0	Depr.—Equip., Furn. & Fix.	7961-0	Conference Apportionment—Reg.
7032-0	Depr.—Home & Cottage Furn.	7962-0	Conference Apport.—Special
7033-0	Depr.—Apartment Furn.	7963-0	Special Gifts—All Other
7034-0	Depr.—Office Equipment	7964-0	Donated Royalty Income
7035-0	Depr.—Transportation Equip.	7965-0	Bake Sales & Bazaars
7096-0	Depr.—Cost Allocation	7966-0	Advanced Special—Ind. & Conf.
7311-0	Interest Exp.—Notes Payable	7970-0	Rental Income—Beauty Shop
7312-0	Interest Expense—Mortgage	7981-0	Gain/Loss—Sale of Securities
7313-0	Interest Expense—Bonds	7991-0	Miscellaneous Income

Other Operating Expense

7901-0	Gain/Loss—Sale of Cap. Assets	

APPENDIX 2
Medicare Reimbursement

Optimization of Facility Bed Size for Medicare Reimbursement Purposes

A 25 percent difference in occupancy is the point at which Medicare will say occupancy is being artificially reduced in certified section. Therefore, this equation will determine the correct number of beds to certify as Medicare to optimize the reimbursement of space-related expenses.

Assume: Total beds = 100
Certified days (actual or projected) = 4,000
Noncertified days (actual or projected) = 23,000
Available days = 36,500

Let: C = certified beds
N = noncertified beds

Then: $C + N = 100$ [A]

or $C = 100 - N$

and $\dfrac{23,000}{65N} - \dfrac{4,000}{365C} = .25$

Substituting [A] above: $\dfrac{23,000}{365N} - \dfrac{4,000}{365(100-N)} = .25$

× 365

$\dfrac{23,000}{N} - \dfrac{4,000}{(100-N)} = 91.25$

× N

$23,000 - \dfrac{4,000N}{(100-N)} = 91.25N$

× (100 − N) $23,000(100 - N) - 4,000N = 91.25N \cdot (100 - N)$

or: $2,300,000 - 23,000N - 4,000N = 9125N - 91.25N^2$

Gathering terms: $91.25N^2 - 36,125N + 2,300,000 = $ zero

Using Quadradic Formula:

$$ax^2 + bx + c = 0$$
$$x = \dfrac{-\sqrt{b} \pm b^2 - 4ac}{2a}$$

or

$$N = \dfrac{36,125 \pm \sqrt{(-36,125)^2 - 4(91.25)(2,300,000)}}{2(91.25)}$$

Simplified:

$$N = \dfrac{36,125 \pm 21,575.811}{182.5} \quad \dfrac{36,125 + 21,575.811}{182.5}, \quad \dfrac{36,125 - 21,575.811}{182.5}$$

$= 316.16883, 79.72$

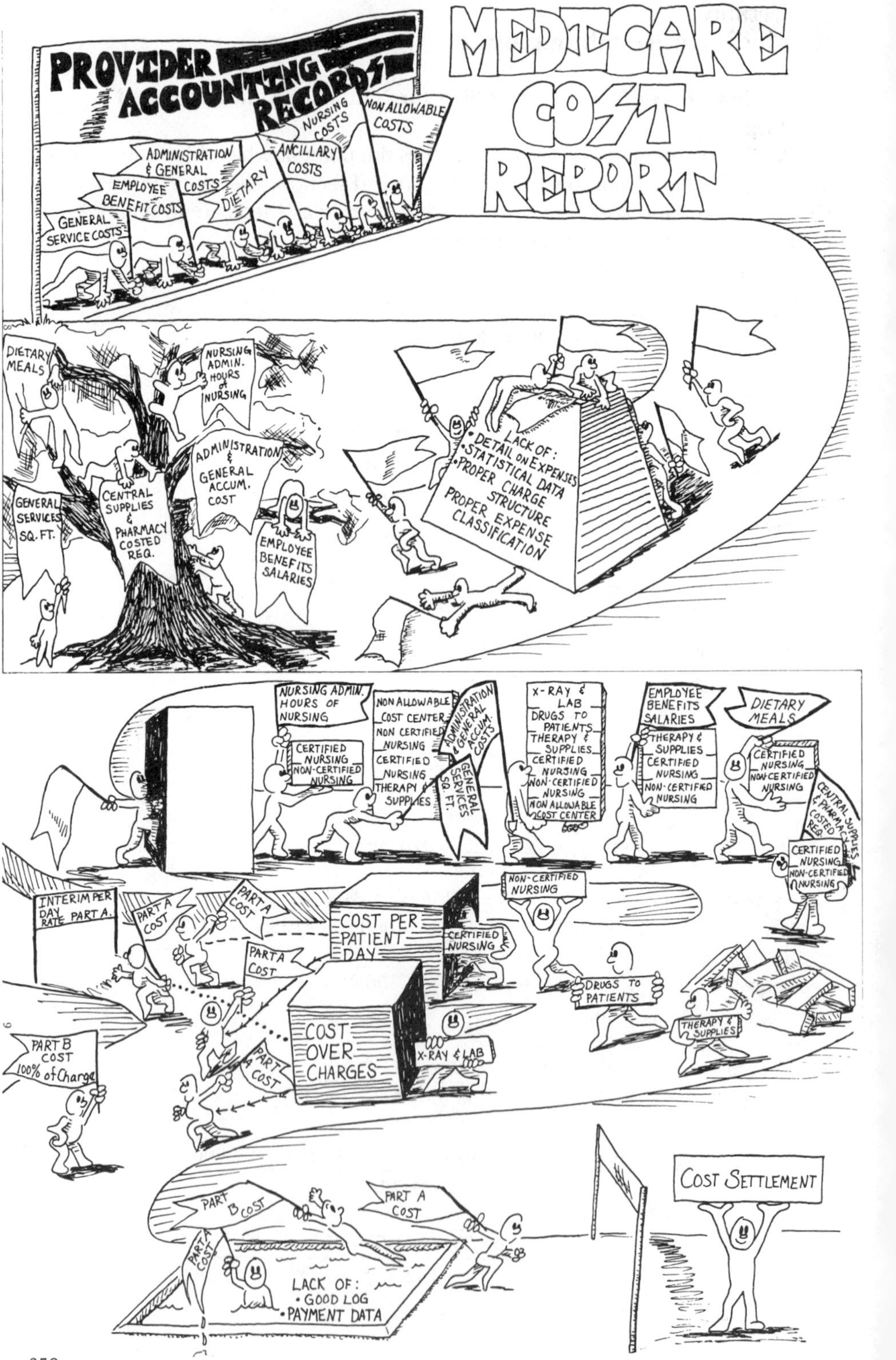

MEDICARE COST REPORT
PROVIDER ACCOUNTING RECORDS
GENERAL SERVICE COSTS
EMPLOYEE BENEFIT COSTS
ADMINISTRATION & GENERAL COSTS
DIETARY
ANCILLARY COSTS
NURSING COSTS
NON ALLOWABLE COSTS
DIETARY MEALS
NURSING ADMIN. HOURS of NURSING
ADMINISTRATION & GENERAL ACCUM. COST
CENTRAL SUPPLIES & PHARMACY COSTED REQ.
GENERAL SERVICES SQ. FT.
EMPLOYEE BENEFITS SALARIES
LACK OF: • DETAIL ON EXPENSES • STATISTICAL DATA • PROPER CHARGE STRUCTURE PROPER EXPENSE CLASSIFICATION
NURSING ADMIN. HOURS OF NURSING
CERTIFIED NURSING NON-CERTIFIED NURSING
NON ALLOWABLE COST CENTER NON CERTIFIED NURSING CERTIFIED NURSING THERAPY & SUPPLIES
ADMINISTRATION & GENERAL ACCUM. COSTS
GENERAL SERVICES SQ. FT.
X-RAY & LAB DRUGS TO PATIENTS THERAPY & SUPPLIES CERTIFIED NURSING NON-CERTIFIED NURSING NON ALLOWABLE COST CENTER
EMPLOYEE BENEFITS SALARIES
THERAPY & SUPPLIES CERTIFIED NURSING NON-CERTIFIED NURSING
DIETARY MEALS
CERTIFIED NURSING NON-CERTIFIED NURSING
CENTRAL SUPPLIES & PHARMACY COSTED REQ.
CERTIFIED NURSING NON-CERTIFIED NURSING
NON-CERTIFIED NURSING
INTERIM PER DAY RATE PART A.
PART A COST
PART A COST
PART A COST
COST PER PATIENT DAY
CERTIFIED NURSING
DRUGS TO PATIENTS
THERAPY & SUPPLIES
COST OVER CHARGES
X-RAY & LAB
PART A COST
PART B COST 100% of Charge
PART B COST
PART A COST
PART A COST
LACK OF: • GOOD LOG • PAYMENT DATA
COST SETTLEMENT

Obviously, 316 N-certified beds is not the correct solution since there are only 100 total beds, so 79.72 N-certified beds is the solution. Let's test the following:

	C	N−C	Total
Proposed beds	20.28	79.72	100
X days in period	365	365	365
Days available	7402.2	29097.8	36500
Actual/assumed days	4000	23000	27000
Occupancy %	.5404	.7904	.7397
% Difference in occupancy		.2500	

Since we cannot select fractional beds, we would therefore select 20 beds as the proper number of beds for the certified section. To be safe always round down to the number of noncertified beds.

Compliance Checklist (Adapted from a number of sources)

HIM-15 Principles of Reimbursement (Medicare and Medicaid Programs)

	Yes	No
Allowance for depreciation:		
(a) Is depreciation based on historical cost?	_____	_____
(b) Has a thorough search been made for donated depreciable assets?	_____	_____
(c) If donated assets are in use, have they been recorded on the general ledger at their estimated fair market value at date of donation?	_____	_____
(d) Has depreciation been separated for depreciable patient-related assets which are owned by other related organizations?	_____	_____
(e) Has consideration been given to the use of accelerated depreciation where it can be justified?	_____	_____
(f) Has consideration been given to the use of straight-line depreciation when it is more than accelerated depreciation?	_____	_____
(g) If any depreciable assets were sold or retired during the reporting period, has the depreciation been adjusted in the cost report for Medicare's portion of the gain or loss?	_____	_____
(h) Is depreciation being funded?	_____	_____
Interest expense:		
(a) What is the facility's policy regarding interest during construction?		
Capitalize	_____	_____
Expense	_____	_____

	Yes	No
(b) Has interest during construction been treated in accordance with GAAP?	_____	_____
(c) Has interest expense been eliminated where it does not relate to patient care?	_____	_____
(d) Has income earned on unrestricted investments been offset against interest expense (but not in excess of the interest expense)?	_____	_____
(e) Has interest expense been recognized on loans from funded depreciation?	_____	_____

Bad debts, charity, and courtesy allowances:

	Yes	No
(a) Are all revenues recorded on a gross basis and discounts recorded in a separate account?	_____	_____
(b) Are bad debts for deductibles and coinsurance due from Medicare patients offset against discounts and claimed on the cost report?	_____	_____
(c) Are payments received from Medicare patients applied first to coinsurance?	_____	_____
(d) Have adequate efforts been made to collect the patient's amounts?	_____	_____
(e) Are adequate records maintained on bad debts?	_____	_____

Cost of inservice education activities:

	Yes	No
(a) Does the facility engage in any inservice educational programs?	_____	_____
(b) If the facility is engaged in inservice programs, has the expense been recognized as an allowable cost and conducted in accordance with the Medicare principles?	_____	_____
(c) Has the cost of reimbursable programs been reduced by grants, tuitions, etc.?	_____	_____
(d) Has the direct cost and overhead of nonapproved programs been eliminated from allowable costs?	_____	_____

Value of services of nonpaid workers:

	Yes	No
(a) Does the facility receive any services from nonpaid workers?	_____	_____
(b) Is the agreement between the facility and the organization in writing?	_____	_____
(c) Does the facility have a legal obligation to pay the contracting organization?	_____	_____
(d) Is the liability for such services recorded in the accounting records?	_____	_____

(e) Was the value paid before the end of the next cost reporting period? _____ _____

(f) Are the services rendered by the workers necessary for patient care? _____ _____

(g) Are the positions filled customarily held by full-time employees? _____ _____

(h) Are the services performed on a regularly scheduled basis? _____ _____

(i) Is the amount paid employees at least as much as the value of the services of the nonpaid workers? _____ _____

(j) Does the facility maintain adequate records on each of these workers to document the services rendered and the hours worked? _____ _____

Purchase discounts, allowances, and refunds:

(a) Does the facility receive purchase discounts, allowances, rebates, or refunds? _____ _____

(b) Where the discount applies to a specific department, has the discount been offset against that department's allowable cost? _____ _____

(c) Where the discount does not apply to a specific department, has the discount been offset against allowable administrative cost? _____ _____

(d) Have discounts, allowances, and refunds received by a related organization also been deducted from allowable cost? _____ _____

Compensation of owners:

(a) Are there compensation and fringe benefits attributable to owners? _____ _____

(b) Was the value of the services paid to the owner within 2-½ months after the close of the reporting period? _____ _____

(c) Are the services rendered by the owners necessary for patient care? _____ _____

(d) Is the amount paid employees for similar services as much as the amount paid the owners? _____ _____

(e) If the owner does not work on a full-time basis, has appropriate recognition been given to this in the amount of expense included in cost? _____ _____

(f) If the owner is assisted by other employees, has recognition been given to this in the amount of compensation included in allowable cost? _____ _____

	Yes	No

(g) Does the facility maintain adequate records on the compensated owners to document the services rendered and the hours worked? _____ _____

Services received from related organizations:

(a) Does the facility receive services from a related organization which is commonly owned or commonly controlled by the facility's shareholders? _____ _____

(b) Are the services received necessary for patient care? _____ _____

(c) Is the amount paid to the related organization(s) eliminated from allowable cost and the related organization's actual cost substituted in its place? _____ _____

(d) Does the fair market value of the services exceed the costs included in allowable cost? _____ _____

(e) Have all costs applicable to patient related services, been included in allowable cost even where the related organization did not directly charge the facility for the services (for example, clerical and administrative services performed at a home office)? _____ _____

Return on equity capital of proprietary facilities:

(a) Does the net equity capital include those assets and liabilities which are related to patient care? _____ _____

(b) If there are loans outstanding to owners which were entered into after June 30, 1966, have the loans been excluded from liabilities and included as equity capital? _____ _____

(c) If there are loans outstanding to owners which were entered into on or before June 30, 1966, and the terms altered after June 30, 1966, have the balances been excluded from liabilities and added to the allowable equity capital? _____ _____

(d) Has the net equity capital of related organizations, applicable to patient care, added to the allowable equity capital? _____ _____

(e) Is the return on equity based on the average *monthly* balance of allowable equity capital? _____ _____

(f) Is the rate of return in agreement with the rate authorized by the Social Security Administration? _____ _____

Cost related to patient care:

- (a) Did the facility engage in any nonpatient related activities?
- (b) Is the cost, including applicable overhead, eliminated from allowable cost?
- (c) If the cost is not identifiable, are the revenues offset against allowable cost?
- (d) Did the facility receive income from nonpatients which arose from patient-related activities (e.g., sale of meals)?
- (e) Is the lower of the revenue or expense of these activities deducted from allowable cost?

Adequate cost data and cost finding:

- (a) Is the revenue and expense reflected in the cost report based on the accrual accounting?
- (b) Are patient days reflected in the cost report based on a daily census?
- (c) Did the facility take and record physical inventory of drugs, supplies, food, and linen at the beginning and end of the reporting period?
- (d) Are the allocation statistics based on actual measurements and tests in the current period?
- (e) Are documents supporting the bases available for testing by the auditors?
- (f) Has consideration been given to the use of alternative statistical bases?
- (g) If statistical bases have been changed, was intermediary approval received?
- (h) Has consideration been given to the use of weighted statistics?

III General Accounting Terms

Accelerated Depreciation A method of computing depreciation, such as sum-of-years'-digits or double-declining-balance, which results in the write-off of the cost of a depreciable asset at a more rapid rate than would occur by the straight-line method.

Accounting The accumulation and communication of historical and projected economic data relating to the financial position of an enterprise and the results of its operations, and the interpretation of the results thereof for purposes of managerial planning and control and for use by decision-making groups external to the enterprise.

Accounting Cycle The procedures involved in maintaining a set of accounting records throughout an accounting period.

Accounting Equation An equation which is both the basic formula for the balance sheet and the foundation of double entry accounting. Assets = Liabilities + Fund Balances (stockholders' equity or capital).

Accounting Period A period of time covered by an income statement. This period generally is not less than one month or longer than one year.

Accounting Principles A body of rules, standards, and conventions which determines the manner in which transactions are recorded and in which data are presented in financial statements.

Accounts Payable Liabilities arising from the purchase of goods and services from suppliers on credit.

Accounts Receivable Assets arising from the provision of services or the sale of goods to patients or other parties on credit.

Accounts Receivable Aging Schedule An analysis of accounts receivable by length of time the accounts have been outstanding.

Accounts Receivable Turnover Charges to patients' accounts during a given period divided by the amount of accounts receivable.

Accrual Basis of Accounting A method of accounting by which revenues are recognized when earned and expenses are recognized when incurred, regardless of actual cash received or disbursed.

Accrued Expenses Expenses that have been incurred but not yet paid.

Accrued Income Income that has been earned but not yet received.

Accumulated Depreciation The accumulation to date of depreciation expense, or the total portion of the original cost of depreciable assets which already has been allocated to expense in prior and current periods.

Adjusting Entry An entry that is necessary to adjust book account balances to conform with the actual balances and accrual basis at the end of the accounting period.

Allowance for Uncollectible Accounts A balance sheet valuation account reflecting the estimated amount of accounts and notes receivable which will prove to be uncollectible such as courtesy discounts and bad debt losses.

Amortization The systematic allocation of an item to revenue or expense over a determined number of accounting periods.

Annuity Rents (receipts or payments) to be received or paid periodically in the future.

Assets The tangible and intangible economic resources of a nursing home enterprise that are recognized and measured in conformity with generally accepted accounting principles.

Balance Sheet A statement of financial position showing the nursing home's assets, liabilities, and fund balances (stockholders' equity or capital) at a given date.

Board-Designated Funds Unrestricted funds set aside by action of the nursing home's governing board for specific purposes.

Bond A written promise under seal to pay a sum of money at some definite future time.

Bond Discount or Premium The difference between the par or face value of a bond and the amount received (by the issuer) or paid (by the investor) when a bond is issued or purchased.

Bond Indenture The contract between the bondholders and the nursing home issuing the bonds.

Bond Sinking Fund A fund in which assets are accumulated in order to liquidate bonds at their maturity date, or earlier.

Book Value The amount at which a specific asset or liability is carried in the accounting records of the nursing home.

Break-Even Point The volume of revenue where revenues and expenses are exactly equal, i.e., the level of activity at which there is neither a gain nor a loss from operations.

Budget A financial projection for future operations using the home's historical data as well as current nursing industry data.

Capital Expenditure An expenditure chargeable to an asset account where the asset acquired has an estimated life in excess of one year and is not intended for sale in the ordinary course of operations.

Capital Expenditure Budgeting The process of planning and controlling expenditures for property, plant, and equipment items.

Cash Basis of Accounting A method of accounting by which revenues are recognized only when cash is received and expenses are recorded only when cash is disbursed.

Cash Budget A projection of cash receipts, disbursements, and balances for a given future period of time.

Cash-Flow Statement A statement of actual or projected cash receipts and disbursements for a given period of time.

Chart of Accounts A listing of account titles, with account numbers, indicating the manner in which transaction data are to be classified in the accounting records.

Chattel Mortgage A mortgage on personal property, excluding real estate.

Closing the Books The process of transferring the balances in the revenue and expense accounts, including revenue deductions, to the fund balance account at the end of the fiscal year.

Coinsurance Clause An insurance policy clause which limits the liability of the insurance company to a determinable percentage of the loss suffered by the insured.

Collateral Assets that are pledged to secure a loan.

Compensating Balances Cash deposits required by a bank as partial compensation for lending and other services it provides to a nursing home.

Compound Interest Interest that is computed on the principal amount invested or borrowed and on any interest earned (on such principal) that has not been paid.

Contingent Liabilities Possible future liabilities which may arise due to some future event that is considered possible but not probable.

Contra Account An auxiliary account which is an offset to a related account, i.e., allowance for uncollectible accounts offset accounts receivable.

Contributed Capital Amounts paid into the nursing home by donors.

Contribution Clause An insurance policy clause which limits the liability of the insurance company to a pro rata portion of a loss of property insured by more than one company.

Contribution Margin The excess of revenues over variable costs.

Control Account A general ledger account, the detail of which is contained in a subsidiary ledger, e.g., accounts receivable.

Controllable Cost A cost whose amount is controllable by someone in the organization (usually a variable cost).

Controller The title usually given to the executive responsible for the accounting function in the organization.

Cost The present value surrendered, or promised to be surrendered in the future, determined at the time of sale, in exchange for goods and services received. Expired costs are expenses; unexpired costs are assets.

Cost Basis The use of historical, objectively determined cost as the basis of accounting for most assets.

Cost Center An organizational unit whose costs are separately accumulated in the accounts.

Cost Control The attempt to maintain actual costs at, or below, budgeted levels.

Cost or Market, Lower of A valuation basis for inventories and temporary investments.

Credit As a noun, an entry, or balance on the right-hand side of an account. As a transitive verb, to make an entry on the right-hand side of an account.

Current Assets Those assets which are cash and will be converted into cash or consumed in the normal operations of the nursing home within one year from the balance sheet date.

Current Liabilities Those liabilities which will be discharged with current assets in the normal course of business within one year from the balance sheet date.

Current Ratio The ratio of current assets to current liabilities.

Days' Revenue in Receivables The average number of days of billings in accounts receivable and uncollected at a given point in time.

Debenture Bond A bond not secured by specific assets but only by the general credit standing of the issuer.

Debit As a noun, an entry or balance on the left-hand side of an account. As a transitive verb, to make an entry on the left-hand side of an account.

Deferred Revenue Future revenue which has been collected or billed but not yet earned.

Depreciation That portion of the original cost of a fixed asset to be expensed and allocated to a particular accounting period.

Discounting of Receivables A method of short-term financing where patient receivables are used to secure a loan from a financial institution.

Economic Order Quantity (EOQ) The optimum (least cost) quantity of goods which should be purchased in a single order.

Equity Capital investment in business.

Expenses Costs that have been used up or consumed in carrying on some activity and from which no measurable benefit will extend beyond the present. Expenses are expired costs and ordinarily are accompanied by the surrendering of an asset or by the incurring of a liability.

Extraordinary Gains and Losses Gains or losses unusual in amount and nonrecurring in nature.

Factoring The process of selling or assigning receivables to a factor as a means of obtaining short-term financing.

FICA Federal Insurance Contributions Act, commonly known as Social Security.

FIFO First-in, first-out. A method of inventory costing.

Flexible Budget A budget prepared in such a manner that it can be adjusted by interpolation to reflect what expenses should be at any level of activity within a relevant range.

Functional Classification The grouping of expenses according to the operating purposes (administrative, property, and related, etc.) for which costs are incurred. Revenues also are classified functionally.

Fund A self-contained accounting entity set up to account for a specific activity.

Fund Balance The excess of assets over liabilities (net equity). An excess of liabilities over assets is known as a deficit in fund balance. Term is used for tax exempt entities.

Funded Debt Long-term debt.

Funds Held in Trust by Others Funds held and administered, at the direction of the donor, by an outside trustee for the benefit of a tax-exempt institution.

Governing Board (Board of Directors) The policy-making body of the nursing home.

Gross Margin Method A method of estimating the amount of inventory at a given point in time.

Gross Revenues The value, at the nursing home's full established rates, of services rendered and goods sold to patients during a given time period before any deductions from revenue.

Imprest Cash Fund *See* Petty Cash Fund.

Income Statement A financial statement indicating the results of operations of an enterprise in terms of revenues earned and expenses incurred for a given period of time. Also referred to as an operating statement, a statement of income and expense or a profit and loss statement.

Insolvency The inability to meet matured obligations.

Installment Note A method of financing the acquisition of new equipment by installment payments over a period of months. The seller retains title until all payments have been completed.

Intangible Asset An asset not having apparent physical existence, e.g., patents, copyrights, and goodwill.

Interest A charge for the use of money.

Interim Financial Statements Financial statements prepared at a date other than the end of the fiscal year, e.g., monthly balance sheets and income statements.

Internal Control The plan of organization and all the coordinate methods and measures adopted within a nursing home to safeguard its assets, check the accuracy and reliability of its accounting data, promote operational efficiency, and encourage adherence to prescribed managerial policies.

Inventory The aggregate of those items of tangible personal property which are held for sale in the ordinary course of business, are in process of production for sale, or are to be consumed currently in the production of goods or services to be available for sale.

Inventory Control The process of regulating the amount and types of supplies in inventory.

Inventory Turnover Cost of supplies used divided by the average inventory for the period.

Journal A book of original entry wherein transactions are recorded in chronological sequence.

Land Improvements Improvements made to land, including sidewalks, parking lots, driveways, fencing, and shrubbery, which are depreciable.

Ledger The group of accounts used in recording the transactions of the nursing home. A book of secondary entry.

Liability The financial obligations of the nursing home as recognized and measured in conformity with generally accepted accounting principles.

LIFO Last-in, first-out. An inventory costing method.

Line of Credit An arrangement whereby a financial institution commits itself to lend up to a specified maximum amount during a specified period.

Liquidity A nursing home's financial position and its ability to meet currently maturing obligations.

Long-Term Investments Investments, generally in securities, which the nursing home intends to hold for longer than one year from the balance sheet date.

Long-Term Liabilities Liabilities that are not payable within one year from the balance sheet date.

Management The direction of resources to the attainment of desired objectives through planning and control.

Marketable Security Short-term financial instruments which can be readily purchased or sold without loss in principal.

Matching An accounting principle which requires the recognition of related revenues and expenses in the same period.

Mortgage A pledge of designated property as security for a loan, e.g., mortgage bonds.

Natural Expenditure Classification A method of classifying expenditures according to their natural classification such as salaries, utilities, and supplies.

Net Assets The excess of assets over liabilities, i.e., fund balance (stockholders' equity or capital).

Net Income The excess of revenues over expenses for a given period of time as presented in the profit and loss statement.

Net Loss The excess of expenses over revenues for a given period of time as presented in the profit and loss statement.

Net Revenues The excess of gross revenues from patient services over contractual discounts and allowances.

Notes Receivable Discounted Notes receivable which have been discounted with recourse at a financial institution.

Operating Ratio Total operating expenses divided by total operating revenues.

Opportunity Cost The measurable advantage foregone in the past or that may be sacrificed as a result of a decision involving alternatives.

Organization Chart A diagrammatic illustration of the manner in which a nursing home is organized internally.

Periodic Inventory System A system of accounting for purchased goods and supplies by which items purchased are charged to expense accounts rather than to inventory.

Perpetual Inventory System A system of accounting for inventories under which a continuous, day-to-day record is kept of inventory levels.

Petty Cash Fund A small fund of cash maintained for the purpose of making minor disbursements for which the issuance of a check would be impractical.

Physical Inventory The actual inventory as determined by physical count, usually at the end of a reporting period.

Planning The process of establishing programs for the achievement of objectives.

Plant Physical properties used for nursing home purposes, i.e., land, land improvements, buildings, and equipment. The term does not include real estate or properties of restricted or unrestricted funds not used for nursing home operations.

Plant Replacement and Expansion Funds Funds put aside for renewal or replacement of the nursing home plant.

Position Control Plan A management tool for controlling the number of employees on the nursing home payroll and for assuring the utilization of each employee to the point of maximum effectiveness. Also termed a staffing plan.

Posting The process of transferring the information in the journals to the ledger.

Preemptive Right The right of existing stockholders to purchase a new issue of capital stock before it is offered to the general public.

Preferred Stock A type of stock which has preference over common stock with respect to dividends or to assets in case of liquidation, or both.

Prepaid Expense An expense-type outlay which benefits (is applicable to) subsequent accounting periods and therefore is an asset.

Present Value The value today of a future receipt or payment or successive receipts or payments, discounted at the appropriate discount rate.

Purchase Order A business document used in purchasing of goods or services.

Qualified Audit Report An audit report including one or more qualifications or exceptions.

Quantity Discount A reduction in unit purchase cost received by those who purchase supplies in a quantity in excess of a certain amount.

Responsibility Accounting A system of accounting which accumulates financial and statistical data according to the organizational units producing the revenues and responsible for incurring the expenses. The purpose is to attain optimum management control.

Restricted Funds Funds restricted by donors for specific purposes. The term refers to specific purpose and endowment funds. This term applies specifically to tax-exempt organizations.

Retained Earnings That portion of stockholders' equity attributable to profitable operation.

Revenue Operating revenue results from the sale of goods and the rendering of services and is measured by the charge made to patients or tenants for goods and services furnished to them. Nonoperating revenue includes gains from the sale or exchange of assets, interest, and dividends earned on investments and unrestricted donations of resources to the nursing home.

Revenue Expenditure An expenditure charged against operations, as opposed to capital expenditure.

ROP Reorder point. In inventory management, the point in time at which a new order should be placed for supplies.

Salvage Value The estimated amount for which a plant asset can be sold at the end of its useful life. Also called scrap value.

Self-Pay Patient A patient who pays either all or part of his bill from his own resources as opposed to third-party payment.

Semivariable Costs Costs that are partly variable and partly fixed in behavior in response to changes in volume.

Sinking Fund Funds required by external sources to be used to meet debt service charges and the retirement of indebtedness on plant assets.

Specific Purpose Fund Funds restricted by donors to tax exempt organizations for a specific purpose. Board-designated funds do not constitute specific purpose funds.

Statement of Changes in Financial Position A financial statement summarizing the movement of funds (working capital) within a nursing home for a given period of time.

Statement of Changes in Statement of Retained Earnings or Fund Balances A financial statement setting forth the changes that have occurred in the amount of retained earnings or fund balance during a given period of time.

Stock Dividend A dividend paid in the form of additional shares of stock.

Stockholders' Equity The excess of assets over liabilities, consisting mainly of invested capital and retained earnings.

Stock Right A transferable subscription warrant issued by a corporation in connection with sale of a new issue of stock.

Stock Split An action taken by a corporation to increase the number of shares outstanding, other than by sale, in order to reduce the market price of the stock to a level more attractive to investors.

Straight-Line Method A method of depreciation. Also a method of amortizing bond premium and discount.

Subordinate Debentures Bonds having a claim on assets only after the senior debts have been paid off in the event of liquidation.

Subsidiary Ledger A group of accounts which is contained in a separate ledger and which supports a single account (a control account) in the general ledger.

SYD Sum-of-years'-digits. A method of accelerated depreciation.

Tangible Asset An asset having physical existence, e.g., equipment.

Temporary Investments Investments, generally in marketable securities, which a nursing home does not intend to hold for more than one year from the balance sheet date.

Term Loan A loan generally obtained from a bank or insurance company with a maturity greater than one year. Term loans are generally amortized.

Trade Credit Debt arising from transactions in which supplies and services are purchased on credit from suppliers.

Trial Balance A list of the accounts in a ledger, with their balances, at a given date.

Unamortized Bond Discount (or Premium) That portion of bond discount (or premium) that has not yet been amortized.

Unemployment Taxes Taxes levied by federal and state governments to finance payments to the unemployed.

Unrestricted Funds A term used in tax exempt organizations for funds which bear no external restrictions as to use or purpose, i.e., funds which can be used for any legitimate purpose designated by the governing board as distinguished from funds restricted externally for specific operating purposes, for plant replacement and expansion and for endowment.

Useful Life An estimate of the number of years an item of plant and equipment will be used by a nursing home.

Voucher System A system for the processing and control of cash disbursements.

Weighted-Average Costing A method of determining the cost of supplies used and the valuation of inventory.

Working Capital Generally, the excess of current assets over current liabilities.

Yield The actual rate of return on an investment as opposed to the nominal rate of return.

Accounting and Finance Terms for Long-term Care Facilities

Accommodation The type of room a patient occupies. It can be a one-bed private room, a two-bed semiprivate room and a three- to six-bed ward. In nursing homes the two-bed room is generally the accommodation provided.

Allowances (sometimes called Contractual Discounts or Deductions from Revenue) In nursing homes the primary deduction from operating revenue to arrive at net operating revenue is the contractual discount. The discount results from the signing of cost reimbursement contracts with third-party payers—mainly Medicare and Medicaid. The theory is that if Medicare and Medicaid are paying for their beneficiaries at a price less than the amount a self-pay (private) patient pays, a discount is being given. To account for the amount of the discount for an operating period, the customary self-pay rate is recorded for *all* patients. Then for those programs paying less than the customary charge a discount is recorded to reduce the amount billed to the amount to be paid. This theory was developed for retrospective cost reimbursement contracts. However, under negotiated prospective reimbursement contracts that do not pay on a cost that is specifically attributed to each facility, the accounting for the discount may have to take a different form. For example, if a target price, independent of each facility and including a factor for profit, is less than the private pay rate, a discount may not exist. The negotiated price with the third party is probably the best price available for the bed and there is no intent to charge more. To assume that a discount is being given when the bed would be empty otherwise is not appropriate. In these circumstances the negotiated price would be the customary charge that is recorded as revenue and no discount would be recorded. In some cases, if a discount were recorded, it more than likely would not be realistic because the customary self-pay rate is subsidizing the lower third-party price. That is, the difference between the self-pay rate and the third-party rate is not a discount; it is merely the difference between prices based on market conditions.

Ancillary Services Restorative, diagnostic, and therapeutic services performed by specially trained personnel. These are distinguished from daily or routine nursing care, including room and board, in that the purpose is to rehabilitate the patient. These services are generally provided outside the patient's room (except for the use of medical supplies and medications administered in the room). Services include, for example, physical therapy, occupational therapy, orientation, laboratory tests, and x-rays.

Apportionment (Allocation) This is a term coined by the Medicare program. It is the term used for describing a cost accounting procedure that distributes overhead costs to the departments producing revenue.

Bad Debts, Charity, and Courtesy Allowances Bad debts are accounts receivable from patients that are not collectible. In nursing homes bad debts are not prevalent in the self-pay market because the room and board and routine nursing services are due at the beginning of the month. If the amount is not paid, the patient usually is discharged. However, in circumstances where the patient has expired or an estate is being settled, bad debts do occur. They also occur, in increasing amounts, from coinsurance and deductibles that Medicare patients are to pay, but do not. In accounting terms, bad debts are operating expenses and should be recorded as an administrative cost, not a deduction from revenue. The generally accepted accounting principles for general business specify that bad debts are period costs and should be reported as such. The conflict arises when Medicare and Medicaid principles do not allow these costs in determining reimbursement. However, GAAP prevails for the accounting records and bad debts should be recorded and reported as an operating expense.

Charity and courtesy allowances are not too prevalent in nursing homes. This type of item results from a facility, normally tax-exempt organization, providing free or discounted care to charity cases or employee and employee family members. Theoretically, there was no intent to collect the full charge so the item is a discount and not an expense. Therefore, the discount is recorded to reduce the customary charge to the net amount to be collected.

Bed Turnover Rate The number of times the bed complement of a facility changes patients during a given period of time. This is determined by dividing the average occupied beds by the total discharges, for the same period of time.

Cost Reimbursement The procedure used by the Medicare Program to pay providers for the services provided to their beneficiaries. It determines the costs incurred and pays on a basis specified by law.

Chain Organization An organization of any form that owns, leases, or manages a group of two or more facilities. Normally, the entity is a taxable corporation that owns, leases, and manages a number of nursing homes.

Community Care Facility A facility that normally provides nonmedical residential care, day care, or agency services to the developmentally disabled, physically handicapped, and mentally disordered. These facilities are many times expanded into full-time nursing care centers, for rehabilitative purposes, if the needs justify the programs and the cost.

Cost Center This is a cost accounting term that designates a distinct service unit that has specific costs assignable to it. For example, the housekeeping department is a cost center because it is a distinct service unit that has specific salaries and supplies assigned to it. It is also called a support or overhead department because it does not, in itself, produce revenue. The nursing department is also a cost center because it is a distinct service unit that has specific salary, space, and supply costs attributable to it. It is also called a revenue department because its service directly benefits the patient and is the basis for producing revenue.

Department A distinct service unit that is designated as such for the purpose of assigning costs and/or management responsibilities.

Developmentally Disabled A person with a disability attributable to mental retardation, cerebral palsy, epilepsy, or other neurologically handicapping condition. Such disability originates before a person is eighteen and continues indefinitely.

Direct Cost The cost of providing the services that can be assigned to a specific department without cost finding. For example, payroll costs are assigned to a specific department based on the actual staff assigned. No assumptions or cost spreading are required.

Distinct Part A term coined by the Medicare program to designate a distinct part of a nursing home for their beneficiaries. To be a distinct part the nursing home must certify a portion of the facility for Medicare coverage by meeting certain life safety, fire safety, and nursing standards. Other programs are picking up on the term to segregate sections of a nursing home for specific purposes.

Donated Services The value attributed to services provided to a facility by employees who receive no compensation or only part compensation. The concept is usually applied to services rendered by members of religious orders to tax-exempt institutions.

Facility The term used to describe a nursing home or similar type of long-term care provider. The term institution is normally confined to tax-exempt organizations.

Fixed Cost (or Expense) An operating or capital expense that does not vary with business volume, for example, interest on mortgages, rent, real estate tax, and depreciation. Costs are not fixed in the sense that they do not increase but in the sense they do not increase from variations in volume.

Indirect Cost An overhead cost that is not directly assignable to the production of the service, but a cost that must be allocated to various services based on their assumed contribution to the production of revenue.

Inpatient A patient who is provided with room, board, and nursing supervision or nursing care as prescribed by a physician in a long-term care facility.

Inpatient Admission The formal acceptance of an inpatient by a long-term care facility for an overnight stay.

Inpatient Bed Count The number of beds available for admission of inpatients as specified by license.

Inpatient Bed Days Available The unit of measure designating the potential number of patient days that could be serviced in a 24-hour period.

Inpatient Occupancy Rate The number of beds occupied in relation to the number of beds available. Calculated by dividing the inpatient bed days occupied by the inpatient bed days available, in the specified period.

Inpatient Census The number of patients occupying beds at midnight.

Inpatient Discharge The formal release of an inpatient from the facility by physician's order.

Intermediary The paying agent for the Medicare program. Normally an insurance company, such as Blue Cross, Aetna, Continental, or National.

Intermediate Care Facility A licensed facility that provides inpatient care to ambulatory or semiambulatory inpatients who have recurring need for nursing supervision and care and continuous need for the activities of daily living.

Level of Care The degree of nursing supervision or nursing care required by an inpatient.

Long-Term Care Facility Any facility licensed as a nursing home, residential facility, shelter care home, convalescent home, intermediate care facility, skilled nursing facility, and extended care facility.

Luxury Items Items not related to general patient care. This is a phrase coined by the Medicare and Medicaid programs to designate items that are not reimbursable, for example, telephones and televisions.

Medicaid The state-administered health program for the indigent. The reimbursement is shared by the state and federal government, and is required to be cost-related effective July 1, 1976.

Medical Services The services provided by physicians, dentists, optometrists, nurses, and other medical professionals.

Medicare The federally administered health program for the elderly and disabled. The program pays certain medical, hospital, and nursing home costs of persons sixty-five and over and certain persons under sixty-five. The patients are responsible for paying the deductibles and coinsurance. Part A covers hospital and skilled nursing inpatient services and Part B covers outpatient hospital and certain skilled nursing services and home health services.

Mentally Disordered Patient A patient with chronic psychiatric impairment whose adaptive functioning is impaired. This patient requires continuous supervision and normally will benefit from rehabilitation.

Nonoperating Revenue Revenue received from sources other than from operations.

Nonrevenue Producing Cost Center These are support departments that represent overhead costs for the production of revenue. For example, dietary, housekeeping, laundry, maintenance, and administration.

Occasion of Service The output unit of production in the ancillary department.

Occupancy Expense Expenses related to use of property. For example, rent, utilities, depreciation, maintenance, and real estate taxes.

Operating Cost (or Expense) An expense incurred in providing the patient care services.

Outpatient A patient that is provided with services without being admitted as a bed patient.

Overhead A cost of doing business that does not contribute directly to the production of revenue, such as, housekeeping, laundry, and maintenance.

Patient Care Services General nursing care including nursing services, activities, social services, disability services, and ancillary services.

Patient Care Point The use of a relative value method of determining level of care. Nursing time is converted to point values for various patient care needs. The criteria for valuing level of care normally relate to aides to daily living and administration of medications.

Patient Day Care of one patient for one 24-hour period starting and ending at midnight. In maintaining statistics, the day of admission is counted as a day of care but the day of discharge is not. A bed that is reserved and held for later occupancy is not included as a regular inpatient day. They are accumulated separately and called bed-hold days. If the bed-hold days are paid for by someone they are then included in the inpatient day statistics.

Provider A long-term care facility certified for purposes of providing Medicare and Medicaid beneficiaries with services.

Replacement Cost The cost of an asset that replaces a retired asset. The replacement asset is recorded in the records, at its acquisition cost, in place of the retired asset. Another definition is the current price that it would cost to replace an existing asset with current features and specifications. This is a contrast to reproduction cost which updates the cost of the existing assets with its existing features without regard to current specifications.

Residential Facility A facility that provides room and board with personal services, protection, supervision, assistance in transportation, guidance, and training to sustain the person in the activities of daily living. Medications and nursing are not provided.

Revenue-Producing Cost Centers Departments providing direct service to patients for which they are charged, such as, nursing, physical therapy, medications, and medical supplies.

Skilled Nursing Facility A nursing home or distinct part of a hospital that provides continuous nursing care to patients that are primarily immobile, needing medications and restorative therapies. The intensity of licensed nursing care and medication is more than that provided in an intermediate care facility. The specifications for the minimum standards of nursing care are regulated by law.

Stepdown Method of Cost Finding A method of cost finding to ultimately assign overhead costs to the revenue production departments. The departments that support the patient care departments are allocated in a rational and systematic manner to the nursing and ancillary departments.

Value of Services of Unpaid Workers
The value of work performed by volunteers in positions normally held by employees. The cost shall be the amount identifiable in the facility's records, which would have to

be paid to a regular employee for such services, including customary fringe benefits. The Medicare program only recognizes costs paid to religious organizations for volunteer workers, but the Medicaid programs have varying methods of valuing volunteer services.

Variable Costs Operating costs that vary in direct proportion to changes in volume. In nursing homes these costs are normally nursing salary costs and supplies. The costs of establishing a staff level to meet minimum standards may be fixed until a certain level of occupancy is attained.

Index

Accelerated depreciation, 69, 256
Accommodation, 263
Accountability, *ix, x,* 77
Accounting, 1–3
   accrual. *See* Accrual accounting
   budgeting, 35–36
   cash flow, 37
   check writing and, 38, 39*t**
   control, 29–44
   cycle, 256
   double entry, 6, 48–49
   equation, 5–6, 256
   payroll, 38, 39*t*
   period, 256
   principles. *See* GAAP
   records, 6–28, 35
   reporting, 36, 37*t*
   write-off method, 54, 60
Accounts payable, 42, 57, 256
   journal, 7, 12–13*t*
   ledger, 7, 14*t,* 42
Accounts receivable, 48–50, 256, 258, 259
   aging schedule, 256
   ledger, 38, 40*t*
   turnover, 256
   uncollectible, 194
Accrual, 57, 204, 256
   accounting, 4–5, 48, 54, 62–64, 195, 224
   vs. cash flow, 145–146
Accrued expenses, 256
Accrued income, 256
Accrued interest, 134
Accrued liability, 4
Acid test, 179
Activities of daily living, *vii,* 266
Adjusting entry, 256
Administrative expenses, 197, 213, 215
Administrative services, 102–119
Admission, patient, 265, 267
Aging schedule, accounts receivable, 256
Agreement to repurchase, 71
Aides, staffing budget for, 106–107
Allocation, 264
Allowances, 196–197, 263–264. *See also* Discount
American Institute of Certified Public Accountants (AICPA), 75, 205
Amortization, 66, 79, 88, 256
Ancillary services, 100–101, 264, 267
Annuity, 256
Apportionment, 264

Asset, 1, 6, 57–61, 256, 259, 260, 263, 267
   current, 57–58, 185, 187–188, 258
   depreciation as, 55
   flexibility, 131
Audit report, qualified, 261
Average earnings, 194, 195*t*

Bad debts, 51, 54, 141, 181, 195, 264
Balance, compensating, 257
Balance sheet, 27–28, 85, 89, 149, 150, 151, 152, 162–163*t,* 180, 181, 185–187, 192–193*t,* 199, 205, 216, 257
Bankers, 187, 206
Bankruptcy. *See* Business failures
Beauty shop income, 141
Bed
   days available, inpatient, 266
   occupancy, 32, 266
   size of facility, optimum, 249, 251
   turnover rate, 264
Bed-hold days, 267
Billings, 48–50
   and accounts receivable, 38, 40*t*
   journal, 6–7, 8–9*t*
Bonds, 252, 257, 258, 262
Book value, 182, 251
Borrowed capital. *See* Debt capital
Break-even point, 201, 257
Budget, *x,* 35–36, 210, 216
   analysis, 120–126
   capital expenditure, 257
   control, 184, 209
   flexibility, 259
   operating, 89–130 *passim,* 204
   plan, 92–94
   report, prospective, 150
   revision, 94
Burial fees, 88
Business cycle, 5, 68
Business failures, 89–91, 201, 223
Business risks. *See* Risks

Capacity extension, 132
Capital, 6, 47, 205
   assets, 58–61
   budgeting, 131–140
   contributed, 69–70, 258
   cost of, 48, 75–76, 111, 134, 187, 197, 226, 227
   debt. *See* Debt capital
   excess over par value, 206

*A page number with the suffix *t* represents a table, graph, or exhibit.

270 Index

Capital *(cont.)*
  expenditure, 251
  owners'. *See* Owners' capital
  stock, 69–70
  working. *See* Working capital
Care, minimum standards of, *viii,* 267
Care point, 267. *See also* Level of care
Cash
  basis of accounting, 195, 257
  budget, 141–146, 257
  control, 29
  disbursements journal, 15, 20–21*t*
  discounts, 90
  management of, 210
  position, 47
  receipts journal, 11, 15, 18–19*t*
  report, 149, 150
  reserves, 90
Cash flow, 5, 46–48, 67, 90, 191
  accounting, 37
  vs. accrual, 145–146
  budget, 140–148
  and investment evaluation, 132–133
  statement, 89, 149, 150, 152, 167–169*t,*
    190–191, 194*t,* 206, 257
Cashiering, 38–39
Catastrophes, 71. *See also* Risks
Census, patient, 31–32, 33*t,* 151, 154–155*t,*
  160*t,* 266
Central store, 31, 42
Charge slips, medical, 30, 31*t*
Charity, 264
Chart of accounts, 22, 57, 216, 242–248, 257
Check (bank)
  endorsement, 11
  register, 15, 20–21*t*
  writing, 38, 39*t*
Classification, functional, 217, 218–220*t*
Closing ledger accounts, 27, 257
Coinsurance, 51, 257
Collateral, 257
Collectibility of receivables, 71
Collection, 72, 90, 181
Combination method, reimbursement, 73
Community care facility, 265
Compensating balance, 257
Competition, 209
Competitive rates, 118
Consistency, accounting, 2–3
Construction-in-progress, 61–62
Consumer demand, 131
Contingencies, predictability of, 71
Contingent liabilities, 70–71, 258
Contra account, 258

Contractual allowances, 196–197. *See also* Discount
Contributed capital, 69–70, 258
Contribution margin, 258
Control, 29–44, 150–151, 226
  account, 258
  budget, 184, 209
  cost. *See* Cost control
  inventory, 181, 260
  in rate-setting, 224
Control functions
  accounting, 35–38
  administration, 32–34
  business office, 38–40
  medical, 30–32
  purchasing, 41–42
  support services, 42–44
Controllable expenses. *See* Variable expenses
Controller, 258
Corporation, 183
Cost, 258, 262, 265, 267, 268
  accounting, 207–220
  analysis report, 149, 150, 152
  of capital. *See* Capital, cost of
  centers, 216, 224, 228, 258, 265, 266, 267
  classifying, 93, 212–213, 228–242
  control, 92, 209, 223, 258
  of debt, 135
  of equity, 135
  finding, 103, 114, 208–209, 216, 224, 267
  historical. *See* Historical cost
  reconciliation, third-party, 51
  reimbursement. *See* Reimbursement
  replacement, 267
  reports, 149, 150, 197–199, 210
  of services, 218*t*
  stratification, 217
Cost-effectiveness, 124
Costing. *See* Cost finding
Cost-per-patient day, 200–201, 204, 224, 267
Courtesy discount, 264
Court order decreeing trusteeship, 77
Credit, 258
  deferred, 67–69
  policy, too-liberal, 81
Current assets, 57–58, 185, 187–188, 258
Current liabilities, 65–66, 185, 187, 258
Current ratio, 179, 180, 258

Data, cost-accounting, 209–210
Days' revenue in receivables, 181, 258
Death, patient, 77, 84
Debentures, 252, 262
Debits and credits, 6, 258

Debt, 65–66, 205
  capital, 67, 188, 190
  cost of, 135
  financing, 66, 180, 259
  priorities, 143–144
  reduction, 190
  service, 190, 191
Debtsmanship, creative, 42, 143–144
Deferred charges, 57
Deferred credits, 67–69
Deferred revenue, 258
Deficit spending, 144
Delegation of accounting function, 210
Departmental operating costs, 93
Deposit slips, 11, 38–39, 40*t*
Depreciable assets, 58–61
Depreciation, 75, 76–77, 188–189, 198, 199, 207, 258, 266–267
  accelerated, 69, 256
  accumulated, 256
  as asset, 55
  schedule, 58, 59*t*
  straight-line, 69
  sum of years' digits, 263
Developmentally disabled patient, 265
Dietary function. *See* Meals
Direct costs, 211, 265
Direct write-off method (bad debts), 54
Disability services, 267
Discharge, patient, 77, 84, 266, 267
Discount, 47, 134
  bond, 257
  to cash customers, 90
  contractual, 195, 196–197
  courtesy, 264
  Medicaid/Medicare, 50–51, 52–53*t*, 73–74, 93, 196
  for prompt payment, 90
  volume, 196, 261
Discounting of receivables, 259, 261
Distinct part, 265
Diversification, full, 132
Dividends, 188, 206, 262
Donated services, 265
Double entry accounting, 6, 48–49
Drucker, Peter, 90
Drugs. *See* Medications

Earnings
  per share, 182
  retained, 69–70, 189, 262, 267
Economic cost of capital, 226, 227
Economic depreciation, 189
Efficiency, 124, 182

Enforceable obligation, 4
Entertainment expenses, 69
Entity, accounting, 2
Equipment, 188, 189
Equity, 259
  capital, 188, 189–190, 205. *See also* Owners' capital
  cost of, 135
  ratio, 179–180
Error, 23, 212
Escrow account, 55
Estimates, accounting, 5
Evidence, objective, 3
Expansion of services, 227
Expense account, 27
Expense categories, 93, 228–242
Expenses, 259. *See also* Cost
  accrued, 62–64, 256
  fixed, 215, 265
  nondeductible, 69
  occupancy, 266–267
Expropriation of assets, 71
External standards (ratios), 185
Extraordinary gain or loss, 199, 259

Factoring, 259
FIFO (first in–first out), 259
Final entry, 22
Financial Accounting Standards Board (FASB), 199
Financial accounting strategy, 191, 194–201
Financial analysis, 185–204
Financial ranking of investments, 138
Financial reports. *See* Reports, Financial
Financial risks. *See* Risks
Financial statements, 149, 150, 259
Fixed assets, 198
Fixed charges earned, ratio, 183
Fixed costs, 215, 265
Flat rate, 200
Flexibility, 131, 224, 227, 259
Floaters (staff), 11, 124
Food. *See* Meals
Forecast of volume, sample, 106
Full absorption accounting, 216
Full capacity revenue budget, 119
Full diversification, 132
Functional classification, 259. *See also* Chart of accounts
Fund balance, 1, 259
Funded debt, 259
Funds, 262, 263
Funds held in trust, 259. *See also* Patient Trust Fund Account

GAAP, x, 2–4, 45, 66, 75, 191, 199, 224, 256, 264
Gain contingency, 70–71
General journal, 22, 57
General ledger, 7, 22, 35, 260
  expense categories, 93, 242–248
Generally accepted accounting procedures. See GAAP
Goals, revenue budgeting by, 116–117
Government
  as purchaser, x, 92
  regulations, 208, 222–223
Gross margin, 259
Gross revenues, 259
Group rate, 196

Historical cost, 3–4, 60, 209, 215
  of capital, 226, 227
Historical depreciation, 189
Horizontal integration, 132
Hours per patient day, 110, 120
Housekeeping, 43, 121, 150, 157t, 215, 267

Income, 27, 67–69, 256, 260
  statement of, 87, 164–166t, 170–178t, 202–203t, 206, 259
Incomparability of original data, 185
Indenture (bond), 257
Indirect cost, 265
Inflation, 189, 198, 199
Insolvency, 259. See also Business failures
Installment note, 259
Insurance, 54, 55, 79, 266
Intangible asset, 259
Interest, 64, 75, 257, 259
Interim financial statements, 259
Intermediary, 266
Intermediate care facility, 266
Internal control, 29, 260
Internal rate of return, 137–138, 139
Internal Revenue Service, 61, 67
Internal standards (ratios) 184
Inventory, 31, 41, 42, 57, 181–182, 198, 216, 260, 261
Investment, 188–189, 260
  nursing home as, 183
  options, evaluation of, 131–139
  in receivables, 181
  temporary, 263
Investors, 183, 206. See also Bankers
Invoice approval, purchasing, 41

Journals, 28, 260
  accounts payable, 7, 12–13t

  billings, 6–7, 8–9t, 50
  cash disbursements, 15, 20–21t
  cash receipts, 11, 15, 18–19t
  general, 22, 57
  payroll, 7, 11, 31, 38, 42
  purchase, 7, 12–13t, 42, 57

Labor, 120, 187, 198, 210, 211, 213
  staffing plan, sample, 156t
Laundry, 43, 57, 121, 151, 158t, 215
Lawsuits, 62, 71
Lease with ownership conditions, 75
Ledger, 260
  general. See General ledger
  subsidiary, 263
Legal function, 211
Letters of credit, 71
Level of care, 114–115, 151, 266
Level of profitability, 105
Liabilities, 1, 6
  accrued (payable), 4
  contingent, 70–71, 258
  current, 65–66, 185, 187, 258
  deferred, 67–69
  and life care contracts, 80
  long-term, 260
Licensed personnel, 108–109
Life care contracts, 78–88
Life expectancy, 79, 88
LIFO (last in–first out), 260
Linens. See Laundry
Liquidity, 57–58, 65–66, 260
Litigation, 62, 71
Loan, short-term, 144, 191
Long-term care facility, 266
Long-term investments, 260
Loss, 70–71, 261
Lower of cost or market, 258

Maintenance, 43, 121, 150, 157t, 215, 266–267
Management
  decision-making, 209
  information, 32–33. See also Reports
  by Objectives (MBO), 90
Margin of safety, 183
Marketability, 222
Marketable securities, 182, 260
Marketing function, 211
Mark-up, profit, 93
Matching, 5, 260
Materials. See Supplies
Meals, 43, 57, 63, 120, 141, 151, 158t, 215

Medicaid/Medicare, 47–53, 67, 72, 211, 249–255, 263–264, 266
  billings, 38, 141
  carryover of settlement, 62
  cost breakdown, 225*t*
  discounts. *See* Discount, Medicaid/Medicare
  and life care contracts, 80, 88
  reimbursement, 74, 124, 221–227 *passim*
Medical services, 266
Medical supplies, 57
Medicare, 72, 249–255, 263–264, 266. *See also* Medicaid/Medicare
  Principles of Reimbursement, 74, 224, 251–255
Medications, 57, 62, 63, 151, 159*t*, 267
Mentally disordered patient, 265, 266
Mortgage, 65–67, 257, 260

Natural expense classification, 260
Net assets, 260
Net income, 183–184, 260
Net loss, 261
Net present value, 134, 137, 138
Net revenues, 260
Nonfinancial ranking of investments, 138
Nonoperating revenue, 266
Nonprofit organizations, 221
Notes payable, 66–67
Notes receivable, 261
Nursing services, *vii*, 99–100, 150, 157*t*
Nursing staff. *See* Licensed personnel
  hours per patient day, budgeted, 110

Objectives, business, 187
Obsolescence, 131
Occasion of service, 266
Occupancy expense, 266–267
Occupancy rate, inpatient, 266
Operating bank account, 38
Operating budget, 89–130 *passim*, 204
Operating cost, 111–115, 197, 267. *See also* Overhead
Operating ratio, 183, 261
Opportunity cost, 261
Organization chart, 29–30, 94–95, 261
Original entry, 22
Outpatient, 267
Output, 120, 132
Overhead, 128–129, 200, 213, 215, 267
Owners' capital, 1, 58, 135

Paid-in capital, 206
Partnership, 183
Par value, stock, 182

Past due accounts, 90. *See also* Bad debts; Collection
Patient
  census. *See* Census, patient
  funds, 77–78
  ledger cards, 7, 10*t*, 49, 50*t*
  mix, 120, 121, 201
  statistics, 210
Patient care services, 267
Patient day, cost per, 200–201, 204, 224, 267
Patient Trust Fund Account, 77–78
Payable liability, 4
Payables report, 149, 150
Payback method of investment ranking, 133–134, 138
Payroll, 11, 44, 210, 216
  journal, 7, 11, 31
Pension, 68
Per diem reimbursement method, 73
Period accounting, 2
Periodicity, 5
Personnel function, 210
Petty cash, 261
Pharmaceuticals. *See* Medications
Philosophy, business, 93, 187
Physically handicapped patient, 265
Physical therapy, 151, 159*t*, 267
Pilferage and waste, 31, 42
Planning, 223
Plant, 188, 198, 261. *See also* Facility
P/L statement, 23, 27, 89, 149, 150–152, 180, 191, 194–201, 216
Position control plan, 261
Posting, 261
Preemptive right, 261
Preferred stock, 261
Premium, bond, 257
Prepaid expenses, 54–57, 261
Present value, 261
Price and quantity variance, 127, 128
Pricing, 33, 34*t*, 103, 150, 209, 211
Principal, 190
Private patient. *See* Self-pay patient
Product defects and warranties, 71
Production
  cost, 211, 212, 213
  levels, 121, 123. *See also* Productivity
  reports, 43, 120, 149, 150, 152, 153*t*
Productivity, 124
  log, 43–44
  reports, 149, 150, 201
Product line reporting, 201
Profit, *x*, 60, 196, 198, 204, 209, 211, 222
  goals, 104–105

Index

Profit *(cont.)*
  potential, 201
  and revenue, budgets, 116–119
Profitability, level of, 105
Profit and loss statement. *See* P/L statement
Profit center reporting, 201
Profit margin, 33, 34–35t, 93, 208
Profit or loss accrual, 5
Prompt payment discount, 90
Property, 188
  taxes. *See* Real estate taxes
Proprietary ratio, 179, 180
Proprietorship, single, 183
Prospective distribution, capital, 223
Prospective reimbursement, 92, 196, 222, 224
Provider, 267
Public relations function, 211
Purchase journal, 7, 12–13t, 42
Purchase option, 60
Purchase order, 15, 267
Purchases, 57

Qualified audit report, 261
Quality care, *vii–ix,* 226, 227
Quantity discount, 196, 261
Quick current ratio. *See* Acid test

Rate of earnings, 182–183
Rate of return, 152, 181
Rate-setting, 103, 118, 224
Ratio of Charges to Charges as Applied to Costs (RCCAC), 73
Ratios, financial, 152, 179–185, 258, 261
Real estate taxes, 55, 64, 75, 216, 266–267
Reasonable level of profit, *x*
Receivables, 258, 259. *See also* Accounts receivable
Record-keeping, 35–38, 89
Regulations. *See* Government regulations
Reimbursement, *x,* 72–73, 221–227, 264–265
Reinvestment, 206
Rent, 55, 60, 75, 266–267
Replacement cost, 198, 267
Reports, financial, 36, 37t, 93, 120, 149–206, 208
  annual, 205–206
  components of, 149–150
  daily, 150–151
  monthly, 151–152
  objectives of, 149
Requisitions, 31, 42, 210
Residential facility, 267

Responsibility programs, budgeting, 95, 99–119 *passim*
Restorative therapies. *See* Physical therapy
Restricted funds, 262
Retained earnings, 69–70, 189, 262, 267
Retroactive reimbursement, 221, 224
Return of investment, 188
Return on investment. *See* ROI
Return on provider's net equity, 221
Revenue, 71–75, 258, 261, 262, 266
  and profit, budgets, 116–117
  recognition, 5, 194–195
  report, 149, 150
Revenue-producing cost centers, 267
Risks, 71, 131, 135, 212
ROI, 47, 93, 188

Salaries, 201
Salvage value, 76, 262
Scheduling, 210
Securities and Exchange Commission, 67
Security deposit, 55
Self-pay patient, 46, 47, 72, 146, 262, 263–264
Semivariable costs, 215, 262
Senility, 77
Service costs, 212, 213–216
Services, 264, 265, 266, 267. *See also* individual service categories
Short-term credit, 188
Short-term loan, 144, 191
Sinking fund, bond, 262
Skilled nursing facility, 267
Social Security, 11, 92
Social services, 267
Sole proprietorship, 183
Spending variance, 128, 129
Stability of cash position, 148
Staffing costs, sample budgets, 106–110
Staffing plan, sample, 156t
Staffing report, 149, 150
Standard absorption rate, 128
Standard cost system, 215–216
Standard overhead cost, 128–129
Statement of changes in financial position, 262
Statement of income. *See* Income statement
Stock, 182, 183, 206, 260, 262
Stockholders' equity, 179, 262. *See also* Equity; Owners' capital
Straight-line depreciation, 69, 262
Strategy, business, 90–91. *See also* Philosophy, business
Subordinate debentures, 262
Subsidiary ledger, 262

Supplementary Security Income law, 77
Supplies, 31–32*t*, 42, 43*t*, 198, 210
  variance analysis of costs, 127–128
Supply and demand, 209, 222–223
Supply costs, 213, 216
Support costs, 212
Support services, *vii*, 101–102, 109–110
SYD (sum of years' digits), 263

Tangible asset, 263
Taxes, 11, 149, 150, 211
  allocations, interperiod, 55
  estimated payments, 64
  income, 55, 64–65, 68
  payroll, 64
  real estate, 55, 64, 75, 216, 266–267
  unemployment, 263
Tax-exempt organizations, 70, 221, 262, 265
Technological change, 189, 227
Temporary investments, 263
Therapy, physical, 151, 159*t*, 267
Third-party payers, 47, 141, 147, 207, 211, 263–264
Time
  contractual period, life care, 79
  discount, 90
  as useful life of asset. *See* Depreciation
  value of money, 134
Timekeeping, 31, 32*t*, 42–43, 210
Timeliness
  of financial reporting, 149
  of payment, 90, 185
Timing difference, 55, 67, 68–69
Total capital employed, 184
Total cost, 212, 213, 214*t*
Trade credit, 263
Travel expenses, 69
Trial balance, 22, 23–26*t*, 27, 263
Trustee relationship, 77
Turnover
  accounts receivable, 256
  inventory, 181–182, 266
  of total assets, 184

Uncollectible accounts, 141, 194, 256. *See also* Bad debts; Past due accounts
Undercapitalization, 146
Unemployment taxes, 263
Uniform expense classifications, 228–242
Union contracts, 211
Unit costs, use of, 215–216
Unpaid workers, 267–268
Unrestricted funds, 263
Useful life, 263
Utilities, 216, 266–267

Valuation, basis of, 60
Variable expenses, 201, 213, 218, 268
Variable rate, 200
Variance, 93–94, 122, 123, 126–130, 216
  accounts, 215
  definition, 127
  interrelations, 129
  of materials costs, 127–128
  of overhead costs, 128–129
  of price and quantity, 127, 128
Vending machine income, 141
Vertical integration, 132
Volume, 120, 184
  variance, 128–129
Voucher system, 263

Wage and Hour Law, 211
Wages, 107, 123, 211
Waste and pilferage, 31, 42
Weighted average, 135, 263
Windfall profit, 196
"Window dressing," 62, 179
Working capital, 47, 58, 148, 185, 187–188, 205, 263
  ratio. *See* Current ratio
Work program, management, 95–99
Worth-debt ratio, 179
Write-offs, 54, 60

Yield, 263